Recent Results in Cancer Research 54

Fortschritte der Krebsforschung
Progrès dans les recherches sur le cancer

Malignant Bone Tumors

Edited by
E. Grundmann

With 116 Figures

Springer-Verlag
Berlin · Heidelberg · New York 1976

VIth International Symposium of the "Gesellschaft zur Bekämpfung der Krebskrankheiten Nordrhein-Westfalen e. V."
Düsseldorf October 17/18 1974

Prof. Dr. Ekkehard Grundmann, Pathologisches Institut,
4400 Münster, Westring 17

Sponsored by the Swiss League against Cancer

ISBN-13: 978-3-642-80999-6 e-ISBN-13: 978-3-642-80997-2

DOI: 10.1007/978-3-642-80997-2

Library of Congress Cataloging in Publication Data. Gesellschaft zur Bekämpfung der Krebskrankheiten Nordrhein-Westfalen. Malignant bone tumors. (Recent results in cancer research; 54.) Proceedings of the 6th international symposium of the Gesellschaft zur Bekämpfung der Krebskrankheiten Nordrhein-Westfalen held in Düsseldorf, Oct. 17—18, 1974 and sponsored by the Swiss League Against Cancer. Bibliography: p. Includes index. 1. Bones — Cancer — Congresses. I. Grundmann, Ekkehard. II. Schweizerische Nationalliga für Krebsbekämpfung und Krebsforschung. III. Series. [DNLM: 1. Bone neoplasms — Congresses. Wl RE106P v. 54/WE258 M251 1974] RC261.R35 vol. 54 [RC280.B6] 616.9'94'008s [616.9'94'71] 75-33987.

Softcover reprint of the hardcover 1st edition 1976

Contents

List of Participants

L. V. ACKERMAN, Health Sciences Center, Dept. of Pathology, State University of New York, Stone Brook, N. Y. 11790.

M. CAMPANACCI, Istituto Ortopedico Rizzoli, Clinica ortopedica dell'Università, I-40100 Bologna.

L. DMOCHOWSKI, Univ. of Texas, Dept. of Virology, M. D. Anderson Hospital, Houston/Texas 77025.

W. GÖSSNER, Pathologisches Institut, Klinikum rechts d. Isar der TU, Ismaninger Straße 22, D-8000 München 80.

E. GRUNDMANN, Pathologisches Institut der Universität, Westring 17, D-4400 Münster.

W. HOEFFKEN, Strahleninstitut der Allgem. Ortskrankenkasse Köln, Machabäerstraße 19/27, D-5000 Köln 1

R. J. HUEBNER, National Inst. of Health, National Cancer Institute, Viral Carcinogenesis Branch, Bethesda/Md. 20014.

M. IMMENKAMP, Orthopädische Universitätsklinik Münster Hüfferstraße 27, D-4400 Münster.

J. C. IVINS, Mayo Clinic, Dept. Orthopedic Surgery, Orthopedic Oncology, Rochester/Minn. 55901.

R. KOTZ, Orthopädische Universitätsklinik, Garnisongasse 13, A-1090 Wien.

R. C. MARCOVE, 517, East 71st Street, New York/ N. Y. 10021.

H. H. MATTHIASS, Orthopädische Universitätsklinik Münster, Hüfferstraße 27, D-4400 Münster.

W. MILLER, National Inst. of Health, National Cancer Institute, Epidemiology Branch, A 521 Landow Building, Bethesda/Md. 20014.

S. W. NIELSEN, Cornell University, Dept. of Pathology, Ithaca/N. Y. 14850.

J. F. PARK, Battelle Pacific NW. Lab., Battelle Boulevard, Richland/Wa. 99352.

H. Poppe, Radiologische Klinik der Universität, Goßlerstraße 10, D-3400 Göttingen.

D. J. Pritchard, Mayo Clinic, Dept. Orthopedic Surgery, Orthopedic Oncology, Rochester/Minn. 55901.

Ch. A. Reilly, Jr., Argonne National Laboratory, Experim. Radiation Pathology, Building 340, 9700 South Cass Avenue, Argonne/Ill. 60439.

W. Remagen, Pathologisches Institut der Universität, Schönbeinstraße 40, CH-4056 Basel.

M. Salzer, Orthopädische Univ.-Klinik, Garnisongasse 13, A-1090 Wien.

M. Salzer-Kuntschik, (Frau), Pathol.-Anatomisches Institut der Universität, Spitalgasse 4, A-1090 Wien.

F. Schajowicz, WHO/Osteo-articular Pathology Center, Hospital Italiano, Gascon 450, Buenos Aires.

H. A. Sissons, University of London, Institute of Orthopaedics, Dept. of Morbid Anatomy, 234, Great Portland Street, London W1N 6AD.

Ch. M. Southam, Jefferson Medical Center, Dept. of Medicine, Div. Medical Oncology, Philadelphia/Pa. 19107.

E. Uehlinger, Pathologisches Institut der Universität, Kantonsspital, Schmelzbergstraße 12, CH-8006 Zürich.

Bone Tumors – A Challenge for Cooperation

E. GRUNDMANN

Among the wide variety of human tumors, those of the skeletal system have an exceptional position in several respects. Above all, they are comparatively rare, and that is why reliable diagnostic criteria were compiled only recently, that is during the last three decades. It is only five years since the outlines of an international code of classification were traced. The code was applied and discussed critically and with varying results by several international working groups. Certain drawbacks are due to the broad and manifold spectrum of histologic manifestations in neoplastic bone. Even the best experts in diagnostic histology would hardly be able to classify more than 85% of all bone tumors after the proposed code system. For quite a long time the osteoclastic giant cells, observed in almost any kind of bone tumor, have so much fascinated the histologist's eye that he was apt to proclaim the diagnosis "brown giant cell tumor" for almost any osteoclastic tumor regardless of its benignity or malignancy. Nowadays the group of "giant cell tumors" though restricted, still remains disputed in terms of malignancy and benignity. The problem will certainly not be settled in a definite way without extensive follow-up studies. In this context we may see actual progress in new regional bone tumor registries being set up after the American example in many countries, among them the German Federal Republic. The collection and registration of cases will not only facilitate epidemiologic perspectives, but also the convention on a world-wide classification code for frequent tumor types, accompanied by a separate list of rare and exceptional cases. The international exchange of data is called for, and the start has been most auspicious.

The diagnosis of a bone tumor has to be based not only on histology, but also on the roentgenogram. If the pathologist is not well trained in the interpretation of roentgenograms - and this may be normal - close cooperation between X-ray specialist and pathologist are a prerequisite of effective and detailed diagnosis. In many cases cytologic methods will facilitate, accelerate, or verify the results of diagnosis. The additional support of electron microscopy is, for the present, restricted to some very special cases.

An exact and detailed diagnosis is the prerequisite of adequate therapy. Although surgery will always be predominant in therapy, the extent and method of a surgical intervention will depend on the respective diagnosis. As in diagnostics, experience has to set the scale in therapy planning. Surgery must be as sparing as possible and as radical as necessary. In many cases it can be successfully supplemented by radiotherapy and even by chemotherapy in some cases, or by recently developed methods of immunotherapy.

Whereas malignant tumors of epithelial origin tend to occur in persons of advanced age, the most frequent of the primary malignant bone tumors will appear before the age of 40. This was observed especially in osteosarcoma and in Ewing's sarcoma. There is a rule in malignant tumors of the bone: when the patient is younger than 40, you have to look out first for a primary bone tumor, if he is over 40, you have to think of metastases. This preferential manifestation in younger people increases the responsibility with regard to diagnostic and therapeutic measures.

Based upon experiments, the virus hypothesis of tumorigenesis is becoming much more probable with respect to malignant bone tumors. Correspondingly bone tumors may be seen in analogy to hemoblastoses, the origin of which is also found in the skeletal system. The fact that ionizing radiation is a potential cause of bone tumors, has its bearings on another intersting problem: it appears possible that ionizing radiation is able to activate latent tumor viruses. A similar concept is, by the way, discussed for malignant epithelial tumors, and this is how results and conclusions drawn from bone tumor findings, may become paradigmatic for cancer research as a whole.

We are only at the beginning of our research on etiology and pathogenesis of bone tumors. We are still living in the age of the "hunters and gatherers." Therefore the exchange of experience among research groups is of vital importance in the field of bone tumor diagnostics and therapy. Every bone tumor that is not listed in a registry, will be lost forever as far as compilation of diagnostic criteria and, in the end, the improvement of therapy are concerned.

The present volume intends to show some contemporary knowledge about origin, pathology, and clinical management of bone tumors; its additional purpose will be an appeal for international cooperation in all these fields.

Comparative Pathology of Bone Tumors in Animals, with Particular Emphasis on the Dog

S. W. NIELSEN

I. OSTEOSARCOMA

The osteosarcoma is the most frequent bone tumor in dogs (Table 1). It appears characteristically as a localized swelling of long bones in the metaphysis at the junction of the shaft and epiphysis. The overlying skin is usually intact, and there is often subcutaneous and intramuscular edema distal and proximal to the tumor, due to impaired circulation. The degree of bone destruction varies a great deal from tumor to tumor, ranging from a few osteolytic foci (Fig. 1a) to complete destruction (Fig. 1b). Advanced muscular atrophy of the affected leg, resulting from inactivity because of pain or compression of motor nerves, is often present in neglected cases. When the tumor is cut, bone is sometimes felt against the knife. Hemorrhagic areas are scattered among firmer grayish portions that contain yellowish irregular necroses in some cases. Sectioning of the regional lymph nodes often reveals these to be enlarged and moist, due either to tumor invasion or to congestion.

Table 1. Histologic typing of 133 canine bone tumors (LING et al., 1974)

86	Osteosarcomas
15	Chondrosarcomas
12	Fibrosarcomas
8	Hemangiosarcomas
8	Osteomas
4	Chondromas

A high percentage of metastases are present in the dog, approximately 50 percent of cases necropsied having pulmonary metastases. They appear as multiple, firm, grayish nodules ranging from the size of a pea to that of a chestnut. When these are cut, osteoid tissue with varying degrees of calcification can be seen.

Histopathology. It is almost impossible to describe any histologic picture as being characteristic of osteosarcoma. The neoplastic osteoblasts are either round or spindle-shaped cells. They are situated in a loose fibrous or myxoid intercellular substance in which foci of tumor bone are seen. The amount of bone formation varies widely and does not seem to be related to the clinical behavior of the tumor. Other characteristics, which are found to be more closely associated with the speed of growth, are the cellularity, the number of mitoses, and the degree of pleomorphism present (Fig. 2). Multinucleated giant cells are

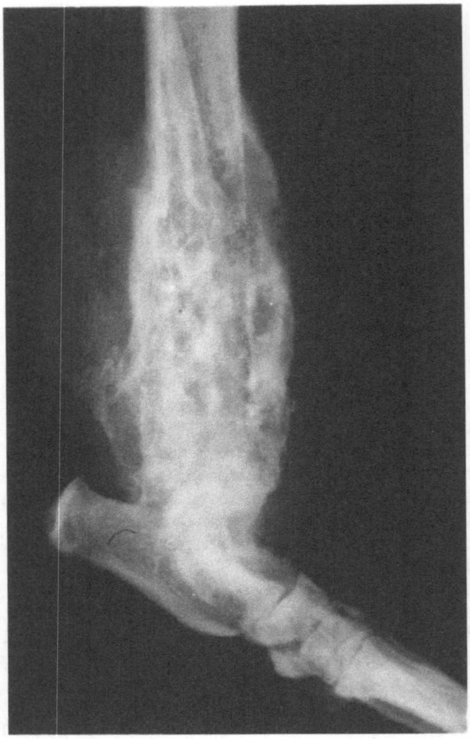

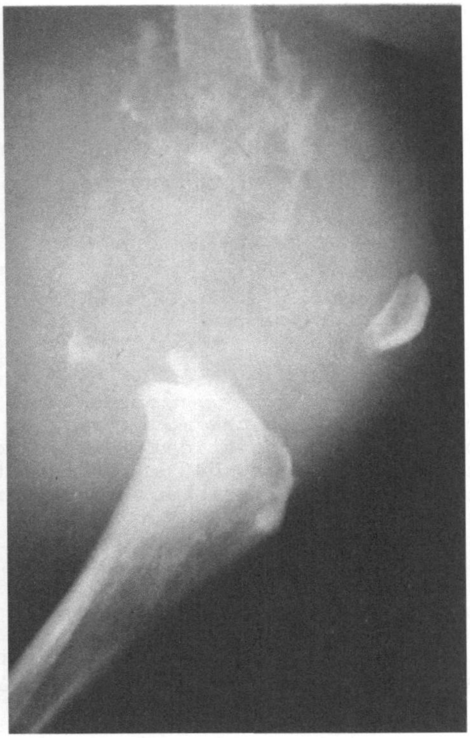

Fig. 1 (a) Osteosarcoma producing a large fusiform swelling of the distal end of the tibia of a 6-year-old female mongrel dog, (b) Osteosarcoma of the osteolytic type with total destruction of the distal third of the femur. Note the round dense soft-tissue swelling, which has displaced the patella. Lung metastases were present

frequently present and are of two types, the tumor giant cell and the osteoclastic cell. In the former type, the cytoplasm stains only faintly with eosin and the nuclei are larger and vesicular, with only a small amount of chromatin. The osteoclasts can be found close to the spicules of necrotic bone. They have a large number of small, dark nuclei situated in a relatively basophilic cytoplasm, and resemble normal osteoclasts or foreign-body giant cells.

Three different kinds of osteoid tissue or bone can be present. The one produced by neoplastic osteoblasts is a more or less unfinished product in which a varying degree of calcification has taken place. This bone, being neoplastic, does not serve any useful purpose. The formation of nontumorous periosteal bone is brought about by the stretching and irritation of the periosteum. Evidence of this periosteal osteogenesis can be seen as reactive cuffings or Codman's triangle in radiographs. Such new bone can sometimes compensate for the deeper-lying, destroyed osseous tissue, and it tends to maintain the strength of the bone. The remaining fragments of the destroyed cortex and cancellous bone are seen as spicules, often surrounded by osteoclastic giant cells.

Discussion. The cause of canine osteosarcomas is not known, but certain factors, such as rapid bone growth, weight-bearing stresses and

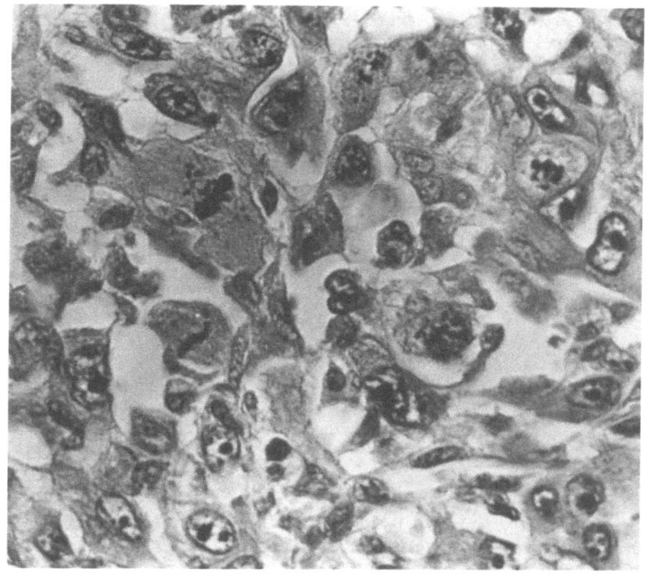

Fig. 2. A rapidly growing osteosarcoma from the proximal metaphysis of a 6-year-old Great Dane, showing pleomorphism and several mitoses. H & E, X 500

also chemical, physical and viral agents must be considered. Pre-existing bone infarcts have been incriminated in the dog (55). The role of trauma as a predisposing factor to osteosarcoma in the dog cannot be properly assessed, since a dog is rarely under observation continuously. An owner often recalls some sort of previous injury to the tumor-affected leg when questioned, but the value of such information is dubious, and no definitive correlations have been made between trauma and osteosarcoma formation in the dog. Trauma, however, has been seen to cause a pathologic fracture of a leg in which an osteosarcoma has rarefied bone. It is difficult to estimate the true breed incidence of canine osteosarcoma, because the normal dog population varies from continent to continent, from country to country, and from decade to decade (60). However, several studies have shown that osteosarcomas of long bones have a definite predilection for dogs of the socalled giant breeds: Great Danes, St. Bernards, Great Pyrenees dogs, and Wolfhounds. The Boxer breed is not one of the giant breeds, but it is also overrepresented in any sample of dogs with osteosarcomas. This, however, is in line with this breed's peculiar susceptibility to sarcomas and endocrine tumors in general (29). This tumor, like its counterpart in man, affects predominantly the metaphyseal end of the shaft of the long bones and has a propensity for certain anatomic locations (Table 2). In man, osteosarcomas occur most often in tall people, and 70 percent of all osteosarcomas occur in the lower limbs which carry great weight and are constantly exposed to small trauma in running and jumping. In dogs, as in the horse, more weight is supported by the front legs than by the hind legs. This fact, together with the finding of a much higher incidence of osteosarcomas in heavy than in smaller breeds and greater frequency, in the front than in the hind leg, suggests that rapid bone growth, heavy weight bearing, and continual slight traumas could be predisposing factors of some significance. WOLKE and NIELSEN (61) found 47 percent of tumors involved the pectoral limb, 29 percent

Table 2. Site of 314 canine Osteosarcomas (WOLKE and NIELSEN, 1966)

Pectoral Limb	149	Pelvic Limb	90
Scapula	3	Pelvis	6
P. Humerus	60	P. Femur	11
D. Humerus	1	D. Femur	26
P. Ulna	3	P. Tibia	12
M. Ulna	3	M. Tibia	1
D. Ulna	7	D. Tibia	31
D. Radius	71	Metatarsals	3
Metacarpals	1		
Skull	20	Rib	34
Mandible	13	Vertebrae	8

D.= distal end; M. = mid-shaft; P. = proximal end.

the pelvic limb, 11 percent the skull and mandible, and 13 percent other areas. The ratio of forelimb to hindlimb involvement was 1.6:1, which corresponds to the ratio of weight distribution between front and hind limb. The sites most often affected were the distal radius (23%), the proximal humerus (19%) and the rib (11%). It is significant that no tumors were reported at the proximal end of the radius and only one of the distal humeral metaphysis, indicating that the humeroradial joint is a highly tumor-resistant site (Fig. 3). Human osteosarcoma occurs with greatest frequency at the distal femur, proximal tibia, and proximal humerus, with approximately 50 percent occurring in the femur. We do not yet understand the reason for the site distribution of osteosarcomas in any species. There is a connection between tumor site and time of epiphyseal closure, the metaphysis with maximum growth and late epiphyseal closure being the area of highest osteosarcoma incidence in the dog. This relationship was observed in the proximal humerus and distal radius, where 60 and 71 tumors, respectively were re-

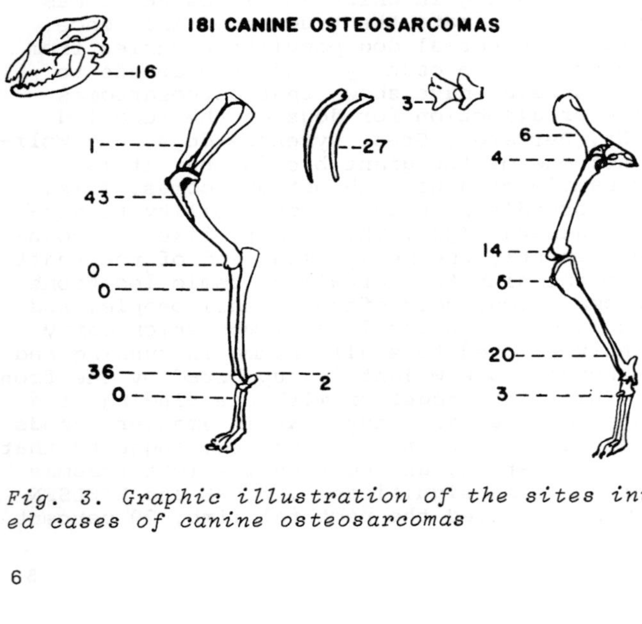

Fig. 3. Graphic illustration of the sites involved in personally observed cases of canine osteosarcomas

corded. Epiphyseal closure is late at both these sites in the dog, taking place at approximately 12 months of age (27). Further evidence of this relationship was observed in the proximal radius and distal humerus, which are rarely affected and in which epiphyseal closure is early, at 8-9 months, and there are correspondlingly fewer tumors. In the dog, 70 percent of longitudial growth takes place in the distal metaphysis (54). The mean age of 255 dogs affected with this neoplasm was 7.5 yr, whereas in man it is approximately 21 yr (61). Data on sample populations of registered dogs indicate that larger breeds have a shorter life span, according to the number of dogs over 20 yr of age. Osteosarcoma in the dog appears to be a disease of the old, while in man it is a disease of the young. Osteosarcomas of the skull appear to affect an older age group of dogs and smaller breeds, and to metastasize less than osteosarcomas of long bones. In one study, the average age of 33 dogs with skull osteosarcomas was found to be 8.8 yr; Boxer dogs were the most frequently affected, and there was a conspicuous absence of St. Bernards and Great Danes (26).

To make a correct clinical differential diagnosis between osteosarcoma and other bone lesions in the dog can be very difficult if only a biopsy section is submitted without adequate radiographs. The anamnesis, clinical, radiographic, laboratory and histopathologic findings must be used in combination if a reliable diagnosis is to be reached.

Osteosarcoma is also the most frequent bone tumor of cats, horses, and cattle, whereas it occurs rarely in other species of animals. The feline osteosarcoma, which is the only one beside its canine counterpart on which adequate information is available, has many similarities to the tumor in dogs. It is primarily a tumor of older cats, most cats affected being over 10 years of age (the normal life span of cats being around 20 years). Long tubular bones and flat bones are affected with equal frequency. The biologic behavior with pulmonary metastases appears similar to that in dog. In horses and cattle the skull appears to be the favorite site, but the information on age and clinical aspects are too incomplete to allow any other statements.

Parosteal or Juxtacortical Osteosarcoma

This entity has been recognized in dogs and cats as having a better prognosis than other osteosarcomas, as in the human counterpart (1, 31, 35). The roentgenographic and macroscopic appearance seem to suggest origin from periosteum with formation of a lobulated, often well delineated, white, firm mass attached to cortical bone (Fig. 4). Histologic examination reveals a mixture of osteoblasts and spindle cells, which may be covered by cartilage, as in osteochondromas. The site most frequently affected is the same as for the other osteosarcomas, namely the metaphysis.

II. CHONDROSARCOMA

This tumor occurs most frequently in dogs and sheep, being the most frequent skeletal tumor encountered in sheep. The unique susceptibility of sheep to this tumor is difficult to explain at present. Chondrosarcomas also have been described in cats, cattle, and horses. It has a predilection for flat bones, particularly the ribs, nose, and pelvis in the dog, and scapula, ribs, and sternum in sheep.

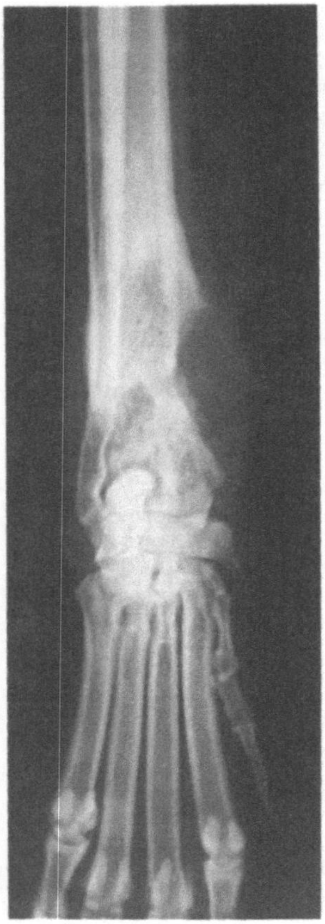

Fig. 4. Parosteal osteosarcoma, showing a localized well-circumscribed lesion on the medial metaphyseal area of the radius in a 7-year-old male Irish setter

In man, 132 of 199 chondrosarcomas observed were in flat bones, in dog 31 of 31 and in sheep 28 of 28.

It is of interest that the two common bone tumors of dogs, the osteosarcoma and chondrosarcoma, not only affect different bones of the body, but also have different predilections for both breeds and age groups. Both tumors are rare in small dogs weighing less than 18 kg; but whereas osteosarcomas occur primarily in the long bones of the so-called giant breeds of dogs (Great Danes, St. Bernards, Great Pyrenees dogs and Wolfhounds) chondrosarcomas have been encountered most frequently in the large medium-sized breeds like Boxers, Alsatians, Setters, Collies, and Airedales (Table 3). The age at which dogs are affected by

Table 3. Biologic data on 35 canine chondrosarcomas (BRODEY et al., 1974)

Frequency:	10% of skeletal tumors
Mean Age:	6 years
Breed:	Boxer, Alsatian, Mongrel > 18 kg
Site:	Flat bones (rib, turbinate, pelvis)

Table 4. Two canine bone tumors: biologic behavior (BRODEY *et al.*, 1974

	Osteosarcoma	Chondrosarcoma
Frequency	84%	9%
Long/Flat	4:1	1:1
Duration (wks)	9	18
Metastasis	47%	18%
8 m. surviv.	15%	71%
Mean age	7.7 y.	5.9 y.
Dogs < 2 yr.	10%	19%
Giant breeds	24%	3%
Alsatian	10%	18%

the two tumors, is also different. The chondrosarcoma affects a younger age group with an average age of 6 years, as against an average age of almost 8 years for the osteosarcoma (Table 4).

Histopathology. The tumor consists of a cartilagenous matrix, containing chondroitin sulfates in which neoplastic chondroblasts are placed. The size, shape, and nuclear configuration of the chondroblasts and the presence of double nuclei and mitoses are helpful criteria for determining whether a chondrosarcoma or one of its benign forms is present. The following benign cartilagenous tumors have been recognized in animals.

1. Enchondromas, originating in the center of short tubular bones;
2. Ecchondroma, developing from the perichondrium of permanent cartilage (costal, sternal, nasal, conchal, laryngeal, tracheal) and from the pelvic symphysis;
3. Osteochondromas or cartilagenous exostose, which consist of an osseous core extending from the cortex, which is covered by a cartilagenous cap. This tumor has two different manifestations, occurring as a solitary growth or in the more frequent multiple form. The latter entity, with a genetic predisposition, has been diagnosed several times in different species of animals, especially dogs, cats, and horses (Table 5). It is furthermore of significance that in the canine species it can transform into chondrosarcomas as in man. Such changes have been described in two dogs (2, 49) (See Table 5).

In addition to the difficulty of distinguishing benign chondromas from chondrosarcomas, there is another difficulty, namely that of distinguishing them from osteosarcomas, which may consist largely of an undifferentiated matrix with only few areas showing maturation with bone formation. The use of Alcian and toluidine blue can be helpful in determinating whether patches of calcified matrix or osteoid material in a sarcoma are formed directly, by tumor cells, or indirectly due to metaplastic changes, sarcoma that produces osteoid or bone by a direct action of tumor cells is an osteosarcoma. The presence of alkaline phosphatase in the tumor cells indicates that they are osteoblasts and not chondroblasts of fibroblasts. Increased serum levels of alkaline phosphatase have not been associated with osteosarcomas in animals. The

Table 5. Multiple cartilagenous exostoses (osteochondromas, aclasis)

I. Cat
1. JUBB & KENNEDY (1963)
2. JACOBSON (1971)
3. BROWN et al. (1972)

II. Dogs
1. BANKS & BRIDGES (1956)
2. CARLSON (1961)
3. OWEN & NIELSEN (1968)
4. DINGWALL (1970)
5. OWEN & BOSTOCK (1971)
6. CHESTER (1971)

III. Horses
More than 6 cases. Exact number not determined

differentiation of a chondrosarcoma from an osteosarcoma is not merely an academic exercise but an important clinical question; recent studies (10) have shown that canine chondrosarcomas, like their human counterpart, have a much better prognosis as assessed both by 8-month survival rates and by rate of metastasis (Table 4). The chondrosarcoma is frequently a large lobulated, radiolucent tumor, mostly of flat bone, that grows slowly and metastasizes only in about one fifth of cases.

III. HEMANGIOSARCOMA

This tumor is rare in all species of animals. Only in the dog has a sufficient number of cases been reported to enable us to draw any conclusion on their appearance and behavior (Table 6). It can be very difficult, even in cases with a thorough clinical work-up and a complete necropsy examination, to decide whether a hemangiosarcoma has originated in bone, or is the result of metastatic spread from elsewhere in the body. There is another possibility which seems more likely, namely that hemangiosarcomas are of multicentric origin, due to multiple, simultaneous attacks of a carcinogenic agent, whether a virus or a chemical or radioactive substance. Hemangiosarcomas can affect any bone in the body, with most cases reported in the ribs, pelvis, and long bones (Table 7). It occurs in older dogs primarily, but a wide range of ages has been reported, from 18 months to 16 years. The mean age is 7 years, which is approximately the same as that of dogs affected with the two common bone tumors, the osteosarcoma and chondrosarcoma. The breeds most frequently affected are Alsatian, Great Dane and Boxer (3). Alsatians have a higher frequency of visceral hemangiosarcomas than any other breed, and Boxers are known to have more neoplasms in general than any other breed of dog.

Histopathology. Histopathologic diagnosis is usually not difficult, except for the differentiation of hemangiosarcoma from aneurysmal bone cysts, which also are found in dogs and cats (Table 8). The presence of blood containing slit-like spaces lined by large endothelial cells, frequently with mitosis, denotes a hemangiosarcoma, whereas large cystic spaces with normal or hyperplastic endothelial lining are indicative of aneurysmal bone cysts.

Table 6. Reports of canine hemangiosarcoma of bone

1.	BRODEY *et al.* (1963) 4 dogs (6-9 y) 2 Boxers, 1 Alsatian and 1 Collie
2.	QUIGLEY *et al.* (1964) 2 dogs (6+8 yr) 2 Terriers
3.	OWEN (1969) 2 dogs (1 1/2 + 8 yr) English Setter, West Highland White Terrier
4.	JACOBSON (1971) 8 dogs (1 1/2 - 11 1/2 yr) 3 Alsatians, 1 Boxer, mongrels
5.	LING *et al.* (1974) 8 dogs (3-16 yr) 5 Alsatians, Hound, Beagle, Spaniel
6.	BINGEL *et al.* (1974) 20 dogs (2-11 yr) Boxers, Great Danes, Alsatians

Table 7. Biologic data on hemangiosarcoma of bone in dogs (BINGEL *et al.*, 1974)

Breeds:	Alsatian, Boxer, Great Dane
Age:	2 - 11 yr (7 yr mean)
Sex:	1.6 male / 1 female
Rate:	2 - 3% of Bone Tumors
Site:	Ribs, Pelvis, Long Bones
Metastatic or Multicentric:	50%

Table 8. Reports of aneurysmal bone cysts in animals

1.	PRICE & SUMNER-SMITH (1966) 1 dog 10 yr male Retriever, Prox. Tibia
2.	JACOBSON (1971) 4 dogs Alsatians (2), Boxer, Great Dane 3 males, 1 female aged 5 to 12 years ribs, mandible, scapula, stifle
3.	LIU *et al.* (1974) 3 cats, female, domestic shorthair sacrum, ileum, coccygeum

IV. FIBROSARCOMA

There are two forms of this tumor, periosteal and medullary depending on the site of origin. Both are rare and occur mostly in dogs (Table 9). The proper diagnosis cannot be made with any degree of confidence in advanced cases where massive bone destruction is present. In animals, as a rule, a bone lesion is frequently not recognized before it produces either lameness or a large swelling, which is possibly why so few medullary fibrosarcomas are reported. The histologic appearance is the same in both types, and only the radiographic and macroscopic findings can determine which type is present. The tumor consists of spindle-shaped

Table 9. Reports of canine fibrosarcoma of bone

1. OWEN (1969) - 3 dogs
   Standard Poodle 9 yr, Wolfhound 2 yr, Greyhound 9 yr
2. JACOBSON (1971) - Boxer 3 yr, M
3. BRODEY <u>et al</u>. (1963) - 3 dogs
   Pointer 4 yr, M, Collie 3 yr, F, Spaniel 3 yr, M

fibroblastic cells arranged in either fascicles or a syncytial pattern, with or without collagen or mucinous ground substance formation. Mitoses are frequent in some cases, bone destruction is usually extensive, and there may be areas of reactive periosteal bone formation, which should not be misdiagnosed as tumor bone. If direct bone formation by the tumor cells is demonstrated the term osteosarcoma should be applied.

V. LIPOSARCOMA

Liposarcoma is an extremely rare neoplasm of bone in animals. Only three cases have been found in which documentation by pictorial and descriptive information is sufficient to warrant the diagnosis (Table 10). It is remarkable that all three occurred in long tubular bones of very young dogs less than two years of age. In all three cases there were marked osteolytic changes in the affected bone; in two cases the tumor had metastasized and in the other amputation was performed.

Table 10. Reports of liposarcoma of bone in dogs

1. D. Femur in 18 mo. Golden Retriever
   (BRODEY and RISER, 1966)
2. D. Tibia in 18 mo. Miniature Poodle
   (OWEN, 1966)
3. D. Radius in 16 mo. Greyhound
   (DAVIS <u>et</u> <u>al</u>., 1974)

VI. GIANT CELL TUMOR (OSTEOCLASTOMA)

At present there are very few reports on dogs and cats in which this diagnosis can be considered. The author has seen sections from one case, occurring in the distal end of the tibia in a mature Labrador Retriever. Other reports concern one case in a dog (<u>31</u>) and a giant-cell tumor occurring in the distal end of the femur in a 1-year-old female cat (<u>28</u>). McCLELLAND reported a case in a cat and one in a dog (<u>37</u>).

VII. RETICULUM CELL SARCOMA

This tumor is extremely rare, only two cases being suggestive for this diagnosis (Table 11). The tumor consists of round or pleomorphic cells with vesicular nuclei that are often ovoid or bean-shaped. The cytoplasm is usually abundant and silver stains may show fine fibers sur-

Table 11. Reports of reticulum cell sarcoma of bone

1.	6 Cases (DRIEUX and VERETENNIKOFF, 1963, 1966)
2.	Prox. Humerus 1-yr m. English Setter (BRODEY *et al.*, 1963)
3.	Thoracic Vertebra (2 and 3) 2-yr m. Springer-Spaniel No Metastases (STEINBERG *et al.*, 1966)

rounding individual cells. Stains for glycogen in the cytoplasm of tumor cells are negative, which is helpful in differentiating this tumor from Ewing's sarcoma.

VIII. EWING'S SARCOMA

There are two descriptions of Ewing's sarcoma in the literature (20, 56).

SUMMARY

A review of bone tumors in animals, based on cases reported in the literature and on personal examination of cases from several universities in the U.S.A. and Europe, has shown that:

1. The following bone tumors occur in decreasing order of frequency in animals: osteosarcoma, chondrosarcoma, osteochondroma, hemangiosarcoma, fibrosarcoma, and liposarcoma;
2. The dog has by far the highest frequency of bone tumors; and osteosarcomas account for approximately 80 percent of bone tumors in dog, followed by chondrosarcomas and hemangiosarcomas;
3. Bone tumors occur less frequently in the cat than in the dog, and are of essentially the same types and incidence as in the dog;
4. Sheep has a unique propensity for chondrosarcoma and primary bone tumors are rare in other species;
5. Giant cell tumors, reticulum cell sarcomas, and Ewing's sarcomas are exceptional findings in animals.

SELECTED REFERENCES

1. BANKS, W.C.: Parosteal osteosarcoma in a dog and cat. J. Amer. vet. med. Ass. 158, 1412-1415 (1971)
2. BANKS, W.C., BRIDGES, C.H.: Multiple cartilagenous exostoses in a dog. J. Amer. vet. med. Ass. 129, 131-135 (1956)
3. BINGEL, S.A., BRODEY, R.S., ALLEN, H.L., RISER, W.H.: Hemangiosarcoma of bone in the dog. J. small Anim. Pract. 15, 303-322 (1974)
4. BRODEY, R.S.: Surgical treatment of canine osteosarcoma. J. Amer. vet. med. Ass. 147, 729-735 (1966)
5. BRODEY, R.S., RISER, W.H.: Liposarcoma of bone in a dog: a case report. J. Amer. vet. radiol. Soc. 7, 27-33 (1966)

6. BRODEY, R.S., RISER, W.H.: Canine osteosarcoma: a clinicopathologic study of 194 cases. Clin. Orthop. 62, 54-64 (1969)
7. BRODEY, R.S., MCGRATH, J.T., REYNOLDS, H.: A clinical and radiological study of canine bone neoplasms. Part 1. J. Amer. vet. med. Ass. 134, 53-71 (1959)
8. BRODEY, R.S., SAUER, R.M., MEDWAY, W.: Canine bone neoplasms. J. Amer. vet. med. Ass. 143, 471-495 (1963)
9. BRODEY, R.S., REID, C.F., SAUER, R.M.: Metastatic bone neoplasms in the dog. J. Amer. vet. med. Ass. 148, 39-43 (1966)
10. BRODEY, R.S., MISDORP, W., RISER, W.H., VAN DER HEUL, R.O.: Canine skeletal chondrosarcoma: a clinicopathologic study of 35 cases. J. Amer. vet. med. Ass. 165, 68-78 (1974)
11. BROWN, R.J., TREVETHAN, W.P., HENRY, V.L.: Multiple osteochondroma in a Siamese cat. J. Amer. vet. med. Ass. 160, 433-435 (1972)
12. CARLSON, W.D.: Veterinary Radiology. London: Bailliere 1968
13. CHESTER, D.K.: Multiple cartilagenous exostoses in two generations of dogs. J. Amer. vet. med. Ass. 159, 895-897 (1971)
14. COTCHIN, E.: Spontaneous sarcomas of bone in dogs: 30 cases. Brit. vet. J. 109, 248-257 (1953)
15. COTCHIN, E.: Further observations on neoplasms in dogs, with particular reference to site of origin and malignancy. II. Male genital, skeletal, lymphatic and other systems. Brit. Vet. J. 110, 274-286 (1954)
16. DAVIS, P.E., DIXON, R.J., JOHNSON, J.A., PARIS, R.: Liposarcoma of bone in a dog. J. small Anim. Pract. 15, 445-456 (1974).
17. DINGWALL, J.S.: Multiple cartilagenous exostoses in a dog. Can. Vet. J. 11, 114-119 (1970)
18. DRIEUX, H., VERETENNIKOFF, S.: Observations de radiologie et de pathologie comparées. II. Etude comparative (Homme-Chien) anatomo-radiologique de l'osteo-chondro-myxo-fibro-sarcome. Rec. Méd. vét. 138, 257-264 (1962)
19. DRIEUX, H., VERETENNIKOFF, S., CÉSAR, R.J.: Observations de radiologie et de pathologie comparées. III. Etude comparative du reticulosarcome osseux de l'Homme et du Chien: histologie et radiologie. Rec. Méd. vét. 139, 523-546 (1963)
20. DRIEUX, H., VERETENNIKOFF, S., CÉSAR, R.J.: Observations de radiologie et de pathologie comparées. IV. Diagnosic radiologique differentiel du sarcome d'Ewing et du sarcome de Parker-Jackson des os longs. Rec. Méd. vét. 142, 37-45 (1966)
21. DRIEUX, H., VERETENNIKOFF, S., CÉSAR, R.J.: Observations de radiologie et de pathologie comparées. V. Etude comparative du chondrosarcome des os longs de l'Homme et du Chien: histologie et radiologie. Rec. Méd. vét. 143, 523-546 (1967)
22. DUNGWORTH, D.L., WILSON, M.R., GRUCHY, C.L., MCCALLUM, G.: Malignant synovioma in a cow. J. Path. Bact. 88, 83-91 (1964)
23. GORLIN, R.J., BARRON, C.N., CHANHRY, A.P., CLARK, J.J.: The oral and pharyngeal pathology of domestic animals. Amer. J. vet. Res. 20, 1032-1061 (1959)
24. GORLIN, R.J., MESKIN, L.H., BRODEY, R.S.: Odontogenic tumors in man and animals. Ann. N.Y. Acad. Sci. 108, 722-773 (1963)
25. HAMILTON, J.M., KNIGHT, D.: Cartilagenous tumors in dogs: a description of two cases and a review of the literature. Vet. Rec. 92, 41-43 (1973)
26. HARDY, W.D., Jr., BRODEY, R.S., RISER, W.H.: Osteosarcomas of the canine skull. J. Amer. vet. radiol. Soc. 8, 5-16 (1967)
27. HARE, W.S.D.: The age at which epiphyseal union takes place in the limb bones of the dog. Wien. tierärztl. Wschr. 1960, 222-245
28. HOWARD, E.B., KENYON, A.J.: Maligant osteoclastoma (giant-cell tumor) in a cat with associated mast-cell response. Cornell Vet. 57, 388-409 (1967)
29. HOWARD, E.B., NIELSEN, S.W.: Neoplasia of the Boxer dog. Amer. J. vet. Res. 26, 1121-1131 (1965)

30. HULSE, E.V.: A benign giant-cell tumor in a cat. J. Path. Bact. 91, 219-271 (1966)
31. JACOBSON, S.A.: The Comparative Pathology of the Tumors of Bone. Springfield, Ill: Thomas 1971
32. JUBB, K.V., KENNEDY, P.C.: Pathology of Domestic Animals, New York: Academic Press 1963
33. LIEBERMANN, L.L.: Synovioma of a dog. J. Amer. vet. med. Ass. 128, 263-264 (1956)
34. LING, G.V., MORGAN, J.P., POOL, R.P.: Primary bone tumors in the dog: a combined clinical radiographic and histologic approach to early diagnosis. J. Amer. vet. med. Ass. 165, 55-67 (1974)
35. LIU, S.K., DORFMAN, H.P., PATNAIK, A.K.: Primary and secondary bone tumors in the cat. J. small Anim. Pract. 15, 141-156 (1974)
36. MCCLELLAND, R.: A giant-cell tumor of the tibia in a cat. Cornell Vet. 31, 86-87 (1941)
37. MCCLELLAND, R.: Giant-cell tumor of the radius in a dog. N. Amer. Vet. 22, 101-102 (1941)
38. MISDORP, W., DEN HELDER, B.A.: Bone metastasis in mammary cancer: a report of 10 cases in the female dog and some comparison with human cases. Brit. J. Cancer 20, 496-503 (1966)
39. MOULTON, J.E.: Tumors in Domestic Animals. Berkeley: University of California Press 1961
40. MULLIGAN, R.M.: Neoplasms of the Dog. Baltimore: Williams and Wilkins 1949
41. NIELSEN, S.W.: Extraskeletal giant-cell tumor in a cat. Cornell Vet. 42, 304-311 (1952)
42. NIELSEN, S.W.: Radiological aspects of bone tumors. J. Amer. vet. radiol. Soc. 2, 1-3 (1961)
43. NIELSEN, S.W., SCHNELLE, G.B.: Primary adamantinoma in the humerus of a dog. J. Amer. vet. med. Ass. 121, 84-88 (1952)
44. NIELSEN, S.W., SCHRODER, J.D., SMITH, D.L.T.: The pathology of osteogenic sarcoma in dogs. J. Amer. vet. med. Ass. 124, 28-35 (1954)
45. OWEN, L.N.: The differential diagnosis of bone tumours in the dog. Vet. Rec. 74, 439-446 (1962)
46. OWEN, L.N.: An account of multiple osteosarcomata of bone in dogs, having multicentric or metastatic origin. Brit. J. Radiol. 38, 520-526 (1965)
47. OWEN, L.N.: Bone tumours in the dog. J. S. Afr. Vet. Med. Ass. 37, 295-401 (1966)
48. OWEN, L.N.: Bone Tumours in Man and Animals. London: Butterworths 1969
49. OWEN, L.N., BOSTOCK, D.E.: Multiple cartilagenous exostoses with development of a metastasizing osteosarcoma in a Shetland Sheepdog. J. small Anim. Pract. 12, 507-512 (1971)
50. OWEN, L.N., NIELSEN, S.W.: Multiple cartilagenous exostoses (diaphyseal aclasis) in a Yorkshire terrier. J. small Anim. Pract. 9, 519-521 (1968)
51. OWEN, L.N., STEVENSON, D.E.: Observations on canine osteosarcomata. Res. Vet. Sci. 2, 117-129 (1961)
52. PRICE, C.H.G., SUMNER-SMITH, G.: "Malignant bone aneurysm" in a dog: an unusual example of osteosarcoma. Brit. vet. J. 122, 51-54 (1966)
53. QUIGLEY, P.J., DESARAM, W., DAWSON, I.M.P., PRYSE-DAVIES, J.: Two cases of haemangiosarcoma of the radius in the dog. Vet. Rec. 77, 1207-1209 (1965)
54. RISER, W.H., SHIRER, J.F.: Normal and abnormal growth of the distal foreleg in large and giant dogs. J. Amer. vet. radiol. Soc. 6, 50-64 (1965)
55. RISER, W.H., BRODEY, R.S., BIERY, D.N.: Bone infarctions associated with malignant bone tumors in dogs. J. Amer. vet. med. Ass. 160, 411-421 (1972)
56. RUDOLPH, R., WEISS, E., BIEL, M.: Multiples Ewing-Sarkom bei einem Hund. Zbl. Vet.-Med. A 16, 426-437 (1969)

57. STEINBERG, S.A., KELLY, A.M.: Clinico-Pathologic Conferences: reticulum-cell sarcoma of bone. J. Amer. vet. med. Ass. 148, 170-179 (1966)
58. SULLIVAN, D.J.: Cartilagenous tumors (chondroma and chondrosarcoma) in animals. Amer. J. vet. Res. 21, 531-535 (1960)
59. SUTER, P.: Klinische und roentgenologische Diagnosen und Fehldiagnosen bei Knochen-Tumoren von Hund und Katze. Schweiz. Arch. Tierheilk. 105, 459 (1963)
60. TJALMA, R.A.: Canine bone sarcoma: estimation of relative risk as a function of body size. J. nat. Cancer Inst. 36, 1137-1150 (1966)
61. WOLKE, R.E., NIELSEN, S.W.: Site incidence of canine osteosarcoma. J. small Anim. Pract. 7, 489-492 (1966)

Bone Tumors Induced by Inhalation of $^{238}PuO_2$ in Dogs

J. F. PARK, J. E. LUND, H. A. RAGAN, P. L. HACKETT, and M. E. FRAZIER

ABSTRACT

Plutonium-238, an alpha-emitting radionuclide, is used as a heat source in thermoeleltric power generators such as have been employed on lunar expeditions or communications satellites and in cardiac pacemakers. It has an 86.4 year half-life and emits 5.5 MeV alpha particles. Beagle dogs were given single 10 - 30 minute exposures to $^{238}PuO_2$ aerosols to study the long-term translocation of plutonium and biological effects. Dogs with a terminal body burden ranging from 7 - 260 μCi were euthanized due to respiratory insufficiency related to plutonium-induced pneumonitis during the first 3 years after exposure. Nine of the 11 dogs euthanized during the 4 - 6 year postexposure period had osteosarcomas. The terminal plutonium body burden in the tumor-bearing dogs ranged from 0.5 - 2.6 μCi with 30 - 55% of the plutonium in the skeleton. Experiments are in progress to further define the dose-effect relationship of inhaled $^{238}PuO_2$ and investigate the mechanisms of plutonium-induced neoplasia.

INTRODUCTION

Plutonium-238 has an 86.4-year half-life. The specific activity of ^{238}Pu is 17.4 Ci/g (one μCi weighs about 0.06 μg). It emits 5.5 MeV alpha particles. The alpha particles penetrate about 25 μm in bone and 37 μm in soft tissues such as bone marrow. Radiation damage is produced close to where the plutonium is located at the time of emission of the alpha particle (VAUGHAN, et al., 1973).

Plutonium-238 is used as a heat source in thermoelectric power generators such as have been employed on lunar expeditions or communication satellites and in cardiac pacemakers (STANNARD, 1973). It has been proposed for powering artificial hearts and cardiac assist devices.

Beagle dogs, with terminal body burdens of 17 - 261 μCi, died 1 - 6 months after inhalation of $^{238}PuO_2$. Death was due to radiation pneumonitis-induced respiratory insufficiency (PARK, et al., 1970). In these acute studies, plutonium was retained primarily in the lungs. The thoracic lymph nodes, liver and skeleton appeared to accumulate plutonium 4 - 6 months after exposure (Table 1). To determine the late effects

---

+ This paper is based on work performed under United States Atomic Energy Commission Contract AT (45-1) -1830.

Table 1. Dog mortality and tissue distribution after inhalation of $^{238}PuO_2$

Dog No.	Survival (days after exposure)	Terminal body burden (μCi)	Plutonium distribution % terminal body burden lungs	Lymph Nodes[a]	Skeleton	Liver
390 M	37	261	92	4	2	1
403 F	30	167	94	2	2	2
408 F	35	168	93	1	3	2
395 M	56	112	92	3	4	1
450 F	56	74	91	4	4	1
393 M	61	140	94	2	3	1
460 M	70	84	90	3	4	2
442 F	76	88	90	4	3	2
449 F	94	44	91	3	4	1
413 F	125	17	80	9	7	3
400 M	180	25	77	4	13	5

[a]Tracheobronchial, mediastinal and sternal lymph nodes.

of inhaled $^{238}PuO_2$, 22 beagle dogs were exposed to $^{238}PuO_2$ aersols and observed for their life span. Table 2 shows the experimental design. Nine of the 16 dogs that have died during the 7-year postexposure observation period had osteosarcomas.

Table 2. Experimental design. (late effects of inhaled $^{238}PuO_2$ in Beagles

	$^{238}PuO_2$ Calcined 350°	$^{238}PuO_2$ Crushed Microspheres	Controls
Number of dogs	10	12	17
Mortalitiy (7 years after exposure)	8	8	0
Bone Tumors	5	4	0

METHODS

Two different $^{238}PuO_2$ materials were used. Plutonium-238 oxide calcined at 350° was used to compare the effects of inhaled $^{238}PuO_2$ with inhaled $^{239}PuO_2$ calcined at 350°C (PARK, et al., 1972). Crushed $^{238}PuO_2$ microspheres were used because $^{238}PuO_2$ microspheres were being used in thermoelectric generators in 1967.

Ten 40 - 42 month-old beagle dogs (9 males and 1 female) were exposed nose-only for 10 - 30 minutes to plutonium calcined at 350°C. Twelve 8-month-old beagle dogs (3 males and 9 females) were exposed to $^{238}PuO_2$-crushed microspheres. Seventeen age-related dogs served as a control group. The count median diameter of the aerosols of both materials was 0.1 μm. The dogs were exposed via a mask from an aerosol exposure chamber as described previously (PARK, et al., 1969).

The dogs, raised in the beagle colony in our laboratory, were immunized annually with canine distemper and hepatitis vaccine. They were housed in inside pens with free access to outdoor runs. They were fed kibbled laboratory diet once each day and water ad lib. Blood samples were collected each 3 months for hematologic and clinical chemistry measurements. They were weighed every 2 weeks. Routine thoracic and skeletal radiographic surveys were completed annually. Minor physical examinations including respiration rate and heart rate were completed once every 3 months.

The dogs were euthanized when clinical signs indicated death was imminent. Representative tissue samples from each organ and samples of gross lesions were collected at necropsy for histopathologic examination. The muscle was manually removed from the skeleton and the disarticulated skeleton was radiographed to detect lesions which may not have been recognized in the live animal. The remainder of the tissues were analyzed for plutonium content by liquid scintillation counting following ashing and dissolution in HNO_3-HF (KEOUGH and POWERS, 1970).

Leukocyte, erythrocyte, and hemoglobin concentration were determined using the coulter counter model S. Smears for leukocyte differential cell counts were made using the Platt blood film centrifuge and stained in Wright-Giemsa stain. The differential cell count was based on a minimum of 200 cells counted by two technicans. Serum constituents were determined by Autoanalyzer II methodology.

Tissue sections, fixed in 10% neutral buffered formalin, were embedded in paraffin and sectioned at 4 - 6 µm thickness. The sections were stained with hematoxylin and eosin (H & E). Autoradiographs of sections adjacent to those examined with H & E were prepared on nuclear track alpha (NTA) plates and stained with methylene blue.

During necropsy suspected neoplasms (based on radiologic evidence and gross pathology) were excised using sterile procedures. Sections were removed from these specimens for histologic examination prior to cell culture. Soft tissues were finely minced and the resultant pieces were explanted into Falcon flasks and incubated in NCTC 135 (EVANS et al., 1967) containing 20% fetal bovine serum, 100 µg/ml gentamycin, and 60 µg/ml tylocine. In one portion of the cultures the explants were immobilized using the plasma clot technique, while in the remaining cultures partial immobilization was obtained by minimal handling and taking extra precautions when changing the medium. The culture medium was changed every 4th or 5th day until a good outgrowth of cells from the explants was achieved (this usually required 2 - 3 weeks). The explants were then removed and the cells trypsinized and reseeded into Falcon flasks and grown as monolayers. Approximately 2 x 10^6 freshly trypsinized cells from fifth passage cell cultures of dog 445 M and dog 469 M were inoculated in utero into 31 - 33 day fetuses of two bitches. The neonates were later sacrificed for histopathologic examination and cell culture when tumor growth was evident.

RESULTS

Mortality and Tissue Distribution of Plutonium

Eight of the 10 dogs exposed to 350°C calcined $^{238}PuO_2$ and 8 of the 12 dogs exposed to $^{238}PuO_2$ crushed microspheres were euthanized when death was imminent during the 7-year postexposure period. The causes of death and the ^{238}Pu distribution in the tissues are shown in Table 3.

Table 3. Mortality and tissue distribution of plutonium in dogs after inhalation of $^{238}PuO_2$

Dog No.	Survival (months after exposure)	Terminal body burden (μCi)	Plutonium distribution % terminal body burden				Cause of death
			Lungs	Lymph Nodes[a]	Liver	Skeleton	
(After inhalation of $^{238}PuO_2$ calcined at 350°C)							
492 F	23	3.0	4	4	23	64	Bone fracture
404 M	36	8.1	32	10	23	32	Respiratory insufficiency
467 M	38	7.0	15	11	13	57	Respiratory insufficiency
469 M	54	2.6	34	5	17	41	Bone tumor
445 M	58	2.5	6	10	23	55	Bone tumor
438 M	60	2.3	7	11	33	43	Bone tumor
453 M	62	2.2	17	9	22	47	Bone tumor
405 M	70	2.6	23	10	28	34	Bone tumor (lung tumor)[b]
(After inhalation of $^{238}PuO_2$ crushed microspheres)							
485 M	22	3.1	72	7	7	12	Encephalitis
500 M	34	1.1	39	21	12	24	Hemorrhage
497 F	52	0.2	16	3	31	46	Intestinal obstruction
481 F	60	0.5	13	23	23	37	Myelogenous leukemia (bone tumor)[b]
489 F	62	2.5	7	26	27	32	Bone tumor (lung tumor)[b]
482 F	70	0.8	8	19	15	47	Bone tumor
494 F	75	0.4	3	9	32	48	Fibrosarcoma
488 F	76	1.4	9	15	29	41	Bone tumor (lung tumor)[b]

[a]Tracheobronchial, mediastinal, and sternal lymph nodes.
[b]Other lesions.

Two of the dogs, 404 M and 467 M, were euthanized because of respiratory insufficiency related to plutonium-induced pulmonary lesions. Three dogs died of causes thought to be unrelated to the plutonium exposures: hemorrhage due to fight wounds (500 M), encephalitis related to ear infection (485 M), and intestinal obstruction (497 F). Three dogs died of causes potentially relatable to plutonium exposure: fractured humerus (492 F), myelogenous leukemia (481 F), and maxillary fibrosarcoma (494 F). Eight of the dogs were euthanized because of plutonium-induced bone tumors. Dog 481 F had a bone tumor, observed at necrospy, in addition to myelogenous leukemia, and dog (405 M) had a lung tumor (bronchiolar-alveolar cell carcinoma) which was evident radiographically 15 months prior to euthanasia because of a vertebral bone tumor. Dogs 488 F and 489 F had small lung tumors which were classified as adenomas.

Four to 6 years after plutonium exposures, the largest fraction of plutonium retained in the body was in the skeleton followed in descending order by liver, thoracic lymph nodes, and lung. The highest plutonium concentration occurred in the lymph nodes followed in descending order by lung, or liver and skeleton (Table 4). The lethal biological effects observed during the 4 - 6 years following exposure to $^{238}PuO_2$ were primarily related to skeletal deposition of plutonium with 9 dogs having bone tumors. In addition to the plutonium-induced lesions causing death, the dogs had fibrotic tracheobronchial and mediastinal lymph nodes, focal pulmonary fibrosis,and nodular hyperplasia in the liver.

Table 4. Plutonium concentration in tissues of beagles after inhalation of $^{238}PuO_2$

Dog No.	Survival time Postexposure (months)	Terminal body burden (μCi)	Plutonium concentration (nCi/g)[a]			
			Lungs[b]	Lymph nodes	Liver	Skeleton
		(After inhalation of $^{238}PuO_2$ calcined at 350°C)				
492 F	23	3.0	2.0	196	3.2	2.3
404 M	36	8.1	7.7	556	5.8	1.9
467 M	38	7.0	13.8	6916	4.0	1.2
469 M	54	2.6	13.7	222	1.6	.8
445 M	58	2.5	2.1	509	1.8	1.0
483 M	60	2.3	1.1	886	3.4	.6
453 M	62	2.2	4.2	229	1.9	1.0
405 M	70	2.6	7.0	179	1.9	.6
		(After inhalation of $^{238}PuO_2$ crushed microspheres)				
485 M	22	3.1	24.9	459	.7	.3
500 M	34	1.1	5.6	1032	.4	.3
497 F	52	0.2	.4	14	.3	.1
481 F	60	0.5	.9	260	.2	.2
489 F	62	2.5	3.2	2282	4.0	.8
482 F	70	0.8	.8	900	.6	.2
494 F	75	0.4	.2	92	.6	.2
488 F	76	1.4	2.2	1609	1.8	.6

[a] nCi/g wet tissues.
[b] Estimated normal weight of lung was used to calculate concentration due to lesions in lung.

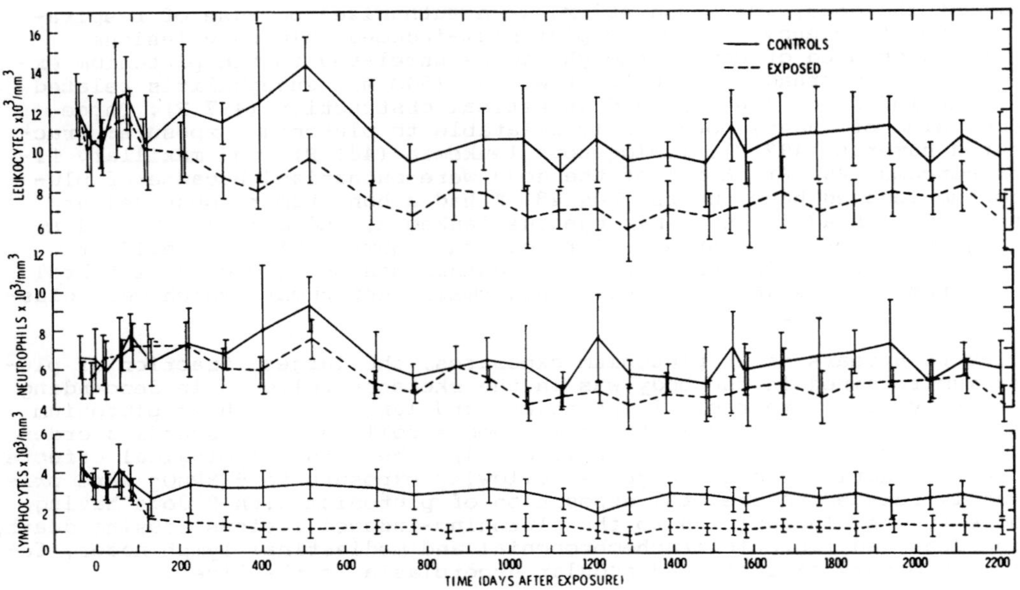

Fig. 1. Leukocyte values of dogs after inhalation of $^{238}PuO_2$ crushed microspheres (means ± 95% confidence interval)

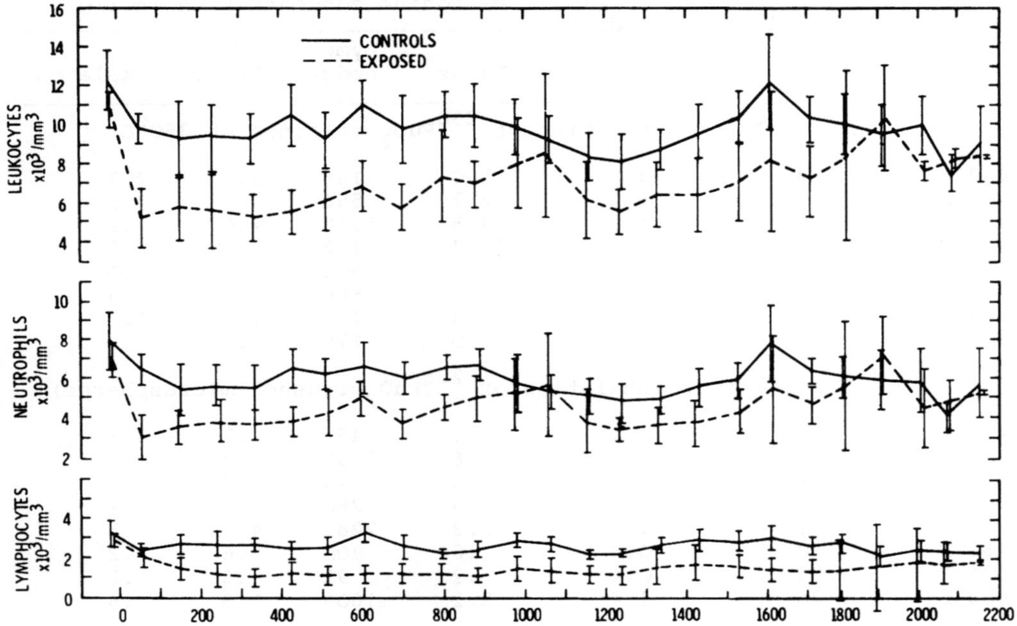

Fig. 2. Leukocyte values of dogs after inhalation of $^{238}PuO_2$ calcined at 350°C (means ± 95% confidence interval)

Hematology and Clinical Chemistry

The dogs had a persistent lymphocytopenia (Fig. 1 and 2) which became apparent in both groups by 200 days after exposure. In the crushed microsphere-exposed dogs (Fig. 1), the mean lymphocyte count of the six surviving exposed dogs was below that of controls at 6 years after exposure. The total leukocyte count of the exposed dogs was frequently lower than that of controls, primarily due to the low lymphocyte counts and a small but consistent reduction in neutrophils. Lymphocytopenia in the 350° calcined plutonium-exposed dogs was evident 5 years after exposure, when only four of the dogs with the lowest body burdens remained alive (Fig. 2). The dogs in this group also had a reduction in neutrophils which was apparent 1 month to 2 years after exposure, when the higher dose-level dogs were still alive. The dogs also showed a leukopenia due to reduction in lymphocytes and neutrophils. No consistent changes were observed in the hemogram for other leukocytes, erythrocytes, or hemoglobin. The lower initial mean lymphocyte values in the dogs exposed to crushed microspheres compared to the 350° calcined plutonium-exposed group may have been due to an age difference. The dogs exposed to 350° calcined $^{238}PuO_2$ were exposed at 3 years of age whereas the dogs exposed to crushed microspheres were 8 months old at the time of exposure. Older dogs generally have lower lymphocyte counts. No consistent differences between control and experimental dogs were observed for serum urea nitrogen, creatinine or glucose. Occasional increases in serum glutamic oxalacetic transaminase (SGOT) activity occurred, but elevations of serum glutamic pyruvic transaminase (SGPT) were most frequently encountered. Percentages of elevated SGPT values (> 55 Wroblewski-LaDue units) in the two treatment groups were 36 and 28, compared with 9 and 10% in the control groups (Fig. 3). The difference between the two treatment groups may have been due to age at exposure or to plutonium dose. Results from SGPT analyses for individual animals reflected the histopathologic findings of hepatic nodular hyperplasia observed in the liver at necropsy.

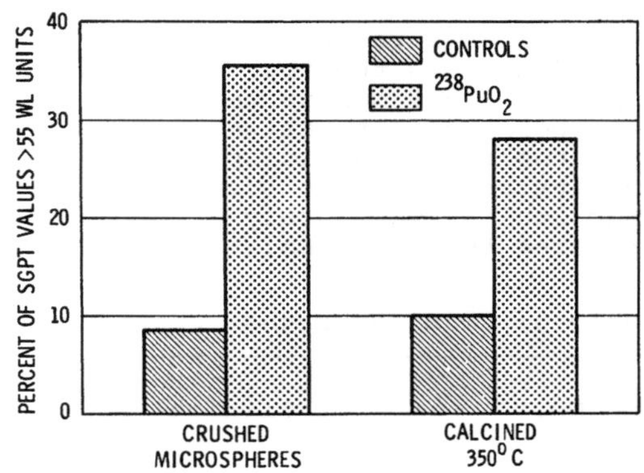

Fig. 3. Percentage of elevated SGPT values (> 55 Wroblewski-LaDue Units) in dogs after inhalation of $^{238}PuO_2$

Increases in alkaline phosphatase activity were moderate, infrequent, and usually paralled the elevated SGPT values. Of the nine dogs with confirmed bone tumors, all but one had occasional aberrant alkaline phosphatase levels. Fig. 4 shows a serum enzyme profile for a dog with osteosarcomas of the scapula, vertebra, and humerus, as well as widespread hepatic nodular hyperplasia. Alkaline phosphatase isoenzyme analyses of the terminal serum sample by means of chemical inhibition

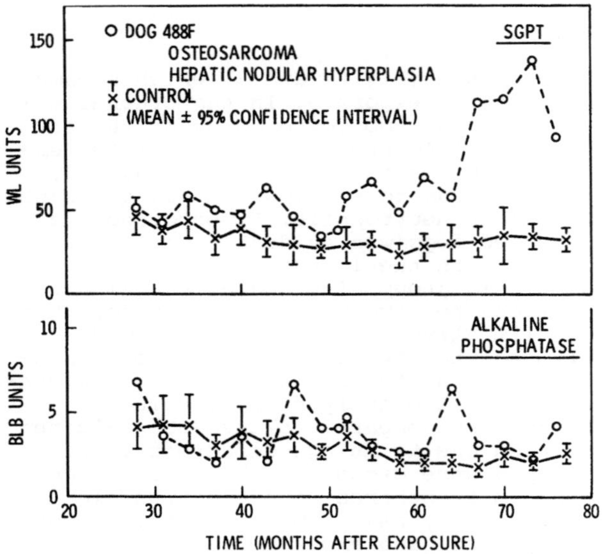

Fig. 4. Serum enzymes in dog 488 F after inhalation of $^{238}PuO_2$. SGPT (Wroblewski-LaDue Units) and alkaline phosphatase (Bessey-Lowry-Brock Units)

yielded values of 43% activity with urea and 47% with L-phenylalanine, indicating the presence of liver isoenzyme.

Bone Tumors

Bone tumors were first detected in four of the dogs during routine annual skeletal radiographic survey (Table 5). At the time of radiographic diagnosis the dogs showed no other clinical signs. The four dogs survived 3 - 7 months before clinical signs of lameness or persistent pain were evident, at which time they were sacrificed. Figs. 5 - 8 show the radiographic appearance of the initial lesions detected on routine radiographic survey of the four dogs compared to the radiographic lesion immediately prior to sacrifice. These radiographic lesions appeared to be osteoblastic.

Table 5. Clinical signs related to bone tumors diagnoses and survival

Dog No.	Clinical sign	Survival after diagnosis (days)[b]
469 M	Radiographic[a]	96
445 M	Radiographic[a]	114
438 M	Radiographic[a]	164
453 M	Radiographic[a]	206
405 M	Lameness	20
481 F	Lameness	20
489 F	Lameness	21
482 F	Lameness	112
488 F	Lameness	7

[a]Routine scheduled skeletal radiographic survey.
[b]All dogs were euthanized when it was evident from radiographic and clinical signs that death was imminent.

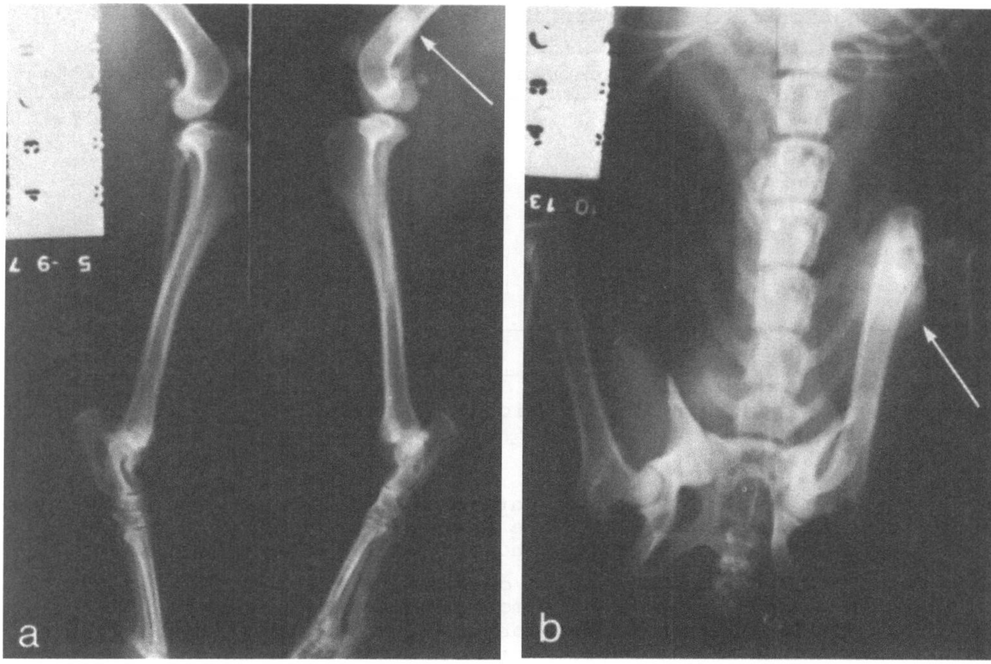

Fig. 5. Radiograph of dog 438 M showing density in the distal right femur (a) and growth of the lesion 157 days later (b)

Bone tumors were first detected in five of the dogs due to lameness and pain. Four of these dogs were sacrificed 1 - 3 weeks after lesions were first detected. In the fifth dog, the lameness and pain subsided and the dog was sacrificed, because of lameness and radiographic evidence of multiple bone tumors, about 4 months after the bone tumor was first detected. Fig. 9 shows the radiographic lesion in the dog sacrificed 112 days after clinical symptoms of lameness and pain were observed. The radiographic lesion appeared osteolytic. In two dogs osteolytic and osteoblastic appearing lesions were present in the same dog.

Table 6. Body weight changes in dogs with inhaled ^{238}Pu induced bone tumors

	Body weight (kg)		
Dog No.	Normal	Diagnosis	Presacrifice
469 M	11.5	11.5	8.9
445 M	13.0	11.7	10.2
438 M	11.5	11.2	7.9
453 M	12.0	12.7	9.9
405 M	12.5	10.0	10.0
481 F	11.0	9.1	8.0
489 F	8.0	7.5	6.5
482 F	9.5	8.3	7.8
488 F	7.5	8.1	6.7

Table 7. Location of bone tumors in dogs after inhalation of $^{238}PuO_2$ [a]

Dog No.	Humerus	Femur	Scapula	Pelvis	Rib	Vertebrae	Tctal
469 M	X			X	XX	XXX	7
445 M		X			X	X	3
438 M		X					1
453 M	X				X		2
405 M						X	1
481 F		X					1
489 F	X					X	2
482 F	X			X			2
488 F	X		X			X	3
Total	5	3	1	2	4	7	22

[a]Radiographic, gross, and histologic diagnosis.

The dogs with bone tumors showed intermittent anorexia and loss of body weight prior to sacrifice. In Table 6 the normal body weight is compared with sacrifice body weight showing a 10 - 20% weight loss.

The location of bone tumors in the dogs are listed in Table 7. Six of the 9 dogs had two or more bone tumor sites in the skeleton. Five dogs had tumors in the humerus. The tumors in the humerus were all in the proximal one-third of the bone. Five dogs had tumors in the vertebrae. In four of the five dogs, the tumors were located in the lumbar vertebrae.

The gross distribution of plutonium in the skeleton was evaluated by plutonium analyses of individual bones or groups of bones. If a tumor occurred in an individual bone, the contralateral or adjacent bone was analyzed. Table 8 compares the plutonium concentration in the individual bones of four dogs with bone tumors. Although plutonium concen-

Table 8. Concentration of ^{238}Pu in the skeleton (nCi/g wet weight)

	Dog Number			
	405 M	453 M	445M	469 M
Pelvis	1.3	1.3	1.3	1.4[a]
Rib	.6	1.4[a]	1.5[a]	1.1[a]
Scapula	.5	1.2	1.8	1.1
Vertebrae	.6[a]	.9	1.4[a]	.8[a]
Femur	.6	.8	1.3	1.1
Humerus	.7	.6[a]	.7	1.5[a]
Cranium	.3	.6	.7	.5
Mandible	.3	.6	.6	.3
Maxilla	.3	.6	.6	.3
Extremities[b]	.2	.5	.8	.4
Total skeleton	.6	1.0	1.0	.8

[a] Bone tumor.
[b] Distal to the humerus and femur.

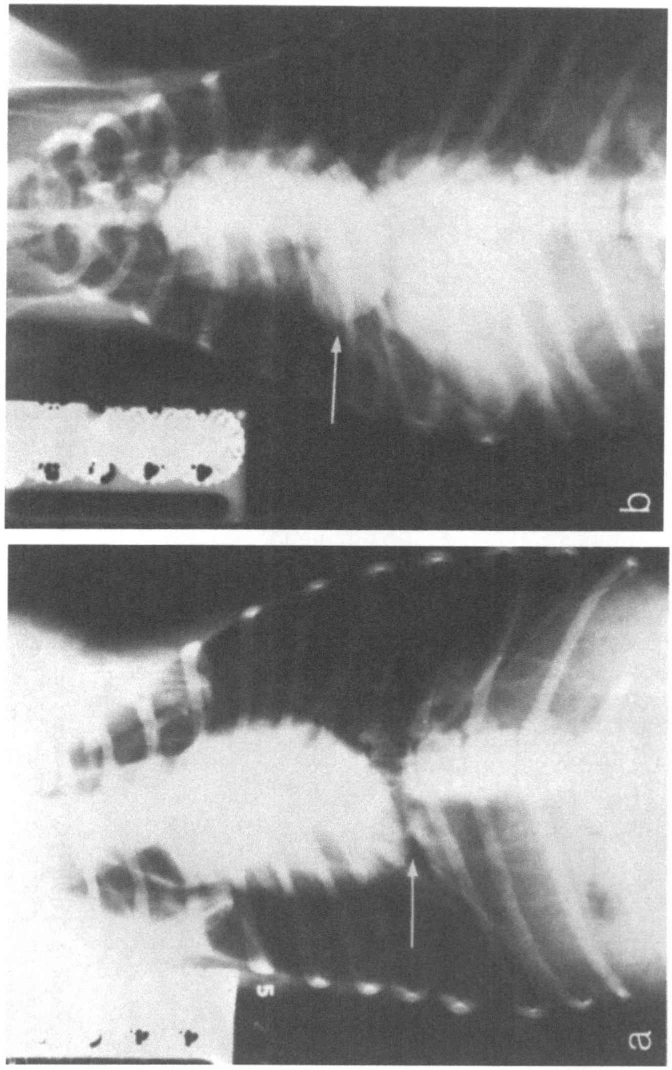

Fig. 6. Radiograph of dog 445 M showing lesion in the left 10th rib (a), and of the tumor 111 days later (b)

tration in the individual bones varied there did not appear to be a consistent trend toward bone tumors in the bones with higher plutonium concentration within the individual animals. Generally, the bones of the extremities (bones distal to the humerus and femur) and the bones of the head had lower plutonium concentrations than the bones in which bone tumors were found.

The neoplastic bone tumor cells were morphologically variable. In areas of the tumors where there was ample tumor bone formation, the cells were polyhedral, with a single nucleus. The cells tended to line the irregular surface of the bone spicules (Fig. 10). In other areas of the tumors, the cells were spindle-shaped, resembling fibroblasts. They were arranged in large bundles and whorls. Tumor bone and/or osteoid was scarce in these areas, which constituted a small part of most tu-

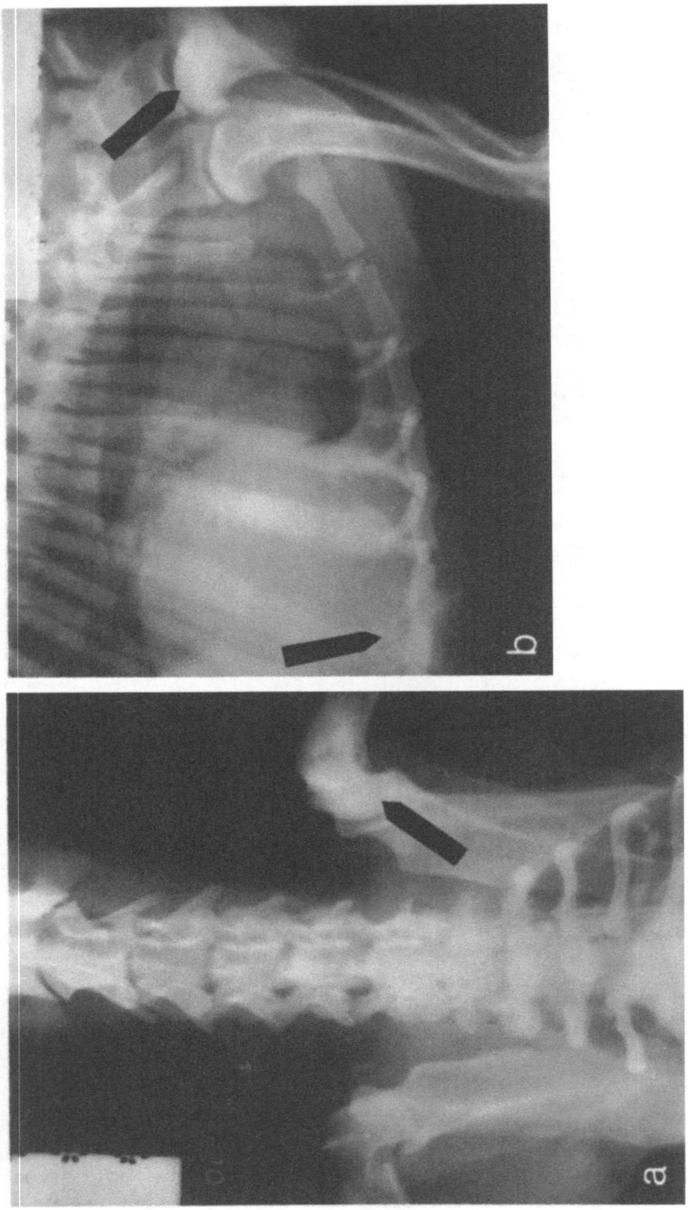

Fig. 7. Radiograph of dog 453 M showing osteogenic lesion in right humerus 114 days prior to sacrifice (a) when radiographic bone lesion was also seen in the sixth sternal rib (b)

mors. Nearly all tumors were characterized by large amounts of tumor bone formation (Fig. 11).

The tumors appeared to grow by expansion and infiltration into adjacent tissues. Blood vessel invasion was common. In two dogs (469 M, and 453 M) there were tumor emboli in the smaller branches of the pulmonary arteries, along with established pulmonary metastases (Fig. 12).

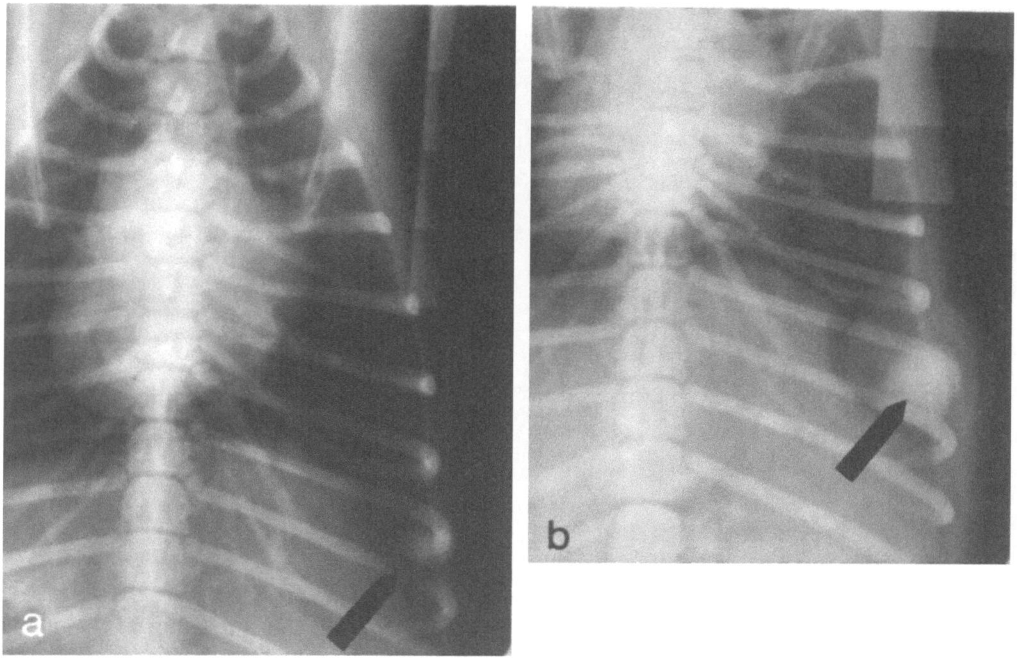

Fig. 8. Radiograph of dog 469 M showing osteogenic lesion originally detected in the right ninth rib (a) and showing growth of the lesion 96 days later (b)

There were numerous single tracts in the photographic emulsion of the autoradiographs over the bone and bone marrow (Fig. 13), indicating deposition of plutonium. The strongest focal activity was observed over hemosiderin granules in the cytoplasm of the marrow macrophages (Fig. 14). Deposition in the bone proper generally appeared uniform. However, occasional focal areas of high activity were observed over bone. The bone tumors contained less activity than the adjacent normal bone.

Fifth passage in vitro cultured tumor cell preparations, obtained from osteosarcomas of dogs 469 M and 445 M, were transplanted in utero into 31 - 33 day beagle fetuses. In vitro, the piling of cells and random growth suggested some loss of normal contact inhibitory growth mechanisms. Of seven puppies born to two bitches, three were dead at birth. Within a few days after birth, rapidly growing nodules developed in two puppies injected with cells cultured from osteosarcomas of dog 445 M and in one puppy injected with cells from the osteosarcomas of dog 469 M. The remaining puppy, now 16 months old, appears normal. The puppies were killed 2 - 8 weeks after birth. Multiple tumors in several organs were present at necropsy. The tumors were characterized by proliferating spindle-shaped cells arranged in large bundles (Fig. 15). Collagen formation was evident in all areas of the tumors. No evidence of bone formation was observed in these tumors. The tumors were classified as fibrosarcomas.

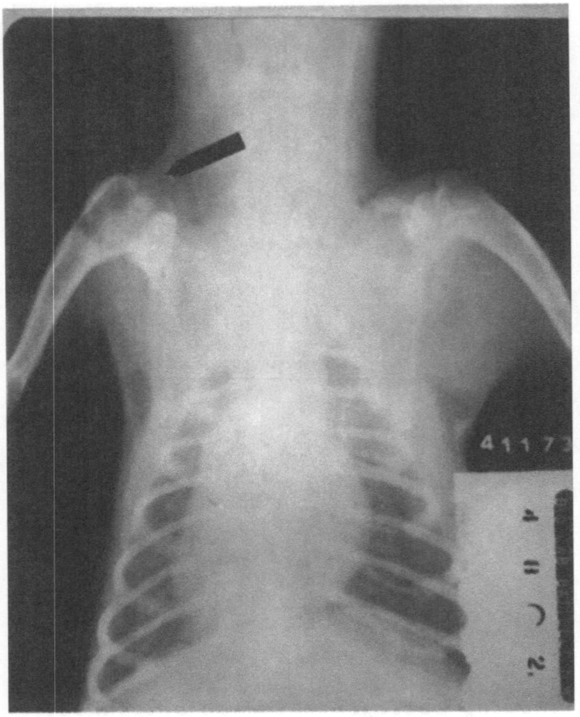

Fig. 9. Radiograph of dog 482 F showing an osteolytic lesion in the humerus

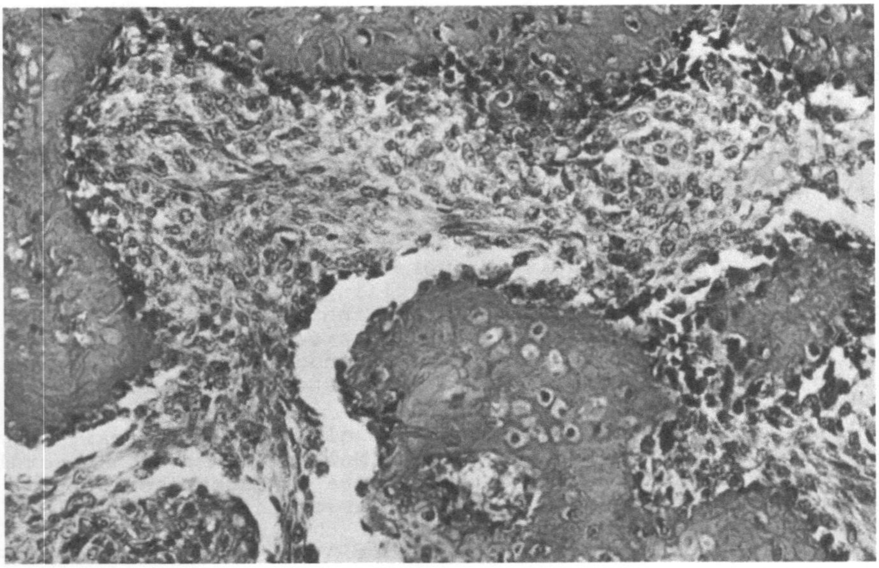

Fig. 10. Area of osteosarcoma where tumor bone formation predominates. Note the irregular surface of the bone spicule, lined by small, polyhedral shaped cells. H & E X 300

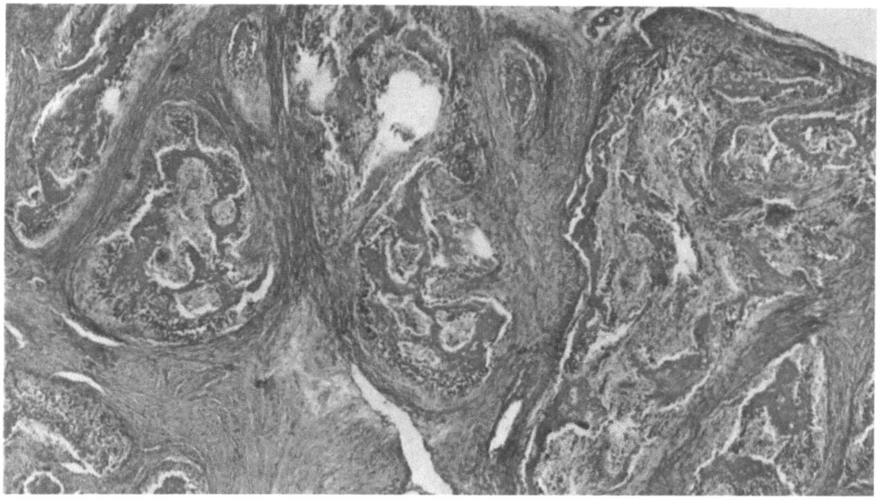

Fig. 11. Osteosarcoma from the rib of a $^{238}PuO_2$ exposed dog. Areas of tumor bone formation are surrounded by large bands of cells resembling fibroblasts. H & E X 50

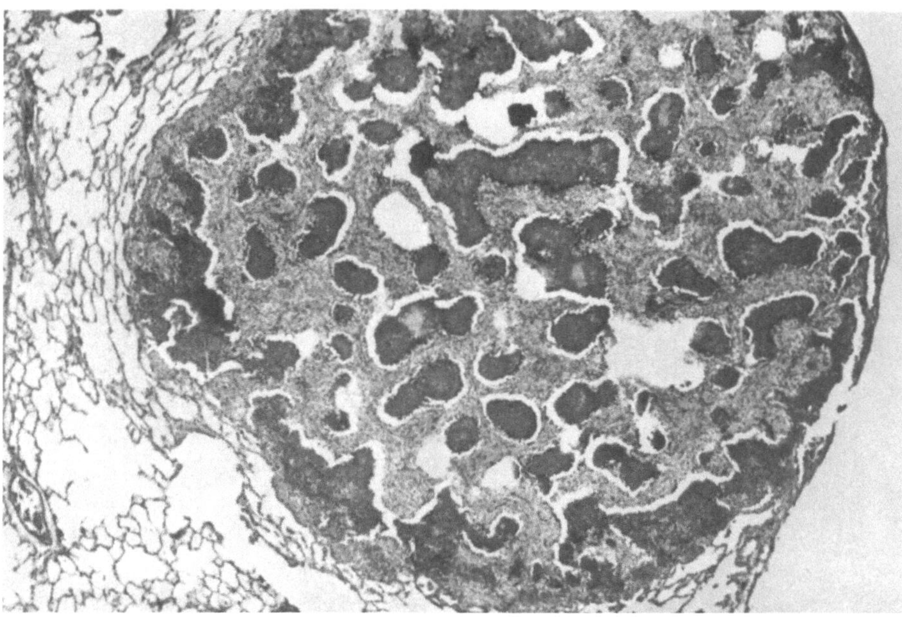

Fig. 12. Metastatic osteosarcoma in the periphery of a lung from a ^{238}Pu exposed dog. H & E X 50

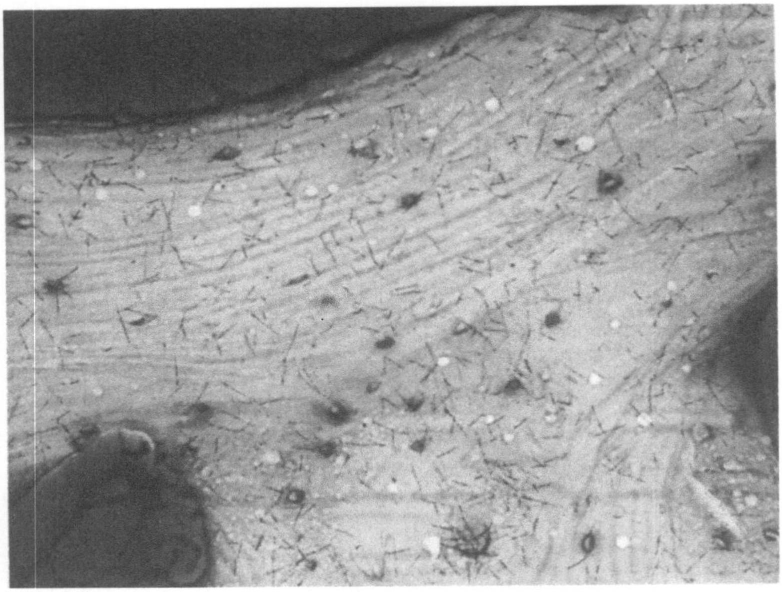

Fig. 13. Autoradiograph of the cortex of the femur of a dog 5 year after inhalation of $^{238}PuO_2$. Note the relatively uniform distribution of silver grain tracts in the emulsion over the bone compared to the distribution in the marrow in Fig. 14. Meythylene blue. X 260

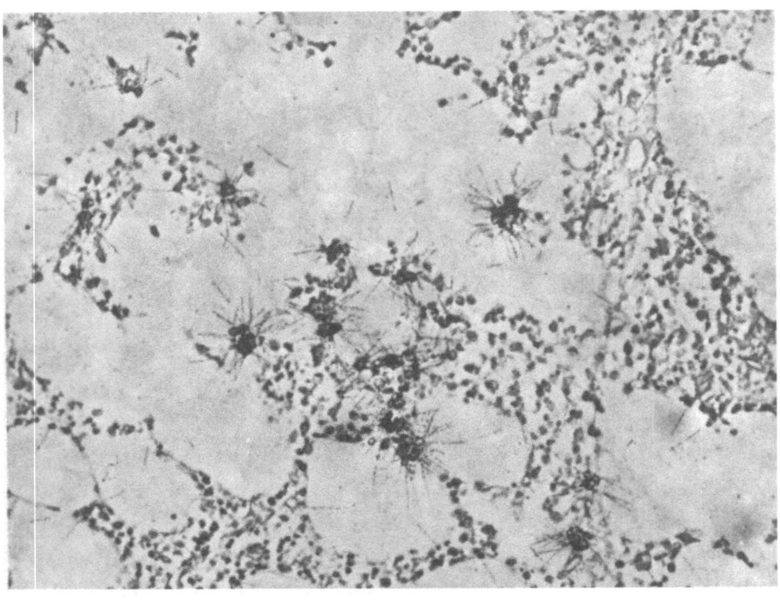

Fig. 14. Bone marrow adjacent to area shown in Fig. 13, illustrating localization of activity over hemosidern containing macrophages. Methylene blue. X 400

DISCUSSION

Bone cancer has a low natural incidence in beagles. MAYS and TAYLOR (1964) estimated a range of natural incidence in beagles of 1 - 100 osteosarcomas per 100,000 deaths. Based on this low natural incidence in beagles, we believe the osteosarcomas observed after inhalation of $^{238}PuO_2$ were caused by the plutonium.

Although the natural incidence of osteosarcoma in beagles is low, the induction of osteosarcoma in beagles by administration of radionuclides has been well documented. MAYS et al. (1969) reported induction of 149 osteosarcoma in beagles given single intravenous injections of ^{228}Th, ^{228}Ra(MsTh), ^{226}Ra, ^{90}Sr, and ^{239}Pu in citrate solution. Induction of osteosarcoma in beagles injected intravenously with ^{238}Pu has not been reported. However, based on reported data in osteosarcoma induction with other alpha-emitting radionuclides, ^{238}Pu would be expected to cause bone tumors if it was retained in the skeleton.

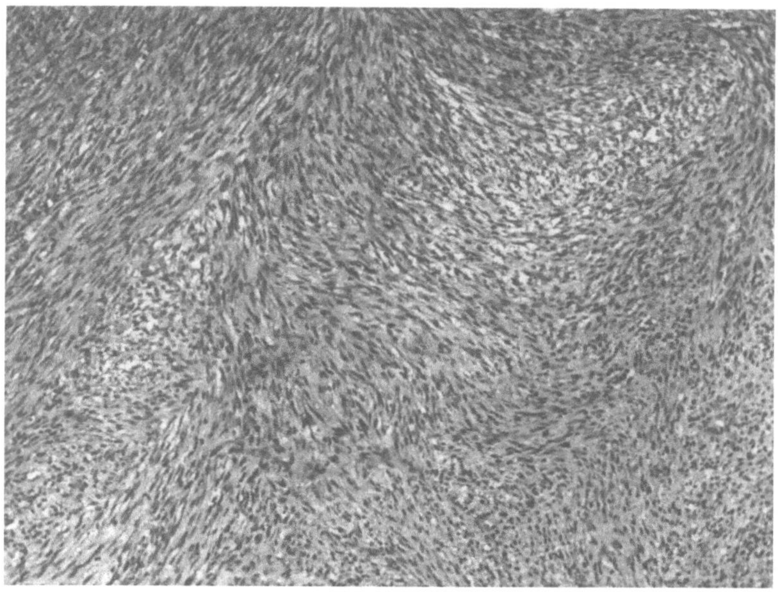

Fig. 15. Tumor removed from muscle of a pup given in vitro cultured tumor cells in utero. H & E X 240

After inhalation of $^{239}PuO_2$ by beagles, plutonium was retained primarily in the lungs and tracheobronchial lymph nodes with less than 10% of the plutonium translocated to the skeleton. Death was caused by sclerosing radiation pneumonitis at high doses and by pulmonary neoplasia at lower doses (PARK, et al., 1972). After inhalation of $^{238}PuO_2$ by beagles, death was due to sclerosing radiation pneumonitis at high doses. (PARK et al., 1969), while at lower doses reported in this paper, osteosarcoma was the primary cause of death. Induction of osteosarcomas by inhaled $^{238}PuO_2$ was apparently related to translocation of ^{238}Pu to the skeleton. Of the plutonium body burden at death 30 - 55% was in the skeleton of the $^{238}PuO_2$-exposed dogs compared to less than 10% in $^{239}PuO_2$-exposed dogs.

Differences in the metabolic behavior of ^{238}Pu and ^{239}Pu have been ascribed generally to the mass effects resulting from the large differences in the specific activation of the isotopes (VAUGHAN, et al., 1973). Plutonium-239 has a half-life of 24,360 years, compared to 86 years for plutonium-238. The energy deposition in the region of a $^{238}PuO_2$ particle will be about 280 times greater per unit time than that deposited in the region of a similar sized of $^{239}PuO_2$. This increased radiation dose could result in greater solunility of $^{238}PuO_2$ particles.

With the dose levels studied to date, bone neoplasia was the primary cause of death 5 - 6 years after inhalation of $^{238}PuO_2$; however, one of the dogs had pulmonary neoplasia in addition to a bone tumor. Experiments were initiated in 1972 to further study the dose-effect relationship of inhaled $^{238}PuO_2$. Table 9 shows the experimental design. None of the dogs in this experiment have died during the first post-exposure year.

Table 9. Dose-effect studies with inhaled $^{238}PuO_2$ in dogs

Dose level group	No. of dogs	Initial alveolar deposition[a] (nCi)[b]
0	20	0
1	20	2.3 ± 0.8
2	20	18 ± 3
3	20	77 ± 11
4	20	354 ± 81
5	20	1308 ± 270
6	13	5192 ± 1372

[a] Estimated from external thorax counts at 14 and 30 days postexposure and estimated lung weights.
[b] Means ± 95% confidence intervals around the means.

The $^{238}PuO_2$-induced osteosarcomas were grown in cultures to determine the feasibility of employing in vitro methods for investigating the cellular aspects of the tumors and host-tumor relationships. Preliminary evaluations of the cell lines arising from the cultures by commonly applied criteria, e.g., cell morphology, lack of contact inhibition, and tumor production in vivo, suggest that the tumors can be cultured in vitro. More work is needed to confirm and clarify the results obtained thus far. The difference in morphology between the donor tumors and those observed in the pups can be explained in several ways, depending on whether the tumor cells in the pups were of donor or host origin. If the cells were of host origin, the passage of transforming agent or factor is likely. If the cells were of graft origin, it is possible that the in vitro culture methods or route of inoculation into the new host may have selected for cells which do not produce tumor bone or osteoid. Analyses of tumor chromosome preparations and assays of reverse transcriptase activity are in progress to clarify the origin of the tumors.

REFERENCES

1. EVANS, V.J., BRYANT, J.C., KERR, H.A., SCHILLING, E.L.: 1964. Chemically defined media for cultivation of long term cell strains from four mammalian species. Exp. Cell. Res. 36, 439-474.
2. KEOUGH, R.F., POWERS, G.J.: Determination of plutonium in biological materials by extraction and liquid scintillation counting. Analyt. Chem. 42, 419-421 (1970).
3. MAYS, C.W., TAYLOR, G.N.: Low natural incidence of osteosarcomas in beagles: Research and radiobiology, Univ. of Utah Report COO - 119 - 321, 70-75 (Sept. 1964).
4. MAYS, C.W. et al.: Radiation-induced cancer in beagles, In Delayed Effects of Bone Seeking Radionuclides. 387-405 (C.W. MAYS et al. Eds.), Salt Lake City: Universitiy of Utah Press 1967.
5. PARK, J.F., BAIR, W.J., BUSCH, R.H.: Progress in beagle dog studies with transuranium elements at Battelle-Northwest. Health Phys. 22, 803-810 (1972).
6. PARK, J.F., HOWARD, E.B., BAIR, W.J.: Acute toxicity of inhaled $^{238}PuO_2$ in beagles. Technical Report No. AFWL-TR-69-75, Air Force Weapons Laboratory, Kirtland Air Force Base, New Mexico (1969).
7. PARK, J.F., HOWARD, E.G., BAIR, W.J.: Acute toxicity of inhaled $^{238}PuO_2$ in beagle dogs. USAEC Document BNWL-1050, Part 1, pp. 3.6 - 3.14 (1970).
8. STANNARD, J.N.: Biomedical Aspects of Plutonium (Discovery, Development, Projections), In Uranium-Plutonium Transplutonic Elements p. 309-322 (HODGE, H.C., STANNARD, J.N., HURSH, J.B.eds.), Berlin-Heidelberg-New York: Springer 1973.
9. VAUGHAN, J., BLEANEY, B., TAYLOR, D.M.: Distribution, Excretion and Effects of Plutonium as a Bone-seeker, In Uranium-Plutonium Transplutonic Elements p. 349-502 (HODGE, H.C., STANNARD, J.N., HURSH, J.B. eds.) Berlin-Heidelberg-New York: Springer 1973.

Experimental Induction of Bone Tumors by Short-Lived Bone-Seeking Radionuclides *

W. GÖSSNER, O. HUG, A. LUZ, and W. A. MÜLLER

The human radium cases based on industrial occupation with ^{226}Ra and ^{228}Ra and medical experience with ^{226}Ra and ^{224}Ra continue to provide basic information on the effects of internal radiation and radiocarcinogenesis in man. The danger of strontium-90 in atomic fall-out and the possibility of industrial accidents with plutonium and other dangerous alpha-emitters have stimulated experimental research in this field. Animal experiments will help to elucidate the problems of radiation hazards and in addition increase our understanding of the mechanisms of radiation carcinogenesis.

Bone tumors have been induced experimentally by internal administration of many bone-seeking radioactive isotopes, including the alpha-emitters radium, mesothorium (^{228}Ra), radiothorium (^{228}Th), americium, plutonium, neptunium and the beta-emitters radiostrontium, radiocalcium, radiophosphorus and radiocerium (9, 14).

Long-term studies of the effects of the short-lived alpha-emitting bone-seekers ^{224}Ra and ^{227}Th have been performed on our laboratory since 1966. (7, 3, 5). This work was initiated in order to investigate the oncogenic effect of short-lived nuclides in dependence on the skeletal dose and its spatial and temporal distribution. In addition, such studies appeared to be relevant to problems of radiation hazard in man since the occurrence of osteosarcomas had been reported in humans after treatment with ^{224}Ra (Peteosthor) (13) and this nuclide is still used in the treatment of ankylosing spondylitis.

^{224}Ra has a short half-life of 3.64 days. The first of the daughter products, ^{220}Rn, is a noble gas which has a short half-life of only 55 seconds. This is followed by ^{216}Po, with a very short half-life of 0.16 seconds, and then by ^{212}Pb, which has a half-life of 10.6 hours (Fig. 1).

The decay scheme of ^{227}Th, which has a half-life of 18.7 days, is shown in Figure 2. It has the relatively long-lived decay product ^{223}Ra which may enter the mineral bone. Therefore the biological effects that may derive from this decay product must be added to those of ^{227}Th per se.

It is usual to divide bone-seeking radionuclides into "volume seekers", such as calcium, strontium, barium,radium, and "surface seekers", such as plutonium, americum, thorium, curium, californium, cerium and yttrium. But this distinction will not be valid if one compares these biological

---

* Herrn Professor Dr. med. Dr. h.c. mult. Erich Letterer zum 80. Geburtstag gewidmet.

Die experimentellen Untersuchungen wurden im Rahmen eines EURATOM-Assoziationsvertrages (090-72-1BIAD) durchgeführt.

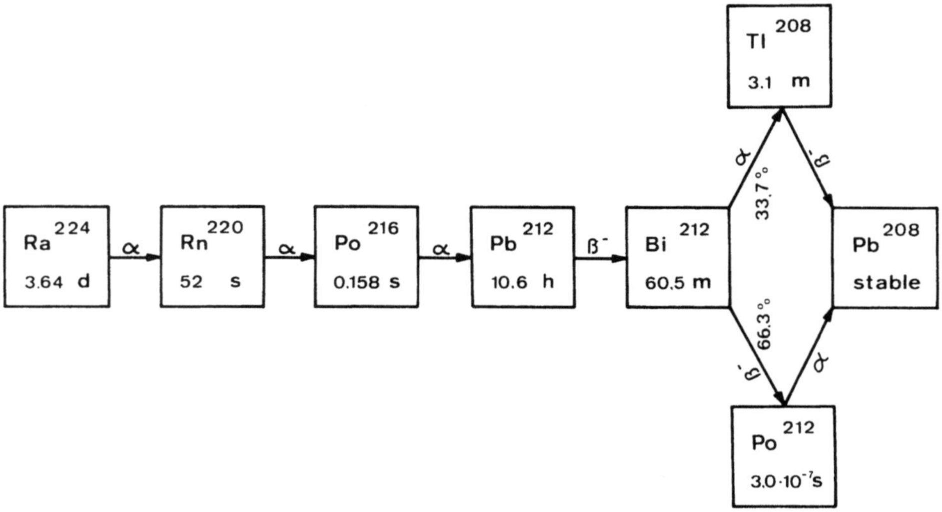

Fig. 1. Decay scheme for ^{224}*Ra and its daughters*

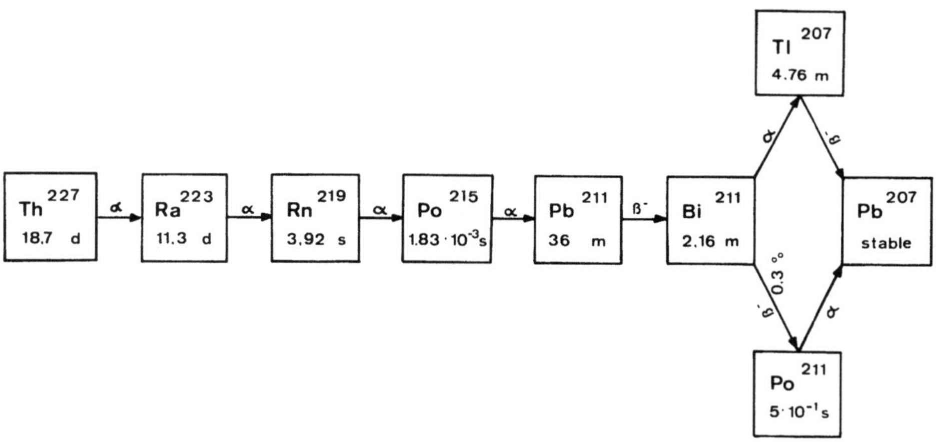

Fig. 2. Decay scheme for ^{227}*Th and its daughters*

characteristics for the short-lived ^{224}Ra and ^{227}Th. Because ^{224}Ra is initially concentrated on bone surfaces, due to its extremely short half-life, most of it will decay on such surfaces before it enters the mineral bone. Figure 3, which shows the autoradiographs of mouse femora 24 hours after injection of ^{227}Th and ^{224}Ra for comparison, illustrates this point.

The purpose of this paper is to summarize some of the data on the incidence of bone tumors after single and repeated applications of ^{224}Ra and single applications of ^{227}Th, the histopathology and anatomical locations of the tumors, and radiographic and histological studies of morphological changes in bone which can be identified in relation to the development of the tumors.

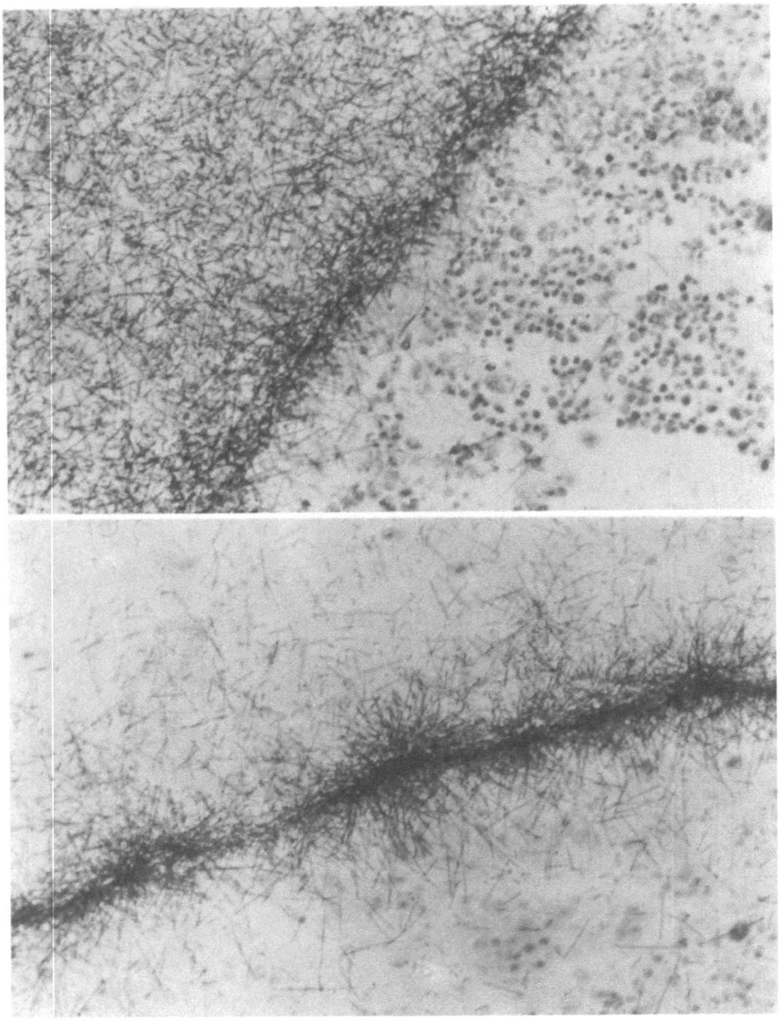

Fig. 3. Autoradiographs of the femur from mice sacrificed 24 hours after injection of ^{224}Ra (above) and ^{227}Th (below) show the trabecular surface concentration of the short-lived radium and thorium and diffuse distribution of radium throughout bone (upper left)

Material and Methods

NMRI female mice 3 to 4 weeks old have been used for most experiments. In addition, some experiments have been performed on male NMRI mice. A series of dose levels was used, each dose group including between 50 and 100 animals. The radionuclides were injected intraperitoneally (10, 11). Nearly 1,000 untreated animals served as controls. The animals were kept under standardized conditions. Experimental routine included sacrifice of moribund animals, gross autopsy, radiography of the skeleton and histopathologic examination of selected tissues.

Dose-Response Caracteristics

The experimental procedures and the bone sarcoma incidences after the single doses of ^{224}Ra and ^{227}Th and the fractioned doses of ^{224}Ra are summarized in the three tables below. After single injections of ^{224}Ra, the highest osteosarcoma incidence in female mice was 22 percent, while in male mice the highest tumor incidence was only 8.5 percent (Table 1). The fact that in the lower dose groups tumors were found to be about 2.5 times as frequent in the females as in the males shows that sex differences are important, at least in mice. Following single injections, ^{227}Th was more carcinogenic than ^{224}Ra, with the highest tumor incidence of 60 percent (Table 2). It is of considerable interest that fractionated application of ^{224}Ra increased bone tumor incidence to 92 percent in the longest protraction period and at low dose rate (Table 3).

Table 1. Incidence of osteosarcoma in female and male mice after single injection of ^{224}Ra in dependence on mean skeletal dose

	μCi / kg inj.	Number of mice	Mice with osteosa.	Incidence	Skel. dose (rads)
Females	50	92	13	14.2%	1500
	36	50	4	8 %	1080
	25	188	27	14.4%	750
	12	49	11	22 %	360
	10	92	14	15.2%	300
	5	91	14	15.4%	150
	2.5	200	21	10.5%	75
	1.0	200	14	7 %	30
	0	460	6	1.3%	0
Males	50	93	7	7.5%	1500
	25	94	8	8.5%	750
	10	98	3	3.1%	300
	5	97	2	2.1%	150
	0	93	0	0	0

Table 2. Incidence of osteosarcoma in female mice after single injection of ^{227}Th in dependence on mean skeletal dose

μCi / kg inj.	Number of mice	Mice with osteosa.	Incidence	Skel. dose (rads)
50.0	100	60	60%	10000
25.0	100	44	44%	5000
10.0	100	47	47%	2000
5.0	100	60	60%	1000
1.0	100	22	22%	200
0.5	100	9	9%	100
0.1	100	3	3%	20
0	200	2	1%	0

Figure 4 compares the patterns of survival, frequency and time of appearance of bone tumors in the single-injection experiments with ^{224}Ra and ^{227}Th and in the fractionation experiment in which 72 doses of 0.5/μCi ^{224}Ra per kg bodyweight were given over a period of 9 months. After incorporation of ^{227}Th with half-life about 5 times longer than

Table 3. Incidence of osteosarcoma in female mice after repeated injections of 224 Ra in dependence on mean skeletal dose, dose rate and treatment period

µCi/kg Total	Scheme of inj.	Treatment period weeks	Number of mice	Mice with osteosa.	Incidence	Dose rate rad/d	Total skel-dose rads
72	48 x 1.5	24	50	40	80%	24.0	2160
36	8 x 4.5	4	50	11	22%	72.0	1080
36	24 x 1.5	12	50	31	62%	24.0	1080
36	72 x 0.5	36	100	92	92%	8.0	1080
12	8 x 1.5	4	49	19	39%	24.0	360
12	24 x 0.5	12	50	23	46%	8.0	360
0	0	-	150	0	0	0	0

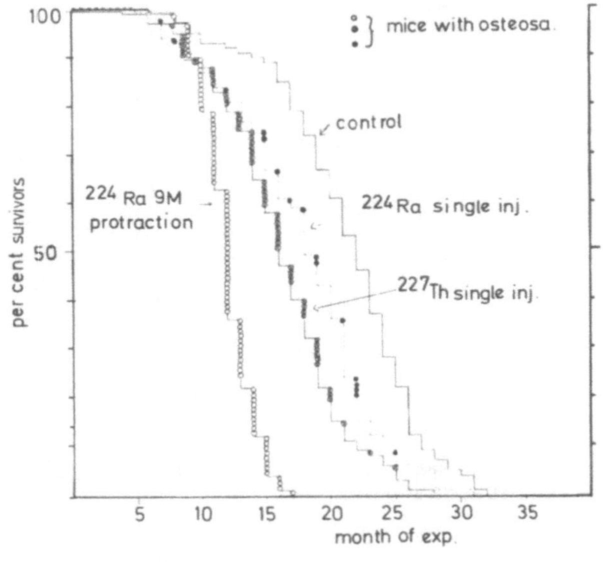

Fig. 4. Patterns of survival, frequency and time of appearance of osteosarcomas in female mice after single injection of 25 µCi/kg ^{224}Ra, single injection of 5.0 µCi/kg ^{227}Th and 72 repeated injections of 0.5 µCi/kg ^{224}Ra over 36 weeks. Mean skeletal dose in all experiments 750-1000 rads

that of ^{224}Ra, and most strikingly after protracted application of ^{224}Ra, the percentage of survivors falls earlier and more steeply than after a single dose of ^{224}Ra, and the tumor frequency is increased. As already mentioned, division of the amount of ^{224}Ra into fractions increased the yield of bone tumors up to 92 percent, and the tumors appeared earlier.

PATHOLOGY

More than 600 radium-and thorium-induced osteosarcomas were available for histologic study, and among 903 control mice there were 8 spontaneous malignant bone tumors that were indistinguishable from the radiation-induced tumors. Less than 10 percent of the mice with osteosarcomas had metastases; most metastases were in the lung, but the spleen, liver and kidney were also affected in some cases.

HISTOPATHOLOGY

Most of the osteosarcomas consisted of more or less well-differentiated bone-forming osteoblastic tissue. The amount of osteoid varied from tumor to tumor and even within the same tumor. The most highly differentiated tumors consist of cells resembling active osteoblasts (Fig. 5). Other morphologic types showed fibroblastic or telangiectatic features and predominance of giant cells of osteoclastic type. The less well-differentiated anaplastic tumors are characterized by pleomorphism and hyperchromaticity. Several different types of cellular components and of differentiation frequently occurred in a single tumor (4). Sometimes islands of newly formed bone marrow occurred within the tumors. The histopathology of the tumors in our experiments corresponds in general to the descriptions given of tumors in mice after ^{226}Ra (2) and after ^{90}Sr (12). The osteosarcomas occurring in the head bones, especially the jaws, showed similar morphologic features as those in other parts of the skeleton. Most of the osteosarcomas studied were very rich in alkaline phosphatase, which confirms that they arise from osteoblasts or precursors of osteoblasts.

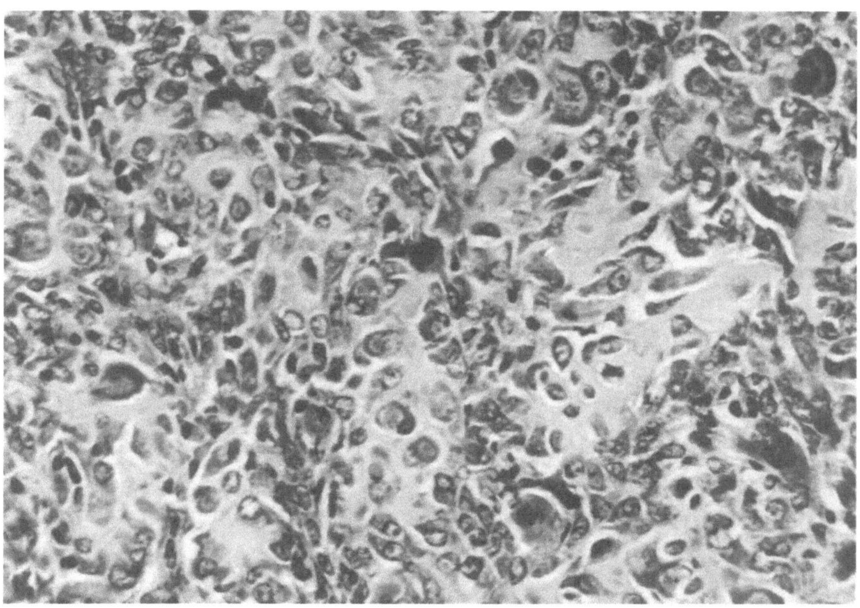

Fig. 5. Typical field of osteoblastic osteosarcoma after administration of ^{224}Ra

In addition to the malignant bone tumors, we observed benign tumors involving the jaws, which are usually solitary, sometimes bilateral and slow-growing. Their histologic appearance corresponds to that of an ossifying fibroma, a fibrous-osseous lesion consisting of bone spicules composed of woven bone, embedded in a fibrous stroma (Fig. 6), and sometimes rimmed with osteoblasts. This basic fibrous tissue of ossifying fibromata failed to react in the test for alkaline phosphatase (8).

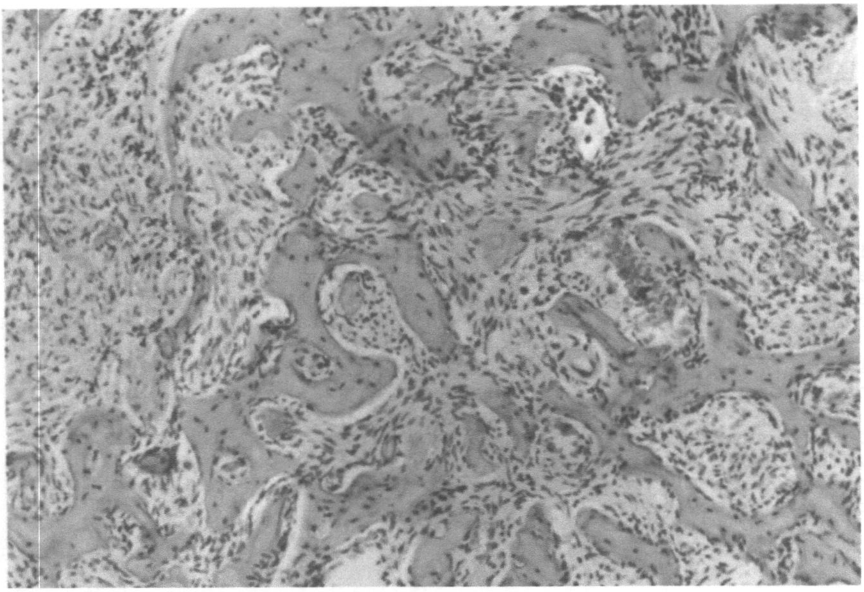

Fig. 6. Ossifying fibroma involving the jaw after administration of ^{224}Ra

ANATOMIC LOCATIONS

About half the ^{224}Ra- and ^{227}Th-induced tumors occurred in the spine, particularly in the lumbar regions (Fig. 7). This corresponds to the findings in the ^{226}Ra mice in FINKEL's experiments and contrasts with the situation in strontium-injected mice, where the majority of tumors occurred in the limbs.

As already reported (2, 12), there is a definite correlation between dose and tumor location, especially with regard to the bones of the head and the other parts of the skeleton.

After single injection of ^{224}Ra or ^{227}Th there is an increased incidence of osteosarcoma of the head in the highest dose groups, which is much more pronounced with ^{227}Th than with ^{224}Ra (Fig. 8). Parallel to this increase in the incidence of osteosarcomas in the head bones in the highest dose groups, there is also a steep increase of the incidence of ossifying fibromata in the jaws in the ^{224}Ra experiments, which is about 6 times higher than the incidence of the head osteosarcomas. After ^{227}Th there is also an increase in the incidence of

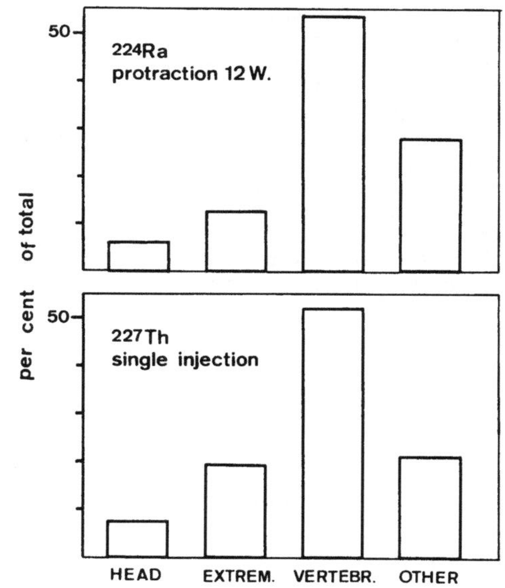

Fig. 7. Anatomic locations of osteosarcomas in female mice after repeated injections of 1.5 μCi/kg ^{224}Ra twice weekly over 12 weeks and single injection of 5 μCi/kg ^{227}Th

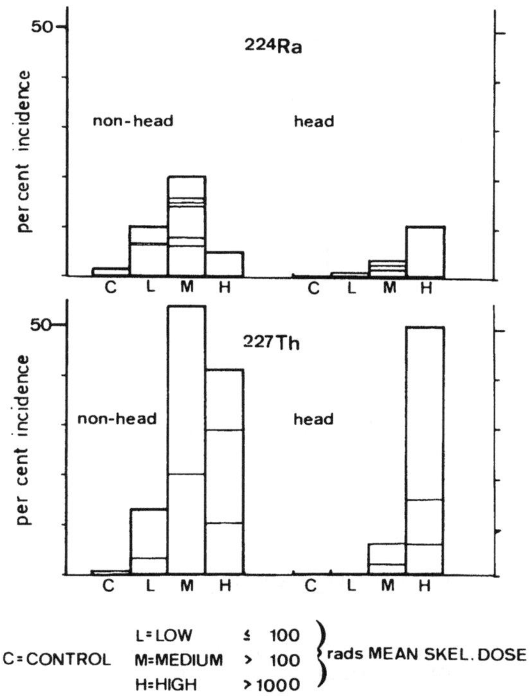

Fig. 8. Incidence of osteosarcomas in the head bones and the other parts of the skeleton in female mice after single injection of ^{224}Ra and ^{227}Th at three levels of mean skeletal dose ranges

ossifying fibroma with dose, but in this case their frequency is exceeded by that of osteosarcomas in the highest dose groups studied (Fig. 9). Dose protraction of ^{224}Ra produces no increase in the incidence of head tumors (Fig. 10). In all experiments with fractionated application of ^{224}Ra, the osteosarcoma incidence in the bones of the head was less than 10 percent. The increase of tumor yield with protraction time is limited to the non-head skeleton. The same is true of ossifying fibromas of the jaws, whose incidence is also not increased by dose protraction (Fig. 11). Four to twelve weeks' protraction yields about the same incidence as a single injection. In the 36 weeks' protraction experiment the ossifying fibromas, which usually do not occur before 9 months after the start of the experiments, have been surpassed by the osteosarcomas.

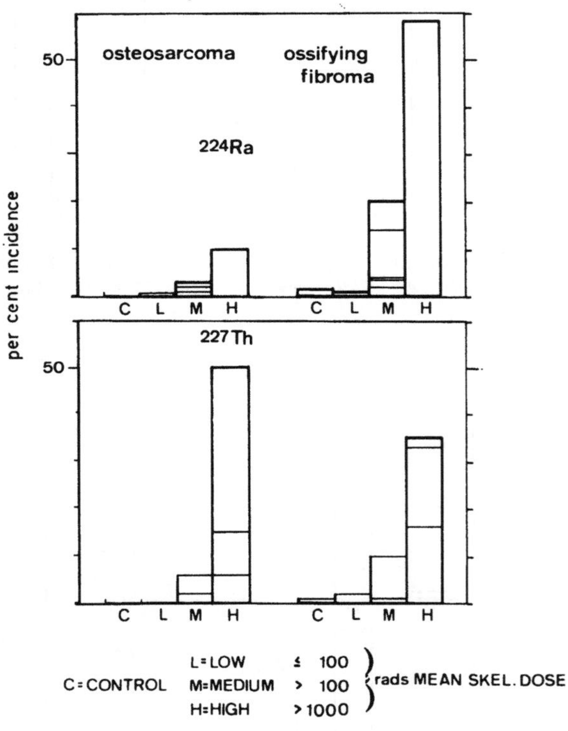

Fig. 9. Incidence of osteosarcomas and ossifying fibromas in the head bones after single injection of ^{224}Ra and ^{227}Th at three levels of mean skeletal dose ranges

MULTIFOCAL OSTEOSARCOMAS AND HYPEROSTOTIC BONE DYSPLASIA

An increase of multifocal osteosarcomas has been observed in the protraction experiments (Fig. 12). With the longest protraction period of 9 months, more than 40 percent of the mice with bone tumor had more than one osteosarcoma. In all other experiments less than 10 percent of mice had multifocal osteosarcomas.

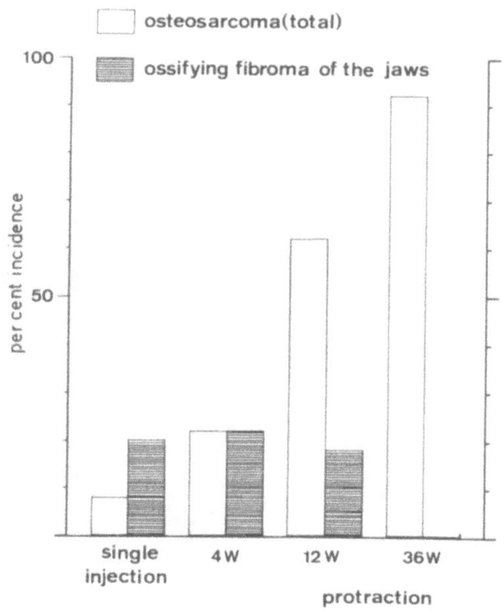

Fig. 10. Incidence of osteosarcomas in the head bones and the other parts of the skeleton in female mice after single and fractionated administration of 36 μCi/kg of ^{224}Ra (1080 rad mean skeletal dose), given as repeated injections of 0.5, 1.5 and 4.5 μCi/kg twice weekly over 4, 12, and 36 weeks

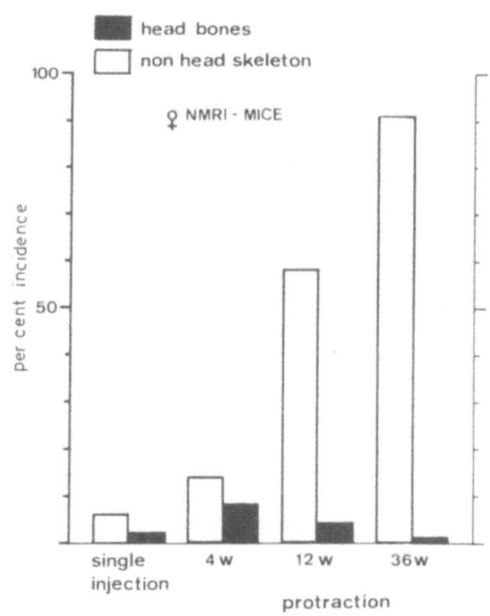

Fig. 11. Incidence of osteosarcomas (total) and ossifying fibromas of the jaws in female mice after single and fractionated administration of 36 μCi/kg of ^{224}Ra (1080 rad mean skeletal dose), given as repeated injections of 0.5, 1.5 and 4.5 μCi/kg twice weekly over 4, 12 and 36 weeks

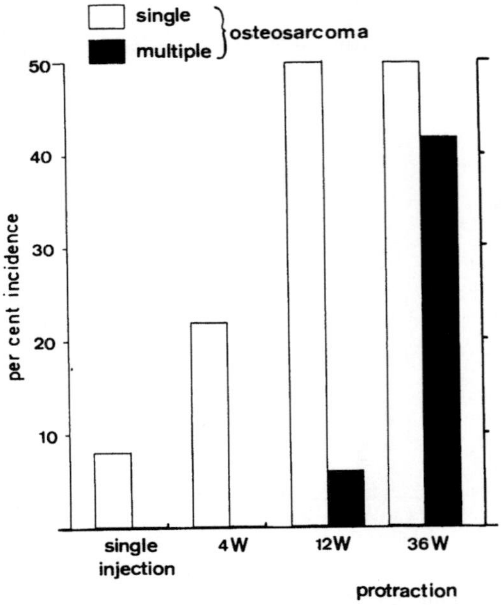

Fig. 12. Incidence of single and multiple osteosarcomas in female mice after single and fractionated application of 36 μCi/kg of ^{224}Ra (1080 rad mean skeletal dose), given as repeated injections of 0.5, 1.5 and 4.5 μCi/kg twice weekly over 4, 12 and 36 weeks

The observation of dysplastic bone changes in this protraction experiment with the high and multifocal osteosarcoma seems particularly interesting. In radiographs these changes are characterized by areas of increased density and histologic examination reveals a proliferation of connective tissue cells, mainly of fibroblasts (Fig. 13), which is followed by the deposition of newly formed bone substance, resulting in osteoclerosis (Fig. 14). A similar finding has been reported in female mice after whole-body irradiation (1). The same lesion occurs in old (over 20 months of age) female mice of our NMRI strain. . The pathogenesis of this lesion is still unknown, but the underlying cause seems to be some metabolic or endocrine disturbance.

A more detailed analysis of this lesion showed that in our protraction experiment with ^{224}Ra this dysplastic lesion was quite constantly observed in mice with osteosarcoma from month 12 of the experiments onward. In these areas of hyperostosis a proliferation of atypical cells has frequently been found, which can be regarded as the early stages of osteosarcomas (Fig. 15). This relation between hyperostotic bone dysplasia and early stages of osteosarcoma formation is quite obvious 12 months after the start of the protraction experiment. But because the first tumor appears after only 9 months without obvious signs of this type of dysplasia it cannot be regarded as an obligatory prestage of osteosarcoma.

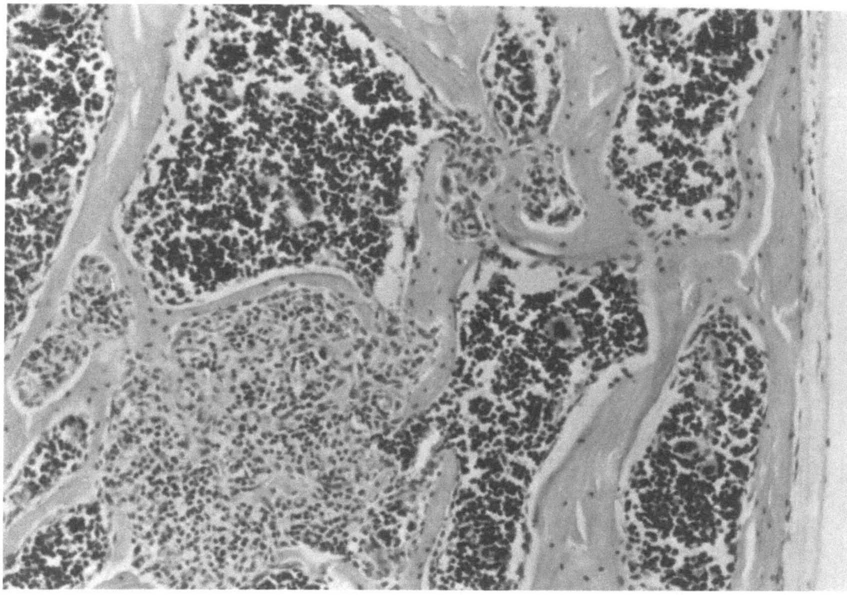

Fig. 13. Typical field of focal dysplasia with cellular proliferation and deposition of new-formed bone substance in the vertebrae of a female mouse after administration of ^{224}Ra

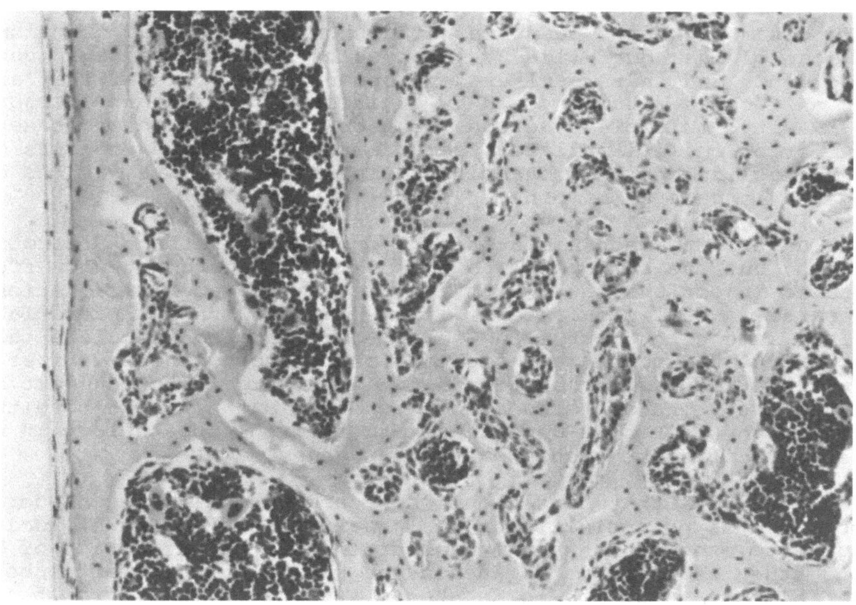

Fig. 14. Focal osteoclerosis in the vertebra of a female mouse after administration of ^{224}Ra .

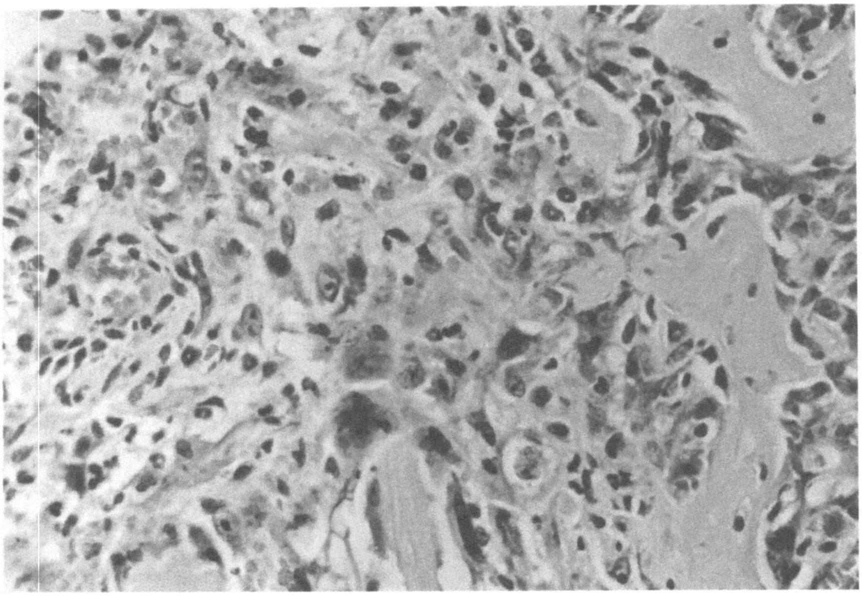

Fig. 15. Profileration of atypical cells in an area of hyperstotic dysplasia which probably represents an early stage of osteosarcoma

DISCUSSION

The data which have been presented show clearly that fractionation of a dose of the short-lived ^{224}Ra results in an increase in bone tumor incidence and in an earlier development of neoplasia. This attainment of an increased tumor yield by division of the amount of short-lived ^{224}Ra into multiple fractions is probably due to an increase in the number of cells irradiated, because the successive deposits of the radionuclide and the concomitant tissue damage move, and so extend over a large area of bone.

The underlying mechanisms of this protraction effect are not yet understood, but one can speculate that this high carcinogenic effect of repeated injections of ^{224}Ra may be due to repeated irradiation of regenerating cell populations during repair, with proliferation of possibly damaged but surviving cells. One can also speculate that with regard to the multistage hypothesis of carcinogenesis, first injections initiate neoplastic change and the following injections act as promotor (2, 6). The differences between head and non-head bone tumors with regard to their dose-dependence and their histopathology in mice may reflect different mechanisms of oncogenesis.

Radionuclides that localize in bone are not only of considerable importance as potential industrial hazards in this era of nuclear energy, but also excellent experimentel tools for the production of bone tumors and study of their pathogenesis and biology. Experimental bone tumors can also serve as models for basic studies on tumor growth and cell kinetics, which are essential to the future development of tumor therapy.

SUMMARY

Single and repeated applications of ^{224}Ra and single applications of ^{227}Th to more than 600 female NMRI mice 3 - 4 weeks old, and to male NMRI mice have led to a high rate of osteosarcomas. Tumor incidence is dose-related. ^{227}Th is more carcinogenic than ^{224}Ra which induced the highest tumor incidence of 60% after a single injection of 5 μCi per Kg body weight or more. Repeated injections of ^{224}Ra to female mice yielded a tumor incidence of up to 92%. Most of these osteosarcomas consist of well-differentiated bone-forming osteoplastic tissue. Half of the tumors occurred in the spine, particularly in the lumbar region. In protraction experiments, multifocal osteosarcomas have been observed. Less than 10% of the mice with osteosarcoma had developed metastases in lung, spleen, liver, and kidney. The possible mechanisms of the protraction effect are discussed.

REFERENCES

1. COTTIER, H.: Strahlenbedingte Lebensverkürzung. Berlin: Springer 1961
2. FINKEL, M.P., BISKIS, B.O.: Progr. exp. Tumor Res. Basel 10, 72 (1968)
3. GÖSSNER, W., HINDRINGER, B., HUG, O., LUZ, A., MÜLLER, W.A.: In: Contamination by Bone-Seeking Radionuclides and Radioprotection, p. 528. Paris: Soc. franc. de Radioprotection 1971
4. GÖSSNER, W., HINDRINGER, B., LUZ, A., SCHWABE, M.: Z. Krebsforsch. 78, 225 (1972).
5. GÖSSNER, W.: Verh. dtsch. Ges. Path. 56, 168 (1972)
6. GÖSSNER, W.: Current Topics in Radiation Research Quarterly 9, 35 (1973)
7. HUG, O., GÖSSNER, W., MÜLLER, W.A., LUZ, A., HINDRINGER, B.: In: Radiation Induced Cancer (Ericson A., Ed.), p. 393 Vienna: International Atomic Energy Agency 1969
8. LUZ, A., HINDRINGER, B.: Verh. dtsch. Ges. Path. 54, 450 (1970)
9. MAYS, C.W., JEE, W.S.S., LLOYD, R.D. (eds): Delayed Effects of Bone-Seeking Radionuclides. Salt Lake City: University of Utah Press 1969
10. MÜLLER, W.A.: Radiochemica Acta 9, 181 (1968)
11. MÜLLER, W.A.: Int. J. Radiat. Biol. 20, 27 (1971)
12. NILSSON, A.: Acta vet. scand. 3, 185 (1962)
13. SPIESS, H.: Dtsch. med. Wschr. 81, 1053 (1956)
14. VAUGHAN, J.M.: The Effects of Irradiation on the Skeleton Oxford: Clarendon Press 1973

Etiology of Childhood Bone Cancer: Epidemiologic Observations

R. W. MILLER

One of the most interesting clues to the origins of bone sarcoma has come from veterinary medicine. Veterinarians have long known that giant breeds of dogs are at much higher risk of bone cancer than smaller breeds. The difference was first quantitated in 1966 (41), and the risk was found to be 185 times greater in giant breeds, such as the Saint Bernard and Great Dane, than in breeds of small or medium size; the frequency of bone sarcoma was found to be 13 times that recorded in smaller dogs (Fig. 1). The histologic type could not readily be studied. It is noteworthy that veterinarians do not use the term Ewing's tumor, perhaps partly because it is a very rare neoplasm in dogs and may not occur at all in other domestic species (2).

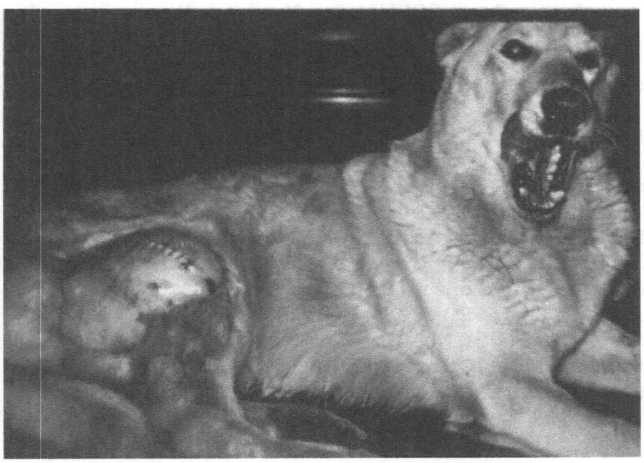

Fig. 1. Large dog (German shepherd) with osteosarcoma. The relative risk of bone sarcoma is 13 times greater in large breeds and 185 times greater in giant breeds than in small or medium-sized dogs (TJALMA, 1966). Photograph by courtesy of Dr. H.W. CASEY, Armed Forces Institute of Pathology

In studies of the etiology of bone cancer in man, it has proved to be extremely important to purify the diagnosis insofar as possible with reference to histology. Marked differences in the distribution of osteosarcoma, as against Ewing's tumor, can be seen when their occurrence in childhood is related to age, sex, race, family aggregation and certain environmental exposures.

A PROBLEM WITH DATA RESOURCES

Childhood bone cancers recorded in population-based tumor registries are usually too few in number to be studied by cell type. If mortality data are used instead, it becomes apparent that the current worldwide method for coding death certificates according to the Manual of International Classification of Diseases (ICD) (24) is unsatisfactory for this purpose. Diagnoses are mostly categorized by site affected (bone in this instance), and not by histologic type. When the ICD is used, osteosarcoma cannot be separated from Ewing's tumor. To circumvent this difficulty, we have recoded the diagnoses on death certificates as to histological type for all children who died of cancer in the United States at under 15 years of age in the period 1960-64 and at under 20 years of age in 1965-68. Altogether 1934 deaths attributed to osteosarcoma or Ewing's tumor were ascertained in this way (29).

RELATION TO AGE AND SEX

Rates, determined by single year of age and sex for white children (Fig. 2), showed a slow climb for each main form of childhood bone cancer. Girls and boys had similar rates until adolescence, when the rates for boys continued to climb, whereas those for girls reached a plateau (osteosarcoma) or declined (Ewing's tumor). Data for the previous decade (1950-59) for all forms of bone cancer combined are shown in relation to stature in Fig. 3 (27). During the first 13 years of life, when boys and girls had about the same stature, they had about the same bone-cancer mortality rates, but in adolescence, as the boys grew taller than girls, a corresponding difference in bone cancer mortality rates developed.

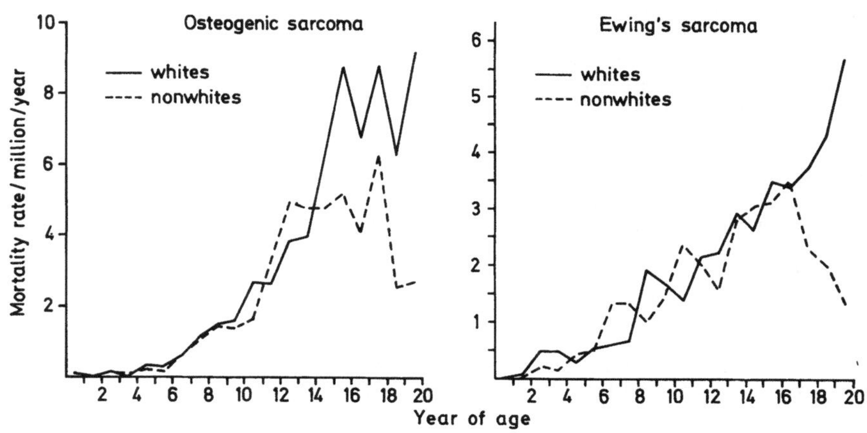

Fig. 2. U.S. mortality rates for osteosarcoma and Ewing's tumor by sex and single year of age in white children under 15 years, 1960-1964, and under 20 years, 1965-1968

These findings are consistent with a general theory proposed by JOHNSON (17). He noted that osteosarcoma occurs in long bones at the points of greatest growth and reconstruction, i.e. at the metaphyseal ends. He

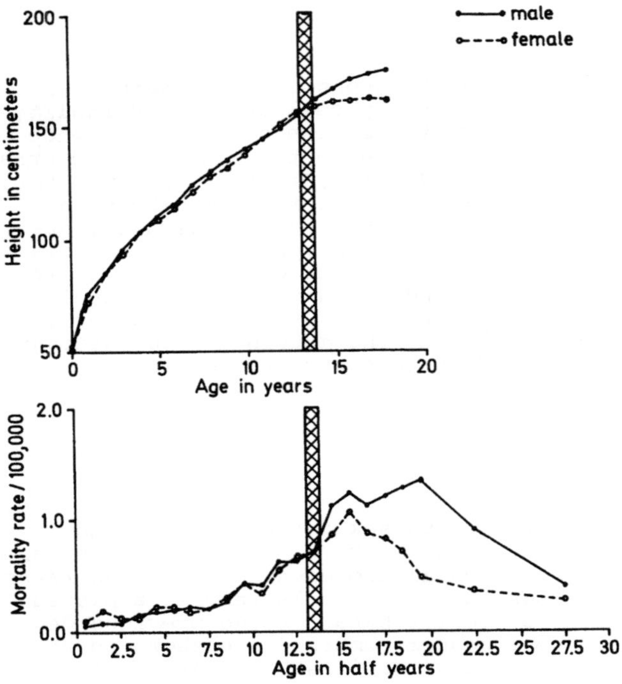

Fig. 3. Comparison of stature with bone-cancer mortality, 1950-1959, by single year of age and sex among U.S. whites (MILLER, 1968)

suggested that the tumors were related quantitatively to the amount of cell activity in the bone, and that diseases characterized by excessive cellularity, e.g. benign fibrous lesions, Paget's disease, organizing bone infarcts, osteomyelitic scars and unresolved calluses, carry an increased risk of bone cancer.

A study of 140 cases of osteosarcoma (32) revealed that tumors arose in the humerus earlier than in the long bones of the legs in both sexes; this difference in age at onset was ascribed to the relatively advanced bone growth in the length of the humerus during the early years of life. WEINFELD and DUDLEY (43) noted that osteosarcoma shifts in its anatomic distribution after the end of the growth period, from long-bone predominance at 15-24 years to an equal division between long and flat bones thereafter.

Further evidence for this relationship was sought in a comparison of the stature of children with bone cancers with that of children with nonosseous cancer, who were measured within one month of the date of diagnosis (6). Children with osteosarcoma or Ewing's tumor were taller on average than the comparison group, but the absolute differences in height were relatively small. Ewing's sarcoma had not previously been related to skeletal growth, but this finding is in keeping with U.S. mortality data for Ewing's tumor by single year of age (Fig. 2).

RACE

U.S. mortality rates for whites vs. nonwhites show a marked deficiency of Ewing's tumor among nonwhites (Fig. 4), whereas no such difference

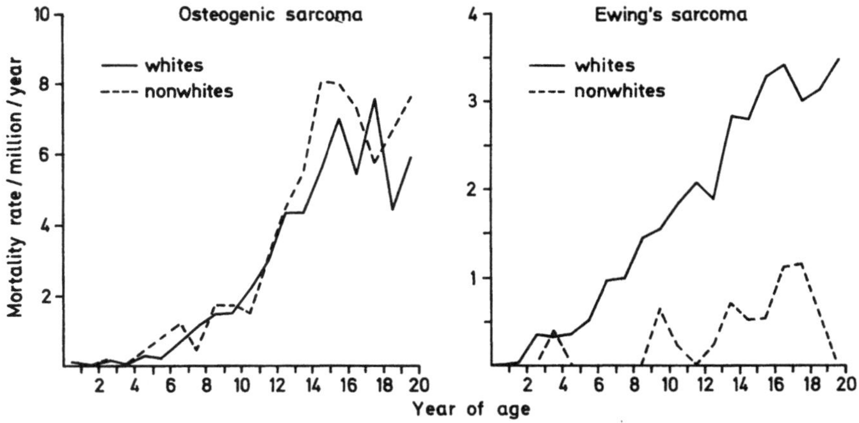

Fig. 4. U.S. mortality rates for osteosarcoma and Ewing's tumor by single year of age, whites vs. nonwhites, under 15 years, 1960-1964, and under 20 years, 1965-1968

applies to osteosarcoma. This discrepancy was first noticed in 1970 (8), and was subsequently demonstrated again by reference to histologically confirmed cases among blacks vs. whites with specimens on file at the Armed Forces Institute of Pathology in Washington, D.C. (15). Data in the California Tumor Registry revealed a similar difference in the incidence rates for Ewing's tumor when the two races were compared (22). Data for blacks in Africa show a similar near-absence of Ewing's tumor (4, 44). Blacks thus appear to be genetically resistant to this form of bone neoplasia - an important point in differential diagnosis and in the etiology of the tumor.

Two independent sources of data on bone cancer in Japanese children show a deficiency of Ewing's tumor as compared with U.S. whites, but it is not nearly as marked as the deficiency among U.S. blacks (Table 1) (20). Misclassification of tumors affecting bone is possible in diagnoses on death certificates or in tumor registries that do not have uniform expert histological review. Such misclassification must be rare in the data from the U.S. Armed Forces Institute of Pathology.

RELATION TO RETINOBLASTOMA

There seems to be an excessive incidence of osteosarcoma of the femur in children with bilateral retinoblastoma (16), a genetically transmitted neoplasm (19). Thus, the retinoblastoma gene may predispose to tumors of other sites, including bone. The risk of osteosarcoma of the orbit resulting from radiotherapy may be greater when retinoblastoma is familial (or bilateral) than when it is unilateral and sporadic. In the future, in-vitro studies of cells from patients with both osteosarcoma and familial retinoblastoma may be of special interest (e.g. with respect to their capacity to repair damage to DNA).

Syndromes Associated with Osteosarcoma

Certain pre-existent diseases of bone, some known to be genetically determined, may predispose to bone cancer in childhood. Among these

Table 1. Ratio of osteosarcoma to Ewing's sarcoma in various racial groups

Race	Source[a]	Age (yrs)	Interval	OS/ET
White	U.S. death certificates	<15 15-19	1960-66 1965-66	521/372 = 1.4 171/ 98 = 1.7
	U.S. tissue registry[b]	?	1940-68	595/237 = 2.5
	California Tumor Registry	<20	?	243[c]/110 = 2.2
Nonwhite	U.S. death certificates	<15 15-19	1960-66 1965-66	99/ 9 = 11.0 28/ 3 = 9.3
Blacks	U.S. tissue registry[b]	?	1940-68	82/ 2
	California Tumor Registry	<20	?	21[c]/ 0
Japanese	Bone tumor registry	<15	1964-69	209/ 34 = 6.1
	Childhood tumor registries	<15	1969-73	42/ 11 = 3.8

[a] See text for references.
[b] U.S. Armed Forces Institute of Pathology.
[c] Bone cancers other than Ewing's sarcoma.

are multiple osteochondromatoses (Ollier's disease), sometimes in combination with hemangiomata (Maffucci's syndrome), and multiple hereditary exostoses (8). Osteosarcoma has been reported in several patients with osteogenesis imperfecta, including one pair of sibs (18). No such syndromes have been associated with Ewing's tumor.

Occasionally osteosarcoma occurs in multiple primary sites. In a series of 600 patients with osteosarcoma seen at the Mayo Clinic (3) from 1909 to 1964, sixteen were found to have this type. Other multicentric tumors of childhood (e.g. retinoblastoma and Wilms' tumor) appear to have a genetic determinant, whereas the same neoplasms usually do not when unifocal (19).

FAMILIAL AGGREGATION

At least 7 families with multiple cases of osteogenic sarcoma have been described (Table 2). In one (5), a man with seemingly separate primaries at 15 and 40 years had a daughter who developed the neoplasm at 13 years and another daughter who died early in life of adrenal carcinoma. At the time of the report there were three normal children and there had been five miscarriages. The father had two sibs. One died at the age of 6 years of spongioblastoma multiforme and the other developed a squamous-cell carcinoma of the forehead at 16 years. Their father died at 29 years of adenocarcinoma of the colon. Taken by itself, this family's experience could be thought to have occurred by chance,

Table 2. Familial cases

Relation	Age at diagnosis (yrs)	References
Osteogenic sarcoma		
Father - daughter	25 / 6	SWANEY (1973)
2 brothers	11 / 4	SWANEY (1973)
Brother - 2 sisters	23/13 /17	ROBERTS and ROBERTS (1935)
2 sisters	3 /11	POHLE *et al*. (1936)
3 brothers - sister	15/20/11 /22	HARMON and MORTON (1966)
2 male first cousins	22 /18	ROBBINS (1967)
Father[a] - daughter	15-40[a]/13	EPSTEIN *et al*. (1970)
Ewing's tumor		
2 sisters	16 /18[b]	HUNTINGTON *et al*. (1960, 1961)
2 sisters	3 /16	HUTTER *et al*. (1964)

[a] Multicentric tumors.
[b] Atypical Ewing's.

but other families are known or have been reported in which osteosarcoma, adrenal cortical carcinoma, rhabdomyosarcoma and/or brain cancer have occurred in various combinations. In some members of these families, double primaries involving these dissimilar cell types have occurred (12, 7, 21, 28).

A study is currently being made, at the (U.S.) National Cancer Institute, of an American Indian family in which three of the nine children have developed osteosarcoma and another child has congenital fusion of the elbow. The father and two children have an unexplained hematologic abnormality (erythrocytic macrocytosis). The family appears to have a cancer/malformation syndrome.

Ewing's tumor has been described in only two pairs of sibs (11, 12, 13), and has not been reported in syndromes with other cancers or congenital malformations.

IONIZING RADIATION

Ionizing radiation in substantial dosage is the only exogenous agent yet known to induce bone cancer in man. The bone tumors induced by external radiotherapy are usually osteosarcomas or fibrosarcomas. In a series of 600 osteogenic sarcomas at the Mayo Clinic, 1909-1964, 23 (3.8%) arose in previously irradiated bone, including the jaws (3). Nine arose at sites that had been irradiated for previous bone disease: giant-cell tumor (3 cases), indeterminate bone lesions (3 cases), aneurysmal bone cysts (2 cases) and fibrous dysplasia (1 case).

In an overlapping series of patients seen at the Mayo Clinic from 1942 to 1969, 34 cases of postradiation sarcoma of bone were ascertained (35). (In 16 the sarcoma arose in pre-existing bone lesions.) The latent period was 5-42 years. Osteosarcoma occurred in eighteen cases, fibrosarcoma in fourteen, Ewing's tumor in one and chondrosarcoma in one. No estimate of dosage could be given.

Among children, internally deposited radioisotopes have also been shown to induce bone sarcomas. Of 220 children given ^{224}Ra intravenously as therapy for tuberculosis, thirty six have developed these neoplasms, in most cases osteosarcoma (36, 37, 38). Most cases with sarcoma had been treated for tuberculosis of bone. In only two cases was there a correlation between the sites affected by both diseases. The isotope, which has a half-life of 3.62 days, was given, usually at weekly intervals, for up to 4 years (average = 11.2 months). The lowest skeletal dose in a child who developed osteosarcoma was 270 rads. The latent period ranged from 4 to 21 years. On average, for each 100 rads received, 1.51 percent of the children have developed bone sarcoma. The effect was related not only to total dose, but also to the interval over which a specific dose was given (38). No substantial difference in susceptibility was observed between children and adults (26).

It is of interest that these patients have not developed an excess of leukemia, in contrast to Portuguese patients treated with Thorotrast (which contains a bone-seeking isotope), who developed an excess of leukemia twenty years later, but not of bone cancer (1).

Benign tumors also occurred excessively in the children who received ^{224}Ra: 18 osteochondromas, 1 chondroblastoma and 1 bone fibroma (37). External irradiation has produced a similar effect: in the latest survey of 2872 persons in Rochester, New York, who received radiotherapy early in life for thymic enlargement, osteoma was observed in eighteen as compared with the expected 2.26 (9).

VIRUSES

There is no convincing epidemiologic evidence in man for horizontal transmission of osteosarcoma or Ewing's tumor. There has been one report (42) of a cluster of musculoskeletal cancers; this was among schoolgirls in a Welsh town. Within an 18-month interval two girls developed osteosarcoma and two developed synovioma. Three of the girls were closely associated as friends and classmates. A feature in common among the four was contact with psittacine birds and other pets. Such coincidences of cancer occurrence, however rare, are bound to happen somewhere at some time by chance, and need not indicate exposure in common or horizontal spread. Such transmission is indicated when clusters occur not once, but excessively in subdivisions of a geographic area, as has been shown for Burkitt's lymphoma (30). It is difficult to study bone sarcomas in this way except perhaps through large registries.

In the United States it has recently become possible to study data from more than 6 million certificates of persons who died of cancer from 1950 to 1969, to determine, among other things, whether site-specific neoplasms cluster geographically according to county (25). The computer tapes containing these data were used to map the counties with the highest bone-cancer mortality (top three deciles) under the age of 20 years according to sex (Fig. 5). Inspection of the maps reveals a seemingly random distribution of counties with high rates, allowing for the fact that the size of counties in the West is often larger than those elsewhere in the nation. There is clearly no concentration

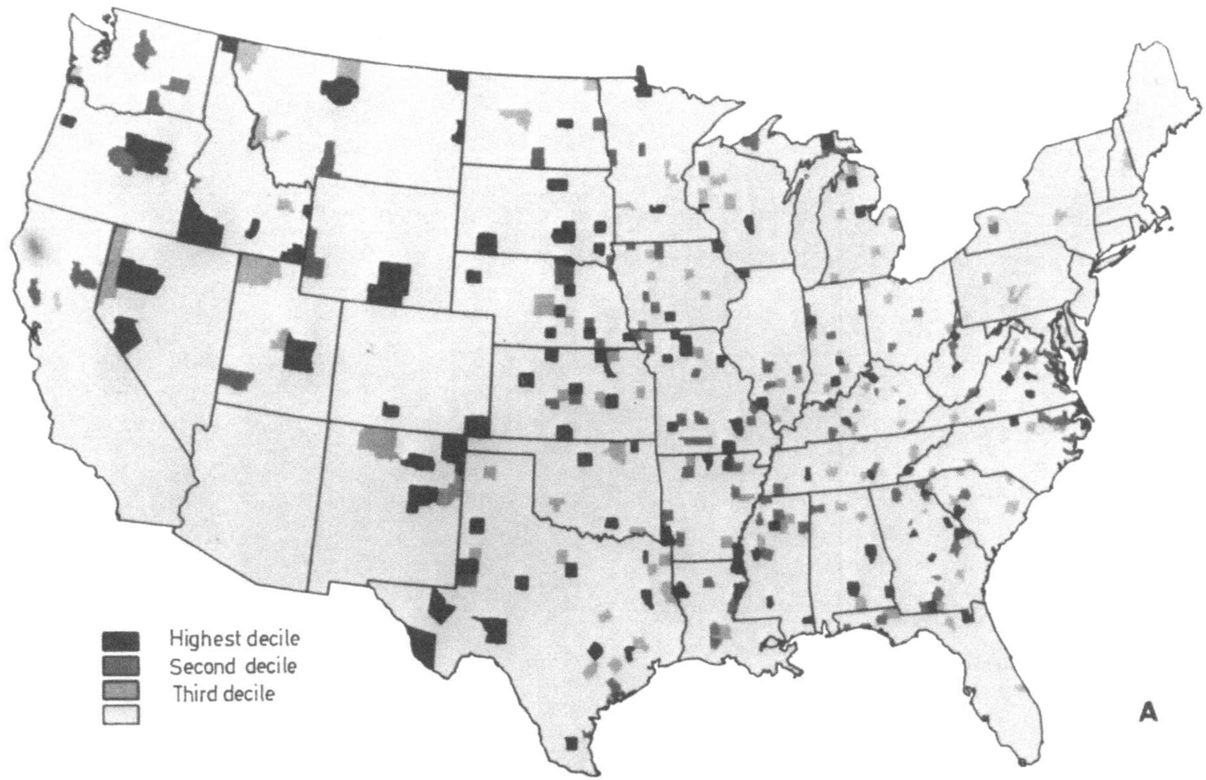

Fig. 5. U.S. counties with the highest mortality from bone cancer among white males (A) and females (B) under 20 years of age, 1950-1969

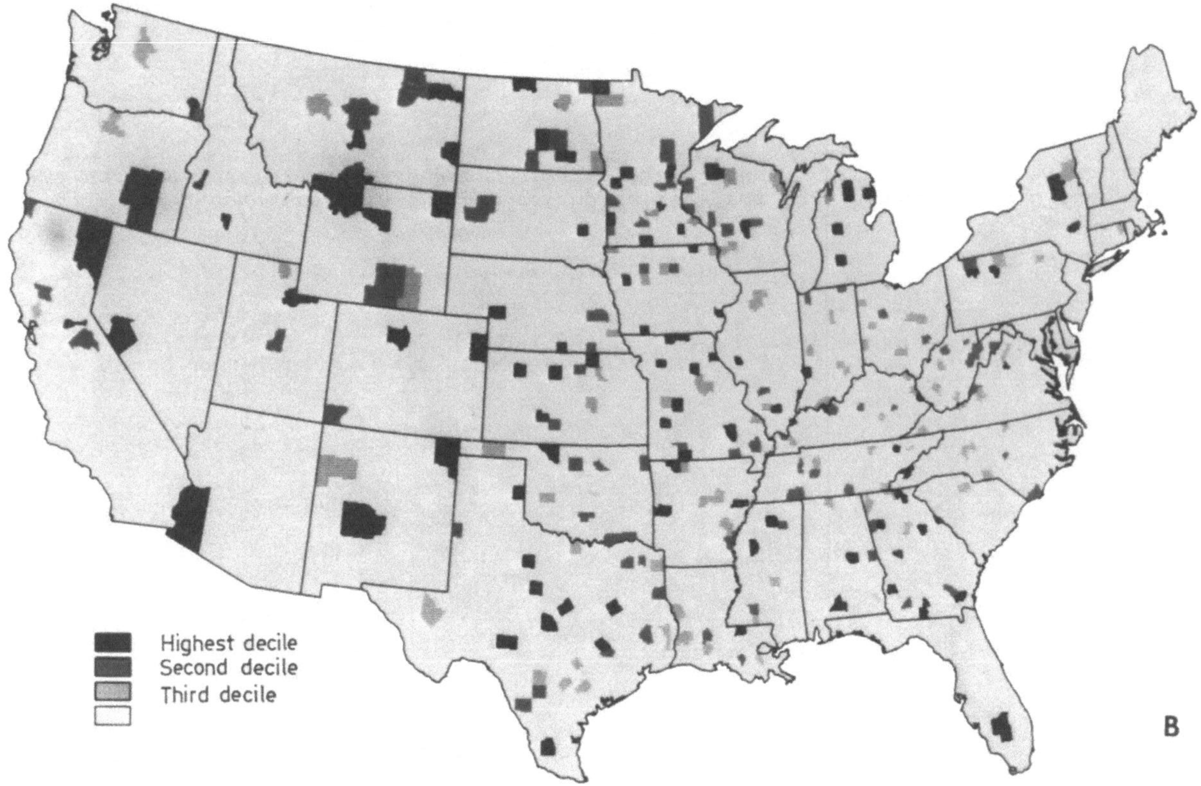

Fig. 5. U.S. counties with the highest mortality from bone cancer among white males (A) and females (B) under 20 years of age, 1950–1969

of counties with high rates to the East of Nevada, where fall-out was heaviest after nuclear-weapons tests in the 1950s. The use of diagnoses of bone cancer derived from death certificates is handicapped because all such tumors are routinely coded under the same rubric (ICD 196), regardless of histologic type. In consequence, fluctuations in mortality rates for osteosarcoma might be masked to some extent by data for other bone tumors with which it is grouped. In addition, the diagnoses on death certificates may vary geographically because of differences in survival or classification of the neoplasm.

EPIDEMIOLOGIC DIFFERENCES BETWEEN OSTEOSARCOMA AND EWING'S TUMOR

Osteosarcoma differs markedly from Ewing's tumor in all epidemiologic characteristics except for a relation to stature during childhood (Table 3). These differences must reflect dissimilarities in the genesis of the two tumors. A propensity for osteosarcoma occurs in certain inborn disorders, or after exposure to ionizing radiation, be it internal or external. Ewing's sarcoma has neither of these characteristics. It is nearly absent in blacks, both in the U.S. and in Africa. Such differences are scarcely surprising, because Ewing's tumor is generally considered to be a diffuse endothelioma of bone, i.e. a primary neoplasm of nonosseous origin involving bone, whereas osteosarcoma presumably arises from malignant osteoid produced by the sarcomatous stroma of bone-forming mesenchyme (39).

Table 3. Epidemiologic summary: osteogenic sarcoma vs. Ewing's tumor in domestic animals or man

Feature	Osteosarcoma	Ewing's tumor
In dogs, incidence related to size	Yes	Rarely if ever reported in domestic animals
In man, incidence related to growth patterns	Yes	Yes (to stature)
Near-absence in blacks	No	Yes
Family aggregation	7 reports published, others pending - up to 4 members affected	2 reports, pairs of sibs (one atypical Ewing's)
Occurrence with other tumors in patient or family	Yes	None as yet
Occurrence with preexistent syndromes	Yes	None as yet
Radiation-induced	Yes	No

Despite the marked epidemiologic and pathologic distinctions between osteosarcoma and Ewing's tumor, there are rare occasions when both histologic types occur in the same neoplasm. Such mixed tumors have been referred to as "primitive multipotential primary sarcoma of bone" (14). These tumors bridge the wide etiologic gap that normally seems to exist between osteosarcoma and Ewing's tumor.

SUMMARY

In dogs, osteosarcoma is markedly more frequent in giant breeds than in small ones. Ewing's tumor rarely occurs in species other than man. In children, both osteosarcoma and Ewing's tumor appear to be related to the rate of bone growth. Nonradiogenic osteosarcoma occurs excessively in persons with the heritable form of retinoblastoma, and in certain malformation syndromes, some of which are known to be genetically induced. Osteosarcoma may also be of the heritable type when it is multicentric or aggregates in families. The neoplasm may occur excessively in certain families with specific cancers not involving bone. By contrast, the only evidence of a genetic influence on Ewing's tumor is its near-absence among blacks in the United States and in Africa. The only exogenous agent known to induce osteosarcoma (but not Ewing's tumor) in man is ionizing radiation in substantial doses. There is no epidemiologic evidence for the virus etiology of bone cancer in man. Despite the epidemiologic differences between osteosarcoma and Ewing's tumor, both histologic types occasionally occur in different portions of the same neoplasm.

Acknowledgment

The assistance of Dr. THOMAS J. MASON, Mr. FRANK W. MCKAY and Mrs. NANCY A. DALAGER in the preparation of the Figures is gratefully acknowledged.

REFERENCES

1. ABBATT, J.D.: Human leukemic risk data derived from Portuguese Thorotrast experience. In: Radionuclide Carcinogenesis (Eds. SANDERS, C.L., BUSCH, R.H., BALLOU, J.E., MAHLUM, D.D.), p. 451. AEC Symposium Series, Vol. 29, 1973.
2. CASEY, H.W.: (Armed Forces Institute of Pathology, Washington, D.C.) Personal communication 1974
3. DAHLIN, D.C., COVENTRY, M.B.: Osteogenic sarcoma. A study of 600 cases. J. Bone Jt Surg. 49A, 101-110 (1967)
4. DAVIES, J.N.P.: Childhood tumors. In: Tumors in a Tropical Country. A Survey of Uganda 1964-1968. (Ed. A.C. TEMPLETON), p. 306. New York: Springer 1973
5. EPSTEIN, L.I., BIXLER, J.E.: An incident of familial cancer including 3 cases of osteogenic sarcoma. Cancer 25, 889-891 (1970)
6. FRAUMENI, J.F., Jr.: Stature and malignant tumors of bone in childhood and adolescence. Cancer 20, 967-973 (1967)
7. FRAUMENI, J.F., Jr.: Unpublished data (1974)
8. GLASS, A.G., FRAUMENI, J.F.,Jr.: Epidemiology of bone cancer in children. J. Nat. Cancer Inst. 44, 187-199 (1970)
9. HEMPELMANN, L.H., HALL, W.J., PHILLIPS, M., COOPER, R.A., AMES, W.R.: Neoplasms in persons treated with x-rays in infancy: fourth survey in 20 years. J. Nat. Cancer Inst. 55, 519-530 (1975)
10. HARMON, T.P., MORTON, K.S.: Osteogenic sarcoma in four siblings. J. Bone Jt Surg. 48B, 493-498 (1966)
11. HUNTINGTON, R.W., Jr., SHEFFEL, D.J., IGER, M., HENKELMANN, C.: Malignant bone tumors in siblings. Ewing's tumor and an unusual tumor, perhaps a variant of Ewing's tumor. A case report. J. Bone Jt Surg. 42A, 1065-1075 (1960)
12. HUNTINGTON, R.W., HENKELMANN, C.R., FRANKLIN, R.: Atypical Ewing tumor in the sister of a patient with Ewing's tumor. Clinical and autopsy findings. J. Bone Jt Surg. 43A, 572-574 (1961)

13. HUTTER, R.V.P., FRANCIS, K.C., FOOTE, F.W.,Jr.: Ewing's sarcoma in siblings. Report of the second known occurrence. Amer. J. Surg. 107, 598-603 (1964)
14. HUTTER, R.V.P., FOOTE, F.W., Jr., FRANCIS, K.C., SHERMAN, R.S.: Primitive multipotential primary sarcoma of bone. Cancer 19, 1-25 (1966)
15. JENSEN, R.D., DRAKE, R.M.: Rarity of Ewing's tumor in Negroes. Lancet 1970 1, 777
16. JENSEN, R.D., MILLER, R.W.: Retinoblastoma: epidemiologic characteristics. N. Engl. J. Med. 285, 307-311 (1971)
17. JOHNSON, L.C.: A general theory of bone tumors. Bull. N. Y. Acad. Med. 29, 164-171 (1953)
18. KLENERMAN, L., OCKENDEN, B.G., TOWNSEND, A.C.: Osteosarcoma occurring in osteogenesis imperfecta. Report of 2 cases. J. Bone Jt Surg. 49B, 314-323 (1967)
19. KNUDSON, A.G., Jr.: Mutation in human cancer. Advanc. Cancer Res. 17, 317-352 (1973)
20. KOBAYASHI, N.: Unpublished data (1974)
21. LI, F.P., FRAUMENI, J.F., Jr.: Rhabdomyosarcoma in children: epidemiologic study and identification of a familial cancer syndrome. J. Nat. Cancer Inst. 43, 1365-1373 (1969)
22. LINDEN, G., DUNN, J.E.: Ewing's sarcoma in Negroes. Lancet 1970 1, 1171
23. LOUTIT, J.F.: Malignancy from radium. Brit. J. Cancer 24, 195-207 (1970)
24. World Health Organization: Manual of the International Statistical Classification of Diseases, Injuries, and Causes of Death, 8th Revision. Geneva: WHO 1967
25. MASON, T.J., MCKAY, F.W.: U.S. Cancer Mortality by County. DHEW Publication No. (NIH) 74-615. Washington D.C.: DHEW 1974
26. MAYS, C.W.: Cancer induction in man from internal radioactivity. Health Phys. 25, 585-592 (1973)
27. MILLER, R.W.: Relation between cancer and congenital defects: an epidemiologic evaluation. J. Nat. Cancer Inst. 40, 1079-1085 (1968)
28. MILLER, R.W.: Deaths from childhood leukemia and solid tumors among twins and other sibs in the United States, 1960-67. J. Nat. Cancer Inst. 46, 203-209 (1971)
29. MILLER, R.W., DALAGER, N.A.: U.S. childhood cancer deaths by cell type, 1960-68. J. Pediatr. 85, 664-668 (1974)
30. PIKE, M.C., WILLIAMS, E.H., WRIGHT, B.: Burkitt's tumour in the West Nile District of Uganda 1961-5. Brit. Med. J. 2, 395-399 (1967)
31. POHLE, E.A., STOVALL, W.D., BOYER, H.N.: Concurrence of osteogenic sarcoma in two sisters. Radiology 27, 545-548 (1936)
32. PRICE, C.H.G.: Primary bone-forming tumours and their relationship to skeletal growth. J. Bone Jt Surg. 40B, 574-593 (1958)
33. ROBBINS, R.: Familial osteosarcoma. Fifth reported occurrence. J. Amer. Med. Ass. 202, 1055 (1967)
34. ROBERTS, C.W., ROBERTS, C.P.: Concurrent osteogenic sarcoma in brother and sisters. J. Amer. Med. Ass. 105, 181-185 (1935)
35. SIM, F.H., CUPPS, R.E., DAHLIN, D.C., IVINS, J.C.: Postradiation sarcoma of bone. J. Bone Jt. Surg. 54A, 1479-1489 (1972)
36. SPIESS, H., MAYS, C.W.: Bone cancers induced by ^{224}Ra (ThX) in children and adults. Health Phys. 19, 713-729 (1970)
37. SPIESS, H., MAYS, C.W.: Addendum. Health Phys. 20, 543-545 (1971)
38. SPIESS, H., MAYS, C.W.: Protraction effect on bone-sarcoma induction of ^{224}Ra in children and adults. In: Radionuclide Carcinogenesis (Eds. SANDERS, C.L, BUSCH, R.H, BALLOU, J.E., MAHLUM, D.D.), p. 437. AEC Symposium Series Vol. 29, 1973
39. SUIT, H.D., MARTIN, R.G., SUTOW, W.W.: Primary malignant tumors of the bone. In: Clinical Pediatrics Oncology (Eds. W.W. SUTOW, T.J. VIETTI, D.J. FERNBACH) p. 473. St. Louis: C.V. Mosby 1973

40. SWANEY, J.J.: Familial osteogenic sarcoma. Clin. Orthop. 97, 64-68 (1973)
41. TJALMA, R.A.: Canine bone sarcoma: estimation of relative risk as a function of body size. J. Nat. Cancer Inst. 36, 1137-1150 (1966)
42. TURNER, R.C.: Unusual group of tumors among schoolgirls. Brit. J. Cancer 21, 17-26 (1966)
43. WEINFELD, M.S., DUDLEY, H.R.: Osteogenic sarcoma. J. Bone Jt Surg. 44A, 269-276 (1962)
44. WILLIAMS, A.O.: Tumors of childhood in Ibadan, Nigeria. Cancer 36, 370-378 (1975)

The Endogenous Origin and Transmission of RNA Viral Genomes that Code for Cancer

R. J. HUEBNER

Perhaps one of the more debilitating factors in cancer research is the widely held notion that the term "cancer" represents 100 quite different diseases with an equal number of different causes, thus requiring a multitude of differing approaches to both prevention and therapy.

In a certain sense this may well be true, but there is a different view of the etiology of cancer which may eventually be found to be more valid or at least more in keeping with natural biology, and at the same time more satisfying and optimistic. However, I will preface this proposition by a number of reflections.

The problem of cancer is obviously not solely one for humans, since virtually all vertebrates (and even lower animals) are liable to a wide spectrum of differing cancers, which are in many instances similar to those in man. It should be pointed out, however, that our information is confined largely to domesticated and laboratory animals, since surveillance of cancer in wild animals is virtually nonexistent; furthermore, many domestic animals are disposed of relatively early, so that incidence information on cancer, which occurs mostly in later life, is very deficient. Thus, experimental studies on the etiology of cancer (other than epidemiological ones) are largely confirmed to available laboratory animals; fortunately such studies have revealed a great deal of valuable information concerning endogenous and exogenous factors involved in the etiology of cancer.

Hundreds, perhaps thousands of different environmental physical and chemical agents, dozens of DNA and RNA tumor viruses, endogenous defective genes, normal permissive genes, abnormal immune and hormone espressions all conspire to produce often essentially the same types of cancer.

Since cancer must begin as a single genetically stable but altered neoplastic cell (102), perhaps it is best explained by endogenous factors such as operon genes that code for the transformed state and regulating genes that determine whether or not the operons go into action (switch on) and, finally, whether or not the host immune surveillance succeeds or fails in attemps to abort or eliminate the initial tumor cells. According to this concept exogenous environmental carcinogens would serve as accelerators of certain cancers by acting as derepressors (at the DNA level) of normal host-cell regulatory systems and inhibitors of the immunological surveillance system.

This is not a new concept. BURNET (19) suggested that cancer was an essentially endogenous disease because in humans and in those animals for which cancer registries are available, cancer incidence is essentially stochastic, i.e. highly predictable in its occurrence. He concluded, therefore, that somatic mutations were etiological factors of cancer. Thus in surveys of cancer death certificates, cancer registries, and multi-city surveys, it appears that approximately 20 percent of the human population dies of cancer each year; it is legitimate therefore to ask why the total incidence does not fluctuate annually, from 20 percent down to 10 percent or up to 50 percent. Burnet insisted that if exogenous causes such as communicable viruses were the major determinants, rather wide fluctuations in total cancers would be expected in the same populations. Similarly, if chemical carcinogens and radiation, which are well known to produce cancer in humans and also in experimental animals, represent ever-increasing risks, this should be reflected in increasing incidences of many different types of cancer, yet this does not seem to happen. Ethnic and racial factors, which are probably genetic in origin, result in variations of the incidences of certain types of cancer in differing genetic groups, but within the groups the total amounts of cancer appear to be relatively predictable. In two studies (82, 92) there were significant specific tumor differences between Jews and Protestants and Catholics, but the total numbers of cancers occurring in one year were highly stochastic over a five-year period (Table 1).

The existence of endogenous cancer-determinating host factors, which is easily demonstrated in inbred animals, does not, of course, detract from the importance of the clear-cut influences that environmental carcinogens have on many cancers. It is possible regularly, to produce nearly 100 percent cancers in some strains of mice and rats with either radiation or chemical carcinogens. Other strains,however, are very resistent to such inductions, and this is known to be due to gene influences. The role of inherited endogenous genes in susceptibility to spontaneous cancer of inbred animals (inbred mice in particular) has been demonstrated, and indeed many of the cancer-controlling genes have been identified and are relatively well known, particularly those involving endogenous as well as exogenous type-C and type-B RNA tumor viruses, a matter to be discussed in some detail in this report.

A study of the modes of action of chemicals in producing cancer in experimental animals (45) suggested that the action of the chemicals on cell DNA led to derepressions of endogenous oncogenic operons by interference with natural functioning of regulatory genes, a conclusion arrived at earlier by LWOFF (81).

The role of endogenous genes in cancer seems quite evident in the case of in-vivo induction of cancer by irradiation and carcinogenic chemicals and in that of in-vitro transformation of cells by a large variety of different carcinogenic chemicals; the stable genetic changes in the transformed cells that readily permit their transplantation as tumors into syngeneic animals simply cannot be attributed to any genetic information carried by the differing chemicals, despite the fact that their action is on the DNA of the cell. Most, if not all, known carcinogens are also mutagens (5), and in the bacterial cell systems the action of mutagens is well known. Mutagens can alter various endogenous genes-operons, regulatory genes, or both.

In 1969, my associates and I proposed that the genomes of endogenous RNA tumor viruses were specific determinants of spontaneous cancers in vertebrates and that the type-C RNA viruses represented endogenous factors in induced as well as spontaneous cancers (56). We postulated that cells of probably all vertebrates contained specific type-C virus genomes that are universally transmitted from parent to offspring (and from cell to daughter cell) as part of normal genetic (DNA) inheritance. Host-cell regulating genes and their repressor proteins, host immune mechanisms, and environmental carcinogens of various types were seen

Table 1. Cancer mortalitiy[c] in New York City

	Catholic	Jewish	Protestant
Cancer of cervix (females)			
a) MacMahon 1955	21/100.000	9/100.000	22/100.000
b) Newill 1953-58	22/100.000	9/100.000	24/100.000
Cancer of breast (females)			
a)	93	98	98
b)	84	96	90
Cancer of prostate (males)			
a)	42	30	50
b)	40	33	51
Cancer of stomach (both sexes)			
a)	51	62	57
b)	52	62	56
Cancer of large intestine (both sexes)			
a)	58	80	58
b)	60	78	60
Cancer of lung (males)			
a)	50	34	56
b)	50	34	60
Leukemias (both sexes)			
a)	13	19	16
b)	13	21	14
All cancers (females)			
a)	437	511	468
b)	430	516	451
All cancers (males)			
a)	585	595	638
b)	578	572	623

a Mac Mahon, B. Acta Unio. Int. Contra Cancrum, 16, 1716-1724 (1960).
b Newill, V.A. J. Natl. Cancer Inst. 26, 405-407 (1961).
Reprinted with permission from Analytical & Experimental Epidem. of Cancer., Univ. Tokyo Press 1973 p. 345-365. (Huebner).
[c] Rates/100.000 among ethnic subgroups; based on comprehensive survey of death certificates.

as important determinants of the expressions of the oncogene(s) and virogene(s) of endogenous viral genome(s), a genome that, in the interests of survival of species, had to be well controlled in early life by genetic and immunological mechanisms in most natural hosts, early cancers being due primarily to genetic or immunologic abnormalities.

This hypothesis therefore stated that cancer was first of all a risk specified by natural biological variation, but also one greatly influenced by the interaction of specific genetic inheritance and exogenous environmental factors; the oncogenic event being determined by spontaneous and/or induced derepression at the molecular level in a manner described by JACOB & MONOD (62). We felt this hypothesis, if true, would provide a useful heuristic basis for a unifying theory of cancer which was consistent with the phenomenon of naturally occurring cancers as well as with that of cancers induced by radiation and chemical and viral agents.

The basic concepts underlying the viral oncogene hypothesis had already been suggested much earlier (24, 81, 62, 4, 113, 42, 66, 102, 131). In our view, the endogenous virus oncogene hypothesis offered, the only satisfactory explanation of the considerable body of data accumulated by 1969 on the natural histories of cancer-inducing RNA tumor viruses in chickens, mice, hamsters, rats and cats. Several critical observations provided the initial basis for the viral oncogene hypothesis. For instance, group-specific (gs) or p30 antigens found in embryonic visceral tissues and in spontaneous and induced tumors were frequently present in the absence of infectious virus; furthermore, significant immunological tolerance to this major species-specific and interspecies-specific antigen provided additional evidence suggesting gene transmission of non-infectious virus rather than the more conventional vertical or horizontal transmission of infectious virus (Tables 2, 3, 4C). This view seemed essential since we knew of no other possibility for transmission of noninfectious viral proteins. Findings 5 years later, as will be discussed below, revealed that in many instances the non-infectious embryonic antigens were expressions of xenotropic type-C viruses that are not infectious for cells of natural species, but do infect cells of other species (Table 4A) (56, 53, 55, 75, 124).

Table 2. Immunological tolerance to gs antigen in mice, chickens, and cats. Reprinted with permission from Perspectives in Virology 7, 55-71 (1971) (Huebner and Igel)

Sera from mice with MSV gs positive tumors		No. tested for gs antibody	
Virus[a]	Mouse strains	Negative	Positive
M-MSV	NIH (Swiss) BALB/c, C57BL	110	0
H-MSV	NIH	10	0
MSV(GL)	NIH	16	0
MSV(RL)	NIH, BALB/c, C57BL	41	0
MSV(FL)	NIH, BALB/c, C57BL	88	0
MSV(KL)	C57BL	16	0
MSV(AKR)	C57BL	14	0
		295	0
C57BL mice injected with RADLV[b]		10	0
Sera from immune chickens			
From Kelloff and Vogt[c]		13	0
From Armstrong ez al.[c]		64	8
Sera from tumored cats			
From Gardner et al. (16)[d]		12	0

[a] M-MSV and H-MSV = Moloney sarcoma virus, Harvey sarcoma virus: MSV ( ) = various pseudotypes of MSV with envelopes provided by Gross, Rauscher, Friend, Kirsten, and AKR leukemia viruses. All were tested by complement-fixation and negative at a 1:10 dilution.

[b] RADLV = Radiation leukemia virus (56)

[c] Chicken sera positive for envelope antibody and/or neutralizing antibody; gs antibody determinations were by fluorescent and gel diffusion tests.

[d] All cats had gs positive tumors; gs antibody tests were done in complement fixation.

Type-C viral antigen expression in BALB/c mice, which was absent at birth and in early months of life, appeared in spleen and thymus tissue at 6 months, and increased with age. This was correlated with increasing incidence of infectious virus and cancer (Table 5). Follow-up observations, continued for several years, established that the pattern of increasing gs, virus and tumor incidence with increasing age was highly stochastic, so that it could not be accounted for by horizontal transmission. It seemed that a predictable pattern of this kind could best be explained, in the case of predictable expression of noninfectious virus in embryos, as overt expressions of endogenous virogenes (56, 96).

Since 1969, studies in experimental animals have greatly strengthened the view that endogenous virogenes and oncogenes of type-C RNA viruses are indeed much involved in the generality of cancers of vertebrates. Continuing studies of endogenous type-C RNA viruses in inbred mice, rats and chickens, and in hamsters and cats, and discoveries of similar

Table 3. Distribution of CF antigens in 10% extracts of mouse embryo tissues from various strains of mice detected by rat antisera to the murine gs anigens. Reprinted with permission from Ann. N.Y, Acad. Sci. 181, 246-271 (1971) (HUEBNER et al.)

Strain Strain	Embryo specimen	Age (days)	No. Pos./No. Tested[a]	Range in Titers
NIH Swiss	Whole[b]	10	47 / 47	1:4 to 1:16
		12	30 / 30	
		14	55 / 60	
	Spleen[c]	18	7 / 11	
	Thymus	18	11 / 11	
	Liver	18	10 / 20	
	Muscle	18	0 / 20	
C3H/Bi	Whole	13	13 / 18	1:2 to 1:16
	Spleen	18	6 / 14	
	Thymus	18	11 / 13	
	Liver	18	14 / 14	
	Intestine	18	7 / 8	
	Muscle	18	0 / 7	
BALB/cCr	Whole	10-11	24 / 24	1:2 to 1: 8
		13	0 / 23[d]	
	Spleen	18	14 / 20	
Thymus	Thymus	18	19 / 21	
	Liver	18	18 / 21	
	Intestine	18	9 / 9	
C57B1	Whole	10-11	16 / 20	1:2 to 1: 8
(Cumberland)	Spleen	17-18	0 / 3	
	Thymus	17-18	1 / 3	1:2 to 1: 8
	Liver	17-18	1 / 3	
	Intestine	17-18	3 / 3	
Wild (feral)	Whole	10-14	2 / 20	1:2 to 1: 4
		16-18	17 / 19	
	Spleen	16-18	3 / 4	
	Thymus	16-18	4 / 4	
	Liver	16-18	3 / 3	

[a] Number with CF antigen titer greater than 1:2/number tested.
[b] Individual embryos.
[c] Pools of five to eight embryos.
[d] Partial reactions less than 3+ at 1:2 observed in most embryos.

transmissible viruses in primates such as gibbon (68) and woolly monkeys (117, 111, 37), and the discovery of xenotropic type-C viruses in baboons (64, 12) and other Old-World monkeys (13) now appear to confirm the general prevalence of type-C viral genomes in the germinal and somatic cells of most if not all animals. Molecular and antigenic relationships of the baboon viral genome to the putative type-C virus observed in human cancer cells (65, 32, 112) offer considerable hope that specific type-C virus will soon be isolated from human tissues and/or cells. The endogenous human virus, like the viruses peculiar to the baboon and other Old-World primates, can be expected to be xenotropic and unable to infect and replicate efficiently in the host species cells.

It might be suggested that the type-C viruses are the prime endogenous viral "causes" of cancer if only because the type-C (and type-B) RNA tumor viruses represent to date the only established natural viral causes of cancer in natural species, i.e. in chickens, mice, cats and hamsters, a statement that I hope to substantiate by attempting to answer the following questions:

1. What are the origins, modes of transmission, and properties of the RNA tumor viruses in their normal hosts; what is the evidence for inheritance of DNA copies in germinal and somatic cells, and finally, how can the known horizontally spread RNA viruses in chickens, cats and baboons be explained?

Table 4. Origins and modes of transmission of natural RNA tumor viruses: examples of endogenous and exogenous viruses

A. Endogenous	Xenotropic type-C viruses	(noninfectious for cells of natural host; infectious for cells of other species. Transmitted genetically?)
Virus Strains		Investigators
Mouse[a]	NZB[b]	LEVY & PINCUS, 1970
	NIH Swiss[b] (AT124)	TODARO et al., 1973
	BALB/c-2	STEPHENSON et al., 1974
	C57L[b]	ARNSTEIN, in preparation
	C57BL/6	LEVY, 1973; BENVENISTE et al., 1974
Hamster	HALV-1	FREEMAN et al., 1974
Rat	RALV-1	KLEMENT et al., 1973
Cat	RD114	McALLISTER et al., 1972; FISCHINGER et al., 1973; LIVINGSTON & TODARO, 1973 SARMA et al., 1973
Chicken	Strain E	WEISS, 1973
Swine[b]	PK15	MOENNIG et al., 1974; TODARO et al., 1974
Baboon[b]	BablV	KALTER et al., 1973; BENVENISTE et al., 1974; TODARO et al., 1974
Human[b]?	Baboon virus-related p30	SHERR & TODARO, 1974
B. Endogenous	**Ecotropic viruses**	**(infectious (tropic) for cells of natural host; some transmitted genetically, others epigenetically**
Virus Strains		Investigators
Mouse	AKR virus	GROSS, 1961
	C57BL/6-RADLV	LIEBERMANN & KAPLAN, 1959
	BALB/c N-tropic	AARONSON et al., 1969; HARTLEY et al., 1970
	BALB/c B-tropic	HARTLEY et al., 1970
	MTV agent	BITTNER, 1936

Wild-mouse	LC & 1504E strains	GARDNER *et al.*, 1971
Hamster	HALV-2 (MSV(HALV))	KELLOFF *et al.*, 1970
Rat	RALV-2 (MSV(O))	TING, 1968; BERGS *et al.*, 1972
Cat	FeLV 1, 2, 3	THEILEN *et al.*, 1968; RICKARD *et al.*, 1969; GARDNER *et al.*, 1970; SARMA *et al.*, 1970

C. Exogenous RNA tumor viruses	(highly infectious for original hosts but often also for heterotypic hosts)
Vertically transmitted through maternal reproductive tract and experimental transmission	Investigators
ALV-avian leukosis viruses: Strains A, B, C, D	RUBIN *et al.*, 1961
MulV-murine leukemia viruses: GLV, FLV, MLV, RLV	GROSS, 1951 & 1958; FRIEND, 1957; MOLONEY, 1960; RAUSCHER, 1962
Horizontally transmitted through excretions and/or nursing of newborns	
Chicken - ALV Strains A und B	BURMESTER & WATERS, 1955; BEARD, 1957
Mouse mammary tumor virus CMTV)	BITTNER, 1936; ANDERVONT & DUNN, 1948; HESTON, 1965
Cat feline leukemia viruses (FeLV's)	HARDY *et al.*, 1973; JARRETT *et al.*, 1973
Gibbon Ape & Woolly monkey viruses	KAWAKAMI *et al.*, 1972; PARKS *et al.*, 1974

Mice, hamsters, rats, cats and chickens have both xenotropic and ecotropic endogenous type-C viruses, many of which appear to be genetically transmitted. Certain cats, chickens and mice, however, also harbor variants of ecotropic viruses that can spread in nature by epigenetic vertical and horizontal modes, particularly in large and dense populations. It is also clear that when strains of mice (both laboratory and wild) are highly permissive to generalized infection with ecotropic viruses, quite high titers of the p30 viral protein and infectious virus can be demonstrated in various tissues (spleens, blood and tails). In virtually all such virus-permissive strains, leukemia and other cancers occur spontaneously during the first year of life, whereas cancer is rare to absent during this period in nonpermissive genetically determined negative strains. When infectious virus is demonstrated in normal and tumerous tissues of "switched-on" mice, it is frequently oncogenic when injected into susceptible mouse strains. However, incubation periods can be quite long (12-20 months), particularly when the virus titer is not augmented by subcultures but given directly as filtered extracts of normal ot tumor tissues (PETERS *et al.*, 1973). Since it is known that serial passages of virus to new host cells or animals results in two or more viral genomes (93, 111), many of the established RNA tumor viruses no longer qualify as natural viruses. The endogenous xenotropic viruses apparently do not produce tumors until relatively late in life, and the endogenous ecotropic viruses often associated with early cancers therefore represent the preferred targets of preventive viral vaccine efforts.

[a] All mouse strains have a serologically very similar xenotropic virus; many have ecotropic viruses also.

[b] Animals in which xenotropic virus is only type of virus demonstrated or suspected.

2. Do the endogenous type-C viruses really carry oncogenes which specify neoplasia *in vivo* and transformation *in vitro*, or do they switch on other, as yet unidentified, host cell genes?
3. How do the endogenous antiviral genetic and immunological factors demonstrated in representatives of various animal species actually regulate virus expression and cancer? Finally, can such factors be exploited in specific fashion to prevent or treat cancer?

Obviously, comprehensive answers are impossible in a single paper, for they would necessitate a review of much of the data accumulated since the initiation of the Viral Cancer Program of the National Cancer Institute.

Any answer to the first question above requires a sound knowledge of the known RNA tumor viruses and their various origins and modes of transmission.

Table 4 (A, B, C) shows the differing categories of these viruses and indicates their relationships to their natural hosts. Recent discoveries of xenotropic type-C RNA viruses (Table 4A) which cannot infect or replicate in the cells of their natural species provides conclusive evidence for genetic transmission of type-C viruses in a wide variety of animals (mice, hamsters, rats, chickens, swine, baboons, other Old-World monkeys and possibly man).

The properties of the xenotropic viruses are very similar to those of other type-C viruses found in many of these animals. The ecotropic viruses (Table 4B) which can replicate in their natural hosts and spread *in vitro* to neighboring host species-type cells are also genetically transmitted (103) and genetically regulated (2, 78, 44, 84) in many cases, but in other instances, particularly in the cat (43, 63) and in the chicken (107), the ecotropic RNA viruses can be transmitted epigenetically through maternal organs and/or milk.

The known exogenous vertically and horizontally transmitted viruses are shown in Table 4C. They include the well-studied and established avian feline and gibbon leukemia viruses which transmit both vertically

Table 5. Incidence by age groups of gs antigens and infectious virus in spleens of normal BALB/c mice: relationship to tumor incidence. Reprinted by permission of Editions du Centre National de la Recherche Scientifique, Paris.

Age groups (months)	CF antigen (% pos.) ([a])	Virus isolation (% pos.) ([b])	Tumor incidence ([c])
< 4	1.7	10.0	0
4 - 6	0	10.0	0.02
7 - 9	17.9	21.4	0.11
10 - 12	26.6	76.5	0.18
13 - 15	39.0	50.0	0.9
16 - 18	55.7	70.6	1.1
19 - 21	63.3	-	4.2
22 - 24	61.5	79.3	10.6
25 - 27	93.3	63.6	13.2
28 - 30	73.5	-	15.4
30 - 32	59.2	-	7.5

[a] At 1:2 dilution of 10% extract: approximately 500 mice tested - range 26 to 91 per group.
[b] Approximately 142 mice tested - range 11 to 29 per group.
[c] Included in tumors are all leukemias and solid cancers; excludes adenomas, hepatomas and other non-malignant tumors. Populations observed include 12,000 at 6 months, 3,000 at 19 months, 200 at 30 months.

and horizontally and the laboratory strains of murine viruses which transmit primarily through the reproductive tract and milk (74, 42).

Thus the horizontally transmitted type-C viruses and most ecotropic representatives have been shown to have definite oncogenic potential *in vivo* and *in vitro*; this has been easily established by preventing infection with virus-specific neutralizing antibodies (31, 26, 89, 59, 70). The oncogenicity of the recently discovered xenotropic viruses has still to be established (see discussion below). The pioneering experiments of various investigators (101, 40, 18, 9, 30, 91, 106, 99, 95) established the oncogenicity of the established horizontally spread RNA tumor viruses in chickens, mice and cats.

Since the widely prevalent endogenous xenotropic viruses (Table 4A) in many classes and species of vertebrates cannot infect and replicate within the individual cells of the species of origin, genetic transmission of these virogenes seems necessary. When grown in cells of other species the xenotropic viruses are bona fide type-C viruses producing appropriate RNA-dependent DNA polymerases and various viral protein moieties such as p30 (the major gs antigen), p15, p12 and p70.

The cat is especially interesting in that while feline leukemia viruses (FeLV) are transmitted to other cats horizontally, producing leukemia (43, 63), its endogenous inherited virus, RD114 (83), which is present as numerous genetic copies in cat cells and is molecularly and antigenically different from FeLV, cannot replicate effectively in its natural host and to date, like other recently discovered xenotropic viruses, has not yet been shown to be oncogenic.

The host-range and viral-envelope (p70 and p15) specificities of the xenotropic viruses are significantly different from those of the endogenous and exogenous ecotropic viruses. The xenotropic viruses of laboratory mice (all strains) have the same neutralizing antigen and antibodies, the latter often produced spontaneously in early life. These facts suggest a profound conservation of the integrity of the p70 envelope antigens of xenotropic viruses. The major internal group-specific p30 antigen (gsl) seems to be same in all mice; the p70 protein antigen specificity varies amongst the epigenetic horizontally transmitted mouse viruses and is significantly different from the genetically conserved envelope antigen of all the xenotropic mouse viruses. Before a conceptual approach to the question as to whether type-C virogenes carry oncogenes which specify induction of cancer is possible, it is necessary to consider that virtually all viral diseases are multifactorial diseases dependent on at least 6 factors such as virulence (pathogenicity of virus), dosage of virus, route of infection, age at infection, host permissiveness (gene restriction), and the quality and quantity of host immune responses. Each of these factors must be on "go" if the disease specified by viral genes is to occur; yet in the final analysis, the virus remains the critical most essential, determinant of the disease; it is impossible to develop poliomyelitis without poliovirus. Thus, with one or two exceptions, the viruses native to natural species rarely produce disease in their natural host. This is true of hundreds of viruses belonging to the entero-, rhino-, adeno-, and myxovirus groups in all mammals; a 1:1 ratio of virus to disease is unknown with these universally prevalent viruses. The mean ratio of virus to disease overall would be closer to 1:100, 1:1000 or even 1:10,000.

It is no different in the case of the RNA tumor viruses; as mentioned above, the replication of infectious RNA viruses and/or their subinfectious expressions are in themselves insufficient to produce cancer. The other factors listed above are just as important for RNA tumor viruses as for the more familiar, conventional, viruses. Again, this does not mean that the RNA tumor viruses are not the critically essential etiological factors in the tumors they are known to produce; they have been proved to be so wherever the transmissible viruses have been adequately tested. From extensive experience with the RNA tumor viruses, I think it can be stated unequivocally that those type-C viruses thus far termed "nononcogenic" are viruses that have not been adequately tested for oncogenesis.

ONCOGENICITY OF ECOTROPIC VIRUSES

Endogenous ecotropic viruses are present in low dosage in natural tumors, and when filtered and transmitted into susceptible newborn hosts they have invariably produced leukemia. This is true for both B- and N-tropic[1] (ecotropic) viruses native to such strains as BALB/c, C57BL/J, AKR, C58, SJL, wild mice, and others: similarly the ecotropic viruses of the hamster, cat, gibbon ape and woolly monkey have been shown to be oncogenic in transmission experiments (77, 42, 7, 21, 63, 98, 10, 52, 67).

Reciprocal virus inhibitors have been reported in extracts of N- and B-type cells (116); the extracts of N cells inhibited B-type virus and those from B-type cells inhibited N-type virus. The extracts were effective after viral penetration and after the virus had been established in the appropriate homologous cells. In each case it seemed clear that the $Fv\text{-}1^{bb}$, $FV\text{-}1^{nn}$ and $Fv\text{-}1^{nb}$ of LILLY et al. (79) were decisive determinants of ecotropic virus expressions (see host-cell regulation below).

Mendelian experiments reveal host genes responsible for regulation of virus and tumor expressions; in backcross progeny of C57L x AKR and BALB/c x AKR, endogenous virus expressions were shown to appear at 30 to 50 days in spleens and/or tail specimens (84, 79). Expression of gs titer in spleens and of the virus in tails of individual mice was qualitatively and quantitatively related to the incidence of cancer during the first and second years of life (Fig. 1, Table 6).

The C57L x AKR cross led to a number of virus antigen-positive nonlymphomatous tumors (carcinomas, etc.) which were not known to occur naturally in the parental lines, and gs antigen was detected in the tumors which occurred late in the lives of the 14 mice that had been free of gs antigen at 30 days. Furthermore, the parental C57L mice (20% of which developed RCS tumors) were later found to have expressions of the xenotropic C57L virus. Studies of congenic lines derived from these experiments now in progress are designed to determine the role of the xenotropic virus in the spontaneous RCS tumors occurring late in life (>500 days).

Activation of previously "switched-off" endogenous type-C RNA tumor viruses has been reported in tissues and cells of mice, hamsters, rats, cats, chickens, swine, baboons and cattle; often both ecotropic and xenotropic viruses are induced in the same animals or cell cultures (see Table 4). The literature on activation of endogenous RNA tumor viruses is voluminous (see Table 7); hence I will only point out certain high-

---

[1] N-type cells are present in NIH Swiss, AKR, SWR, C57L, others; B-type cells are represented by BALB/c and C57Bl and others.

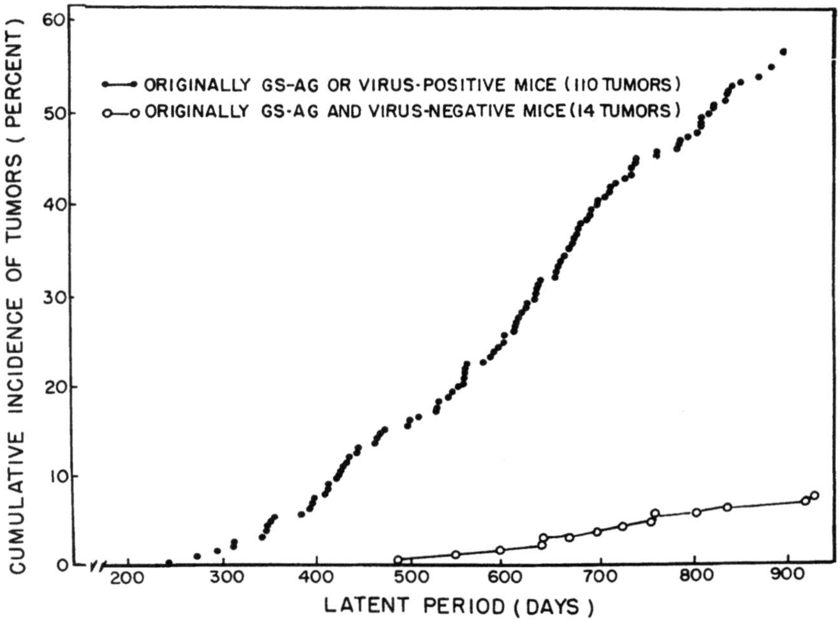

Fig. 1. Development and occurrence of tumors in BC-C57L/J mice segregating for type-C RNA tumor virus or its gs antigen. Tumors of all types occurred in mice that were originally gs-antigen or virus positive; their appearance and incidence were significantly earlier and greater than those developing in mice that were originally gs-antigen and virus negative. Twice as many tumors occurred in mice that were gs-antigen or virus positive before the first tumor developing in mice that were gs-antigen negative than the total cumulative incidence of tumor occurring in them. •, mice that were originally gs-antigen or virus positive (110 tumors); o, mice that were originally gs-antigen and virus negative (14 tumors). Reprinted with permission from Proc. Nat. Acad. Sci. U.S. 70, 1450-1455 (1973) (MEYER et al.)

Table 6. Leukemia incidence among (BALB/c x AKR) x AKR backcross mice, according to MuLV titer at 6 weeks of age. LILLY (1974), in press

Virus titer	$H\text{-}2^k/H\text{-}2^k$	$H\text{-}2^k/H\text{-}2^d$	Total
3.3 - 3.0	11/15 (73%)	7/ 9 (78%)	18/ 24 (75%)
2.9 - 2.0	23/37 (60%)	17/38 (45%)	39/ 75 (52%)
1.9 - 1.0	9/22 (41%)	1/14 (7%)	10/ 36 (28%)
0.9 - 0.3	1/14 (7%)	3/14 (21%)	4/ 28 (14%)
none	6/64 (9%)	1/86 (1%)	7/150 (5%)

lights, particularly the more recent investigations done in vitro. One group reported that type-C RNA viruses could be regularly induced by BrdU and IdU in all mouse cell clones derived from mice having xenotropic and/or N- and B-type ecotropic viruses (1, 2). The cells without treatment generally remained free of type-C virus expressions. These findings demonstrated that the complete type genomes are indeed present in all mouse cells and that often in their natural state in culture and in animal tissues (vide supra) remained switched off for

Table 7. Methods for induction of endogenous ecotropic and xenotropic type-C RNA tumor viruses

Method of induction	Type virus induced	Investigators
<u>In Vivo</u>		
Radiation (mouse)	Ecotropic (RadLV)	GROSS, 1958; LIEBERMANN & KAPLAN, 1959
Carcinogenic chemicals (mouse and hamsters)	Ecotropic & xenotropic	IRINO <u>et al</u>., 1963; IGEL <u>et al</u>., 1969; WHITMIRE <u>et al</u>., 1971; FREEMAN <u>et al</u>. 1974
Immunosuppressants and graft-vs-host reactions (mouse)	Ecotropic & xenotropic	SCHWARTZ <u>et al</u>., 1966; HIRSCH <u>et al</u>., 1970; ARMSTRONG <u>et al</u>., 1972 CORNELIUS, 1972
M-MSV in hamsters & rats	Ecotropic & xenotropic	KLEMENT <u>et al</u>., 1969; KELLOFF <u>et al</u>., 1970
Aging (mouse)	Ecotropic & xenotropic	PETERS <u>et al</u>., 1972; GARDNER <u>et al</u>., 1973; MEIER <u>et al</u>., 1973
Virus permissive cell transplants & antithymocytic sera (mouse)	Ecotropic & xenotropic	TODARO <u>et al</u>., 1973
<u>In Vitro</u>		
Pyrimidine Inhibitors (mouse & rat)	Ecotropic & xenotropic	AARONSON <u>et al</u>.,1971; KLEMENT <u>et al</u>., 1971; ROWE <u>et al</u>.,1971; FREEMAN <u>et al</u>., 1973
Chemical carcinogens (chickens & hamsters)	Ecotropic & xenotropic	WEISS <u>et al</u>., 1971; FREEMAN <u>et al</u>., 1974
Protein inhibitors (cyclohexamide) (mouse)	Ecotropic & xenotropic	AARONSON <u>et al</u>., in press
Co-cultivation of another species with permissive cells (mouse, cat, baboon)	Xenotropic	LEVY, <u>et al</u>., 1973; SARMA <u>et al</u>., 1973; BENVENISTE <u>et al</u>., 1974; STEPHENSON <u>et al</u>., 1974; TODARO <u>et al</u>., 1974
Mixed lymphocyte cultures (mouse)	Ecotropic & probably xenotropic	HIRSCH <u>et al</u>., 1972
Long-term culture (mouse & rat)	Ecotropic & probably xenotropic	AARONSON <u>et al</u>.,1969; KLEMENT <u>et al</u>., 1973; FREEMAN, unpublished observation
Phytohemaglutinin (bovine)	Xenotropic	MILLER <u>et al</u>., 1969; FERRER <u>et al</u>., 1971

long periods. Subsequently similar endogenous type-C viruses were activated in rat, hamster, cat, bovine and baboon cells; the latter having some degree of relatedness to type-C viral protein (p30) and DNA in human tumor cells (112).

It should be stated that many cell lines (mouse, rat, hamster, swine, baboon and chicken) undergo spontaneous derepression in long-term cultures, yielding ecotropic or xenotropic virus and sometimes both viruses; tests of clones show that all the cells have the endogenous genomes.

It would be difficult to explain the evidence for such inducible viruses in any fashion other than that these prevalent noninfectious viral genomes are natural genes resident in animal cells, and that these genes are generally repressed, like most other genes, by other specific regulating genes. Indeed, in the inbred mouse one locus has been shown to contain well-defined gens, most notably the $Fv\text{-}1^b$ and $Fv\text{-}1^n$ genes which specify reciprocal control of N- and B-tropic virus expressions and of course tumor expressions as well (79).

Although most of my evidence in support of type-C RNA virus and viral genomes as likely universal endogenous causes of oncogenesis, is based on studies in inbred and noninbred experimental animals (and some in feral animals), the apparent universality of these viral genomes in animal tissues and cells (see Table 4) suggests that similar viral genes will also be found to be resident in human tissues and cells. There are data which support this; particularly the reports of type-C viral particles and of molecular and protein subunits in human tumors and placentas (65, 12, 112).

Evidence for Oncogenic Behavior of the Endogenous Ecotropic and Xenotropic Viruses. It should be made clear the the endogenous xenotropic and ecotropic viruses are *bona fide* representatives of the RNA tumor virus class having properties found in the established exogenous oncogenic viruses listed in Table 4C. There are no convincing data available as yet which establish the endogenous viruses as oncogenic, but neither are there any suggesting that they lack oncogenes. However, the data clearly show that the oncogenic capabilities of endogenous ecotropic viruses are subject to controls by regulatory genes that specify virus inhibitors and a variety of autogenous virus-specific immune responses which are both antiviral and antitumor. In fact, the increasing evidence for built-in multiple genetic controle for endogenous type-C virus in inbred chickens (22) and in mice (78, 84, 104, 114, 115) is in itself testimony for oncogenic potential. In addition the use of immunosuppressants such as azathioprine, anti-lymphocyte and antithymocyte sera in mice often results in tumors specified by endogenous viruses which are otherwise immunologically suppressed by virus-specific autogenous antibodies (20, 46, 58, 8, 85).

Direct Induction of Cancer by Ecotropic RNA Tumor Viruses. GROSS (41) and LIEBERMAN & KAPLAN (77) reported the production of leukemia in mice injected with filtrates of leukemias induced by total body X-ray radiation. These findings were subsequently confirmed by other groups (61, 123). Subsequently a number of reports described the production of leukemias and other tumors in mice by endogenous viruses activated by the various methods described above and in Tables 4 and 7. Thus when carcinogen-induced endogenous type-C viruses and similar viruses induced by graft-versus-host reactions and integrated defective sarcoma viruses were injected, they readily produced leukemias or lymphomas in the same species (60, 69, 7, 21, 51). Similarly, spontaneous tumors developing with aging in BALB/c mice and cells treated with IdU yielded B-tropic and N-tropic (ecotropic) viruses that induced tumors following injection on newborn mice (98, 39). There are numerous other reports of spontaneous and induced tumors that yielded leukemia-inducing type-C viruses which then were used to produce tumors in natural hosts.

Certain unique demes of wild mice (Lake Casitas, *vide infra*) produce an endogenous type-C virus that result in spontaneous leukemias and motor neuron paralysis within the first year of life (34, 35). It should be mentioned that the demonstration of oncogenic activity on the part of endogenous ecotropic viruses activated in relatively nonpermissive hosts such as mice (C57BL and BALB/c), hamsters and rats has not been a simple matter; after inoculation it may require many months for the viral tumors to appear. The viruses from these hosts are often subject to rigid restrictive gene controls, particularly at the Fv-1 locus in the mouse, and the tumor cells are also often aborted by strong immune responses (*vide supra* and *vide infra*); thus any attempt to prove or disprove oncogenic behavior depends on selection of sufficiently infective virus and appropriate permissive test systems which will allow the virus to replicate. Thus the N-tropic viruses must be injected into N-type newborn mice and B-tropic virus in B-type newborn mice. In order to produce tumors the virus must be infectious in the animal tissues. When this is accomplished the endogenous viruses often cause cancers in mice (98, 39). In some instances the virus produces significant levels of neutralizing antibody when given in high titers, thus aborting the tumor.

If took up to 21 months to demonstrate the oncogenicity of hamster ecotropic virus (HALV-1, derived from tumors induced either by a resident MSV (O) genome or by treatment with DMBA) (Table 8; 52). The table shows that the Graffi inbred and Lakeview strains of hamster were more susceptible to the RCS tumors induced by HALV than were those of the NIH strain.

Table 8. Reticulum-cell sarcomas (RCS) induced by hamster leukemia virus (halv) in newborn Syrian hamsters of three substrains. Paired sera (taken before and after tumors) showed rise in complement-fixation antibodies to banded HALV

	Months			Total
Hamster Strains	7	14	21	RCS
Graffi	1/12	4/12	7/12[a]	58%
Lakeview	1/11	1/11	5/11	45%
NIH	0/13	1/13	3/13[a]	23%
Totals	2/36	6/36	12/36	33%
Controls (3 strains)	0/32	0/32	1/32[b]	3%

[a] One adrenal cortical adenoma observed at autopsy.
[b] Two " " adenomas observed at autopsy.

It has now been demonstrated that the ecotropic gibbon type-C virus (GALV) produces myeloproliferative disease and a granulocytic leukemia in newborn gibbons (67), while earlier studies had established oncogenic effects of the related SSV type-C virus in primates (23). Similarly a baboon virus isolated from a lymphomatous baboon (38) possessed identical properties with the baboon virus demonstrated by other groups

(64, 122, 11) in placentas and normal tissues of baboons. Exceptional studies of the baboon xenotropic virus after it was isolated and grown in dog and human cells have recently been reported. The virus was shown to be very closely related molecularly and antigenically to type-C genomes in a wide variety of old-world monkeys and to a somewhat lesser extent in the more distantly related apes, and man; however, the degree of genetic relatedness was in keeping with expectations based on known evolutionary speciation.

The Role of Endogenous and Exogenous Type-C RNA Viruses in Spontaneous and Chemically Induced Transformation in vitro. When established cultures of mouse and rat cells that were resistant to spontaneous transformation were used, infection with Rauscher murine leukemia viruses (and other viruses) rendered the cells transformable by small amounts of a variety of chemical carcinogens including nitrosamines, hydrocarbons and azo dyes. ZIMMERMANN et al. (32) reported that BALB/c embryo fibroblast cells infected in early cultures with a B-tropic type-C virus (from BALB/c spontaneous tumor), unlike MSV-infected cells, were not immediately sarcomagenic; however, after 20 subcultures 5 of 6 infected sister cell lines became transformed and, as expected, were transplantable as sarcomas in newborn BALB/c mice. Six uninfected sister cell lines carried for subcultures did not transform, nor did the cells transplant successfully in newborn mice (Table 9). LILLY's and MEYER's experiments showing that high level natural expressions of endogenous ecotropic viruses cause leukemia in natural host (discussed earlier) provide convincing evidence in support of the endogenous viral role in cancer.

Table 9. Association of b-tropic virus infection with malignant transformation of BALB/c embryo cultures. (ZIMMERMANN et al., 1974)

Cell strain	Chronic virus carrier	Indefinite continuous growth past P 20-30	Conversion to "wild" state	Tumors in animals
1	-	-	-	NT[a]
1	+	-	-	NT
2	-	-	-	0/5
2	+	+	+	5/5
3	-	+	-	NT
3	+	+	+	NT
4	-	+	-	NT
4	+	+	+	NT
5	-	+	-	0/4
5	+	+	+	5/6
6	-	+	-	NT
6	+	+	+	NT

[a] NT = not tested.

Evidence that leukemia and motor neuron paralysis in wild mice from the Lake Casitas deme in Los Angeles (mentioned above) were due to an endogenous ecotropic virus was established by two methods. In a conventional in-vivo neutralization test, leukemogenic and paralysis-inducing virus strains were inoculated with virus-specific mouse or rabbit neutralizing antisera; both antisera completely prevented leukemia and paralysis in highly susceptible newborn laboratory mice (47, 54).

Recent data show that cross-breeding of the Lake Casitas (LC) wild mice with C57BL/10Sn (B10) mice eliminates (in the F_1's and backcrosses to B10) virtually all evidence of infectious virus normally found in LC mice; preliminary data indicate that the tumors and paralysis expected in the first year of life will also be eliminated (36). The B10 strain is known to carry homozygous dominant genes for the Fv-1 gene, which specifies repression of the LC N-type virus, clearly demonstrating the etiologic role of the endogenous LC virus in both diseases in the natural host.

Evidence for Oncogenicity of Xenotropic Viruses and the Effects of Immune Responses on Virus and Tumor Expressions. Since the new class of xenotropic viruses (75) cannot be successfully used to infect newborns of the host species, their putative role in natural cancer cannot be tested by direct inoculation. Furthermore, the xenotropic viruses of mice do not appear to be regulated by the well-known genes which regulate the ecotropic viruses, and hence the use of genes present in the B10 strain described above does not offer the same solution that it does in the LC wild mouse (54). However, a number of strains of inbred mice have only xenotropic viruses; some are expressed and stimulate strong virus-neutralizing antibodies (NZB is one example); others are not generally expressed and make limited amounts of such antibodies (e.g. NIH Swiss, C57L and SWR). Crossing of the two extremes should elucidate regulating genes which can be expected to segregate high and low expressions of virus and high and low immune responses. Genes in C57BL strains which specify strong immune responses to endogenous ecotropic virus (57) may prove useful in controlling xenotropic virus and tumor expressions; as discussed below, vaccines made from xenotropic virus stimulate specific virus-neutralizing antibodies.

The NZB mouse system deserves special study because it produces large amounts of endogenous xenotropic virus early in life and at the same time correspondingly large amounts of immune globulins which form antigen-antibody complexes that interfere with normal functions of the kidney and bone marrow, thus stimulating the lupus syndrome in man (86, 87, 76, 75).

Azathioprine immunosuppression during early life leads to early lethal leukemias, lymphomas and sarcomas in the NZB mouse, a fact that not only demonstrates the importance of immune responses in the control of the cancer but also rather strongly suggests that the large amounts of the xenotropic virus present in the leukemic tissues may be the actuating cause of the leukemias. Furthermore, the leukemias which occur naturally or are induced in NIH Swiss and SWR/J, and the spontaneous RCS tumors in C57L, appear to be associated with overt expressions of the endogenous xenotropic viruses.

It emerged from a study of the HRS system (46) that the high-titered virus-producing hr/hr hairless mouse developed leukemia at a rate of 50 to 60 percent within 12 months, whereas the hr/+ congenic twin developed leukemia at a rate of 5 to 7 percent, despite the fact that the congenic strains had equivalent amounts of ecotropic type-C virus in their tissues. Treatment of the hr/+ with azathioprine, as described above for the NZB system, led to leukemia rates of 50 to 60 percent within 12 months. This clearly suggested that the hr/hr mice were in some fashion less immunologically competent than the hr/+. This was confirmed by a demonstration that the humoral responses of the hr/hr mice to tetanus toxoid antigens was significantly lower than that of the hr/+. Thus it appears that the hairless gene specifies immune defectiveness, which leads to spontaneous leukemia associated with high-level type-C virus expressions.

Natural and Vaccine-Induced Immune Responses in Control of Endogenous Virus Replication and Spontaneous and Induced Cancers. One of the more conclusive methods for proving the etiologic role of a virus in disease is to prevent or modify virus disease with the use of effective type-specific viral vaccines. Success in similar endeavors with RNA tumor viruses may provide a method for prevention of tumors as well as for conclusively establishing postulated RNA tumor viruses as specific causes.

Since, with some notable exceptions in highly permissive animal systems, most spontaneous cancers in natural species generally occur late in life rather than early, and since effective virus-specific neutralizing and cell-mediated immune responses to endogenous virus can be produced early in life (58, 97) by live attenuated and formalin-killed virus-specific vaccines, prevention of some spontaneous cancers by such vaccines now seems feasible. As mentioned earlier, effective vaccine prevention of cancer-inducing laboratory strains of well-established leukemia and sarcoma viruses has already been achieved.

Evidence supporting these statements is in part published and in part still in press or in preparation. My associates and I believe there is sufficient documentation to justify attempts to explore in depth the possibilities for viral vaccine prevention of spontaneous cancers, of cancers induced or accelerated by chemical carcinogens, and possibly also of those induced by DNA tumor viruses. Recent experience gained during vaccine experiments which resulted in specific induction of viral-neutralizing antibodies in mice and rats (52) should furnish useful background for future efforts to prevent and modify cancer in higher animals and man. Our reasons for selecting mice (inbred, outbred and wild) and rats and hamsters are based on the large amount of information available concerning natural cancer incidence, virus expressions, and immune responses in these animals and, in inbred mice, on well-defined genes which regulate RNA tumor viruses and tumor expressions.

Prevention and/or Moderation of Cancer by Natural Antibodies and by Immune Responses Induced by Specific RNA Virus Vaccines. Virtually all viral vaccines which are successful in preventing diseases in humans have been developed and produced in tissues or cells of experimental animals and tested for protective potency and safety in experimental animals before use in humans. This is not only a humane imperative but is also, scientifically speaking, the soundest procedure for discovery and development of the most effective products prior to human trials. Thus, in 1972, my associates and I, in collaboration with colleagues in a number of Viral Cancer Program contracts, became interested in immune responses and their effects not only on spontaneous and induced lymphomas, but also on other pathogenic manifestations of type-C RNA viruses. For instance, the lupus-like autoimmune disease in NZB mice appears to be due to exaggerated immune responses to DNA, RNA and proteins of fully expressed xenotropic MuLV virogenes. The resulting immune complexes produce malfunctions in kidneys and bone marrow. The recent findings that both lymphoma and paralysis induced by endogenous wild mouse viruses could be prevented with specific antiviral neutralizing antisera produced in mice or guinea pigs (47) led to a systematice study of specific vaccine modification and prevention of not only cancer but other diseases in which expressions of ecotropic and xenotropic type-C viruses are involved.

The Importance of Knowing which Immunotypes of Type-C RNA Tumor Viruses are Involved. In order to hope to modify endogenous RNA virus-induced diseases (including cancer) it is essential to know as much as possible about the natural behavior and immunology of the viruses involved. Fortunately, within the last year it has been possible to characterize the biologic and molecular properties and the immunologic specificities of many of the endogenous and exogenous viruses shown in Table 4. This information, plus detailed information concerning the natural histories of many type-C viruses and of tumors with which they are associated, now provides a rational basis for strategic attempts at vaccine prevention of cancer.

Vaccine Experiments. It has proved possible to produce type-specific viral neutralizing antibodies to endogenous viruses at an early age in inbred and outbred laboratory mice and rats. The neutralizing antibodies were associated with cell-mediated antibodies as well as to various exogenous type-C RNA tumor viruses.

Formalin-inactivated banded type-C virus vaccines produced according to specifications by Flow Laboratories, Inc. and Electronucleonics, Inc., were given to weanling BALB/c, SWR/J, C57BL/Cum, NIH Swiss, and wild mice, and Fischer rats; the vaccines were made from AKR, GLV, RLV, RADLV, SLV, RALV and wild mouse xenotropic AT124 viruses. Except for wild-mouse virus vaccine given to apparently tolerant Lake Casitas wild mice, all produced potent neutralizing antibodies which were type-specific. All the antisera were produced in NIH Swiss mice, since this strain has no ecotropic virus and expresses its endogenous virus (a xenotropic virus) at very low levels and consequently produces relatively little natural antibody to its endogenous virus during early life.

The immune response results shown in Table 10 for four different viral vaccines represent the optimum degree of specificity provided by extremely potent formalin-inactivated preparations, less potent vaccines of the same types as those shown in the table required more inoculations, gave lower type-specific responses and frequently significant amounts of cross-reactivity, the latter most probably representing nonspecific precipitation rather than specific inactivation of virus. Although there is good evidence for virus-specific cell-mediated antibody responses to several of these vaccines (97) the formalin-killed vaccines have had little or no effect on tumors induced subcutaneously by 3-methylcholanthrene with one exception (28).

Live Attenuated Viral "Vaccines" Induce Protection Against 3-Methyl-Cholanthrene-Induced Tumors. Early experiments revealed that specific complement-fixing and neutralizing anibodies to RADLV could be produced in C57BL mice by inoculation of RADLV itself (57) or the MSV(RADLV) pseudotype sarcoma virus (54). Earlier experiments using a variety of MSV pseudotypes revealed high levels of the type-specific neutralizing antibodies in inoculated mice particularly those in which the MSV-induced sarcomas regressed (54). In Table 11 a representative cross-reaction neutralization test illustrates the specificity of such reactions.

Use of RADLV in a low dosage as a live virus "vaccine" in 3 experiments in C57BL/6 mice (127) resulted in significant reductions in the incidence of subcutaneous and intramuscular fibrosarcomas induced by 3-methylcholanthrene (see Table 12). In a fourth experiment also shown in Table 12, the immunologically heterotypic Graffi leukemia virus used in low dosage did not provide protection against 3MC-induced sarcomas (129); the fact that infection with Graffi virus was confirmed suggests that immune responses specifically to RADLV, the natural endogenous virus of C57BL mice, provided the type-specific protection observed.

A critical premise of our vaccine approach postulates that it is likely to be far easier to prevent virus-induced leukemia and other cancers than to attempt therapy after the disease has been initiated. Thus, while we have preliminary evidence that live attenuated MuLV's (RADLV)

Table 10. Neutralization of specific viruses[c]

Vaccine made from	AKR 10	AKR 20	AKR 40[a]	SLV 10	SLV 20	SLV 40	WM 10	WM 20	WM 40	RLV 10	RLV 20	RLV 40
AKR (virus)	100[b]	98	75	6	0	0	0	0	0	0	0	0
SLV	0	0	0	100	99	92		NT		0	0	0
Wild mouse	0	0	0	0	0	0	100	99	70		NT	
RLV	29	0	0	0	0	0	0	0	0	73	41	0

[a] Reciprocal of serum dilution.
[b] Percent foci neutralized.
[c] By pooled sera of mice given 3-4 inoculations as weanlings of formalin-inactivated banded virus vaccines.

Table 11. Type specificity of neutralizing antibodies in sera[a] of mice by gross and FMR pseudotype sarcoma viruses

Virus[b]	Dilution	Serum[c]	Dilution	No. with Sarcomas[d]
GL-MSV	1 : 10	GL-MSV	1 : 10	0/16 (40 days)
GL-MSV	1 : 10	RL-MSV		14/14 (15 days)
FL-MSV	1 : 50	GL-MSV		14/14 (10 days)
FL-MSV	1 : 50	FL-MSV		0/16 (40 days)
ML-MSV	1 : 100	GL-MSV		16/16 (10 days)
ML-MSV	1 : 100	ML-MSV		0/16 (40 days)
RL-MSV	1 : 100	GL-MSV		15/15 (12 days)
RL-MSV	1 : 100	RL-MSV		0/16 (40 days)

[a] All antisera from NIH Swiss mice infected with pseudotype sarcoma virus.
[b] Virus - 10% clarified extract of sarcoma tissue, diluted to contain at least 40 sarcoma-inducing units.
[c] Taken 62 days after injection from mice in which sarcomas had regressed.
[d] Periods of observation.

can produce early antiviral immunity and protection versus chemically induced tumors, convincing evidence that wholly inactivated vaccines will do so has yet to be established.

Use of Both Live and Attenuated Vaccines. Reduction of type-specific virus replication in F_1's of SWR females x AKR males was observed when the maternal SWR mice were vaccinated four times (at 14-day intervals) with banded formalin-inactivated Gross leukemia virus, and F_1's were injected at 10 days of age with a maximum dose of the Gross pseudotype of Moloney sarcoma virus (MSV (GLV)). Neutralizing antibodies to GLV were observed in the SWR females 10 to 14 days after the fourth intraperitoneal inoculation with the GLV banded vaccine. While neutralizing antibody levels in the sera of the F_1 mice (taken at 10 days) were low in titer, all the 10-day-old mice were completely resistant to a maximum dose (10^4) of MSV(GlV) virus, while unvaccinated cohorts died with large sarcomas by 10 to 12 days.

Table 12. Use of infectious RADLV and Graffi virus in newborn C67BL/6Cum mice for protection against chemically (3MC) induced subcutaneous sarcomas. (Published data from WHITMIRE: WHITMIRE & SALERNO)

Viral Dosage	3MC Dosage	(Interval)	Sarcomas/ total	(%)	% Re- duction	Mean latency	Total period of observation
RADLV $10^{1.5}$	150 ugm	10 wks	4/18[a]	(22%)	58%	>4 months	8 months
PBS controls[b]	150 ugm		16/20	(80%)		<4 months	
RADLV $10^{1.1}$	100 ugm	8 days	12/27	(44%)	51%	5 months	8 months
PBS controls	100 ugm		20/21	(95%)		4-1/2 months	
RADLV $10^{1.1}$	25 ugm	8 days[c]	9/31	(29%)	34%	>5 months	8 months
PBS controls	25 ugm		19/31	(63%)		4-1/2 months	
Graffi (LV)[d] $10^{1.1}$	100 ugm	30 days	15/25	(60%)		<5 months	8 months
HBBS controls[e]	100 ugm		15/28	(54%)		5 months	

a Three leukemias of RADLV type also observed; RADLV is the endogenous ecotropic natural virus of C57BL/6 mice.

b PBS= phosphate buffered saline.

c Shorter interval between virus infection and smaller dose of 3MC in Exp 3 possibly led to lesser protection. No leukemias were observed in 8 months.

d Graffi virus is immunologically distinct from RADLV.

e Hanks' balanced salt solution.

Table 13. Titers of type-C virus in tails[a] of vaccinated and unvaccinated SWR x AKR F_1's. 5 of 10 vaccinated mice had one log or less virus.

	Vaccinated	Virus titers		Unvaccinated Controls	Virus titers
Exp 79	TC 1[c]	$<10^{1}$	Exp 80	TC 3	$>10^{4}$
	5	10^{1}		6	$>10^{4}$
	6	$<10^{1}$		7	$>10^{4}$
	8	$<10^{3}$			
	9	10^{3}			
Exp 91	TC 1	10^{4}	Exp 92	TC 1	$>10^{4}$
	5	10^{2}		4	$>10^{4}$
	6	10^{1}		7	$>10^{4}$
	10	$<10^{2}$		9	$>10^{4}$
	12	$<10^{1}$		2	$>10^{4}$
Average		$<10^{2}$			$>10^{4}$

a Tails of F_1's taken at 40 to 58 days of age (10% extracts).
b Three injections, banded formalin-killed (GLV) virus vaccine given to SWR females at 14-day intervals. Vaccinated newborns challenged with MSV(GLV); no tumors produced.
c TC = Toe clip.

Results of XC tests for infectious virus in 2% tail extracts taken from F_1's at 40 to 60 days of age are shown in Table 13. Although all unvaccinated controls revealed $>10^4$ viral content, the vaccinated mice had much lower amounts of infectious virus. This experiment is still in progress and possible vaccine effects on the development of subsequent leukemia or other cancers must still be determined; however, significant numbers of spontaneous leukemias should occur in controls within 18 months, thus providing critical information on possible immunoprophylaxis by this type of immune procedure.

A similar genetic experiment (79) (see Table 9) in BALB/c x AKR x AKR revealed close correlations between leukemia incidence at 18 months with virus titers in tails at 40 to 50 days of age. In this experiment, 75 percent of the mice that had 10^4 or greater virus titers in their tail specimens developed leukemia, while in those with lesser virus titers significantly lower rates of leukemia were recorded.

SUMMARY

In certain experimental animals, type-C virus genomes are universally prevalent. They are mostly but not exclusively transmitted genetically and produce tumors naturally as well as when transmitted experimentally. The spontaneous virus and tumor expressions are regulated and modified by genetic factors; and virus-specific virogenes used as vaccines prior to high-level natural expressions can suppress natural expressions of the virogenes. Application of this significant information to the prevention of cancer in mice now seems quite feasible; however its application to the control of human cancer is still dependent on the isolation of specific human type-C virus(es).

REFERENCES

1. AARONSON, S.A., ANDERSON, G.R., DUNN, C.Y., ROBBINS, K.C.: Cycloheximide induction of type C RNA virus: increased expressions of virus-specific RNA. Proc. Nat. Acad. Sci. (Wash.) 70, 3941-3945 (1974)
2. AARONSON, S.A., HARTLEY, J.W., TODARO, G.J.: Mouse leukemia virus: "Spontaneous" release by mouse embryo cells after long term in-vitro culture. Proc. Nat. Acad. Sci. (Wash.) 64, 87-94 (1969)
3. AARONSON, S.A., TODARO, G.J., SCOLNICK, E.M.: Induction of murine C-type viruses from clonal lines of virus-free BALB/3T3 cells. Science 174, 157-159 (1971)
4. AGEENKO, A.I.: Filtrable virus-like agent isolated from tumors induced by carcinogenic substances. Folia Biologica 8, 7-11 (1962)
5. AMES, B.N., LEE, F.D., DURSTON, W.E.: An improved bacterial test system for the detection and classification of mutagens and carcinogens. Proc. Nat. Acad. Sci. (Wash.) 70, 782-786 (1973)
6. ANDERVONT, H.B., DUNN, T.B.: Mammary tumors in mice presumably free of the mammary tumor agent. J. nat. Cancer Inst. 8, 227-233 (1948)
7. ARMSTRONG, M.Y.K., BLACK, F.L., RICHARDS, F.F.: Tumour induction by cell-free extracts derived from mice with graft versus host disease. Nature New. Biol. 235, 153-154 (1972)
8. ARNSTEIN, P., LEVY, J.A., OSHIRO, L.S., PRICE, P.J., SUK, W., LENNETTE, E.H.: Recovery of murine xenotropic type-C virus from C57/Leaden mice. J. nat. Cancer Inst. 53, 1787-1792 (1974)
9. BEARD, J.W.: Etiology of avian leukosis. Ann. N.Y. Acad. Sci. 68, 473-486 (1957)
10. BENTVELZEN, P., BRINKHOF, J.: Leukaemogenic effect of repeated inoculations with small doses of Tennant virus in BALB/c mice. Nature 251, 155-156 (1974)
11. BENVENISTE, R.E., LIEBER, M.M., LIVINGSTON, D.M., SHERR, C.J., TODARO, G.J., KALTER, S.S.: Infectious type C virus isolated from a baboon placenta. Nature 248, 17-20 (1974)
12. BENVENISTE, R.E., LIEBER, M.M., TODARO, G.J.: A distinct class of inducible murine type C viruses that replicates in the rabbit SIRC line. Proc. Nat. Acad. Sci. (Wash.) 71, 602-606 (1974)
13. BENVENISTE, R.E., TODARO, G.J.: Evolution of type C viral genes: I. Baboon type C viral nucleic acid as a measure of divergence among primate species. Proc. Nat. Acad. Sci. (Wash.) 71, 4315-4318 (1974)
14. BERGS, V.V., PEARSON, G., CHOPRA, H.C., TURNER, W.: Spontaneous appearance of cytopathology and rat C-type virus (WF-1) in a rat embryo cell line. Int. J. Cancer 10, 165-173 (1972)
15. BITTNER, J.J.: Some possible effects of nursing on the mammary gland tumor incidence in mice. Science 84, 162 (1936)
16. BITTNER, J.J.: Mammary tumors in mice in relation to nursing. Amer. J. Cancer 30, 530-538 (1937)
17. BURMESTER, B.R.: Transmission of tumor-inducing avian viruses under natural conditions. Texas Rep. Biol. Med. 15, 540-558 (1957)
18. BURMESTER, B.R., WATERS, N.F.: The role of the infected egg in the transmission of visceral lymphomatosis. Poultry Sci. 34, 1415-1429 (1955)

19. BURNET, R.M.: A modern basis for pathology. Lancet I. 1383-1387 (1968).
20. CASEY, T.P.: Azathioprine (Imuran) administration and the development of malignant lymphomas in NZB mice. Clin. exp. Immunol. 3, 305-312 (1968)
21. CORNELIUS, E.A.: Rapid viral induction of murine lymphomas in the graft-versus-host reaction. J. exp. Med. 136, 1533-1544 (1972)
22. CRITTENDEN, L.B., SMITH, E.J., WEISS. R.A., SARMA, P.S.: Host gene control of endogenous avian leukosis virus production. Virology 57, 128-138 (1974)
23. DEINHARDT, F., WOLFE, L., MASSAY, R., HOEKSTRA, J., McDONALD, R.: Simian sarcoma virus: oncogenicity, focus assay, presence of associated virus, and comparison with avian and feline sarcoma virus-induced neoplasia in marmoset monkeys. In: Unifying Concepts of Leukemia (Eds. DUTCHER, R.M. CHIECO-BIANCHI, L.), p. 258. Basel: Karger 1973
24. DURAN-REYNALS, F.: Realities and hypotheses of viral infection as a cause of cancer. Rev. Canad. Biol. 14, 411-428 (1956)
25. FERRER, F.J., STOCK, N.D., LIN, P.: Detection of replicating C-type viruses in continuous cell cultures established from cows with leukemia: Effect of the culture medium. J. nat. Cancer Inst. 47, 613-621 (1971)
26. FINK, M.A., RAUSCHER, F.J.: Immune reactions to a murine leukemia virus. I. Induction of immunity to infection with virus in the natural host. J. nat. Cancer Inst. 32, 1075-1082 (1964).
27. FISCHINGER, P.J., PEEBLES, P.T., NAMURA, S., HAAPALA, D.: Isolation of an RD114-like oncorna virus from a cat cell line. J. Virol. 11, 978-985 (1973)
28. FREEMAN, A.E., GILDEN, R.V., VERNON, M.L., WOLFORD, R.G., HUGUNIN, P.E., HUEBNER, R.J.: 5-Bromo-2'deoxyuridine potentiation of rat embryo transformation induced in vitro by 3-methylcholanthrene: Induction of rat leukemia virus gs antigen in transformed cells. Proc. Nat. Acad. Sci. U.S. 70, 2415-2419 (1973)
29. FREEMAN, A.E., KELLOFF, G.J., LANE, W.T., CAPPS, W.I., BUMGARNER, S.D., TURNER, H.C., HUEBNER, R.J.: Studies on the prevalence of endogenous type C virus in normal hamster induced by chemical carcinogens, SV40 and polyoma virus. J. Natl. Cancer Inst. 52, 1469-1475 (1974)
30. FRIEND, C.: Cell-free transmission in adult Swiss mice of a disease having the character of a leukemia. J. Exp. Med. 105, 307-318 (1957)
31. FRIEND, C.: Immunological relationships of a filtrable agent causing a leukemia in adult mice. I. The neutralization of infectivity by specific antiserum. J. Exp. Med. 109, 217-228 (1959)
32. GALLAGHER, R.E., TODARO, G.J., SMITH, R.G., LIVINGSTON, D.M., GALLO, R.C.: Relationship between RNA-directed DNA polymerase (reverse transcriptase) from human acute leukemic blood cells and primate type C viruses. Proc. Nat. Acad. Sci. U.S. 71, 1309-1313 (1974)
33. GARDNER, M.B., ARNSTEIN, P., RONGEY, R.W., SARMA, P.S., RICKARD, C.G., HUEBNER, R.J.: Experimental transmission of feline fibrosarcoma to cats and dogs. Nature 226, 807-809 (1970)
34. GARDNER, M.B., HENDERSON, B.E., ESTES, J.D., MENCK, H., PARKER, J.C., HUEBNER, R.J.: Unusually high incidence of spontaneous lymphomas in wild house mice. J. Natl. Cancer Inst. 50, 1571-1579 (1973)
35. GARDNER, M.B., HENDERSON, B.E., OFFICER, J.E., RONGEY, R.W., PARKER, J.C., OLIVER, C., ESTES, J.D., HUEBNER, R.J.: A spontaneous lower motor neuron disease apparently caused by indigenous type C RNA virus in wild mice. J. Natl. Cancer Inst. 51, 1243-1254 (1973a)
36. GARDNER, M.B., MEIER, H., HUEBNER, R.J.: Unpublished data

37. GILDEN, R.V., TONI, R., HANSON, M., BOVA, D., CHARMAN, H.P., OROSZLAN, S.: Immunochemical studies of the major internal polypeptide of woolly monkey and gibbon ape type C viruses. J. Immunol. 112, 1250-1254 (1974)
38. GOLDBERG, R.J., SCOLNICK, E.M., PARKS, W.P., YAKOVLEVA, L.A., DZIKIDZE, E.K., LAPIN, B.A.: Isolation of a primate type C virus from a lymphomatous baboon. Int. J. Cancer 14, 722-730 (1974)
39. GREENBERGER, J.S., STEPHENSON, J.R., MOLONEY, W.C., AARONSON, S.A.: Different hematologic diseases induced by type C viruses chemically activated from embryo cells of different mouse strains. Cancer Res. 35, 245-252 (1975)
40. GROSS, L.: Spontaneous leukemia developing in C_3H mice following inoculation in infancy with Ak-leukemic extracts of Ak-embryos. Proc. Soc. exp. Biol. 76, 27-32 (1951)
41. GROSS, L. : Attempt to recover filtrable agent from X-ray-induced leukemia. Acta Haematol. 19, 353-361 (1958)
42. GROSS, L., DREYFUSS, Y.: How is the mouse leukemia virus transmitted from host to host under natural life conditions? In: Carcinogenesis: A Broad Critique, p. 9, Baltimmore: Williams and Wilkins 1967
43. HARDY, W.D., Jr., OLD, L.J., HESS, P.W., ESSEX, M., COTTER, S.: Horizontal transmission of feline leukaemia virus. Nature 244, 266-269 (1973)
44. HARTLEY, J.W., ROWE, W.P., HUEBNER, R.J.: Host range restrictions of murine leukemia viruses in mouse embryo cell cultures. J. Virology 5, 221-225 (1970)
45. HEIDELBERGER, C.: Some reflections and speculations about chemical carcinogenesis. In: Canadian Cancer Conference, 1966, p. 326. New York: Pergamon 1967
46. HEINIGER, H.J., MEIER, H., KALISS, N., CHERRY, M., CHEN, H.W., STONER, R.D.: Hereditary immunodeficiency and leukemogenesis in HRS/J mice. Cancer Res. 34, 201-211 (1974)
47. HENDERSON, B.E., GARDNER, M.B., GILDEN, R.V., ESTES, J.D., HUEBNER, R.J.: Prevention of lower limb paralysis by neutralization of type C RNA virus of wild mice. J. nat. Cancer Inst. 53, 1091-1092 (1974)
48. HESTON, W.E.: Genetic factors in the etiology of cancer. Cancer Res. 25, 1320-1326 (1965)
49. HIRSCH, M.S., BLACK, P.H., TRACY, G.S., LEIBOWITZ, S., SCHWARTZ, R.S.: Leukemia virus activation in chronic allogeneic disease. Proc. nat. Acad. Sci. (Wash.) 67, 1914-1917 (1970)
50. HIRSCH, M.S., PHILLIPS, S., SOLNIK, C., BLACK, P.H., SCHWARTZ, R.S., CARPENTER, C.B.: Activations of leukemia viruses by graft-versus-host and mixed lymphocyte reactions in vitro. Proc. nat. Acad. Sci. (Wash.) 69, 1069-1072 (1972)
51. HUEBNER, R.J., FREEMAN, A.E., WHITMIRE, C.E., PRICE, P.J., RHIM, R.S., KELLOFF, G.J., GILDEN, R.V., MEIER, H.: Endogenous and exogenous RNA tumor virus genomes in chemical carcinogenesis. In: Environment and Cancer, p. 318. Baltimore: Williams and Wilkins 1972
52. HUEBNER, R.J., GILDEN, R.V., LANE, W.T., CAPPS, W.I. (in preparation)
53. HUEBNER, R.J., IGEL, H.J.: Immunological tolerance to gs antigens as evidence for vertical transmission of noninfectious C-type RNA virus genomes. In: Perspectives in Virology VII. (Ed. M. Pollard), p. 55. New York: Academic Press 1971
54. HUEBNER, R.J., LANE, W.T.: (unpublished data)
55. HUEBNER, R.J., SARMA, P.S., KELLOFF, G.J., GILDEN, R.V., MEIER, H., MYERS, D.D., PETERS, R.L.: Immunological tolerance to RNA tumor virus genome expressions: significance of tolerance and prenatal expressions in embryogenesis and tumorigenesis. Ann. N.Y. Acad. Sci. 181, 246-271 (1971)

56. HUEBNER, R.J., TODARO, G.J., SARMA, P., HARTLEY, J.W., FREEMAN, A.E., PETERS, R.L., WHITMIRE, C.E., MEIER, H., GILDEN, R.V.: "Switched off" vertically transmitted C-type RNA tumor viruses as determinants of spontaneous and induced cancer: a new hypothesis of viral carcinogenesis. In: Defectiveness, Rescue and Stimulation of Oncogenic Viruses. Second International Symposium on Tumor Viruses,p. 33. Paris: Centre National de la Recherche Scientifique 1970
57. IGEL, HUEBNER, R.J., TURNER, H., KOTIN, P., FALK, H.L.: Mouse leukemia virus activation by chemical carcinogens. Science 166, 1624-1626 (1969)
58. IHLE, J.N., HANNA, M.G., Jr. ROBERSON, L.E.: Autogenous immunity to endogenous RNA tumor virus: Identification of antibody reactivity to select viral antigens. J. exp. Med. 136, 1568-1581 (1974)
59. IOACHIM, H.L., GIMOVSKY, M.L., KELLER, S.E.: Maternal vaccination with formalin-inactivated Gross lymphoma virus in rats and transfer of immunity to offspring. Proc. Soc. exp. Biol. 144, 376-379 1973
60. IRINO, S., OTA, Z., SEZAKI, T., SUZAKI, M., HIRAKI, K.: Cell-free transmission of 20-methylcholanthrene-induced RF mouse leukemia and electron microscopic demonstration of virus particles in its leukemic tissue. Gann 54, 225-237 (1963)
61. IRINO, S., SOTA, S., HIRAKI, K.: The role of virus in radiation leukomogenesis. Gann 57, 505-511 (1966)
62. JAKOB, F., MONOD, J.: Genetic regulatory mechanisms in the synthesis of proteins. J. mol. Biol. 3, 318-356 (1961)
63. JARRETT, W., JARRETT, O., MACKEY, L., LAIRD, H., HARDY, W., ESSEX, M.: Horizontal transmission of leukemia virus and leukemia in the cat. J. nat. Cancer Inst. 51, 833-841 (1973)
64. KALTER, S.S., HELMKE, R.J., PANIGEL, M., HEBERLING, R.L., FELSBURG, P.J., AXELROD, L.R.: Observations of apparent C-type particles in baboon (Papio Cynocephalus) placentas. Science 179, 1332-1333 (1973)
65. KALTER, S.S., HELMKE, R.J., HEBERLING, R.L., PANIGEL, M., FOWLER, A.K., STRICKLAND, J.E., HELLMAN, A.: C-type particles in normal human placentas. J. nat. Cancer Inst. 50, 1081-1084 (1973a)
66. KAPLAN, H.S.: On the natural history of the murine leukemias (Presidential address) Cancer Res. 27, 1325-1340 (1967)
67. KAWAKAMI, T., BUCKLEY, P., DePAOLI, A. PULLEY, T. (in preparation)
68. KAWAKAMI, T.G., HUFF, S.D., BUCKLEY, P.M., DUNGWORTH, D.L., SNYDER, S.P.: C-type virus associated with gibbon lymphosarcoma. Nature New. Biol. 235, 170-171 (1972)
69. KELLOFF, G., HUEBNER, R.J., LEE, Y.K., TONI, R., GILDEN, R.V.: Hamster-tropic sarcomagenic and non-sarcomagenic virus(es) derived from hamster tumors induced by the Gross pseudotype of Moloney sarcoma virus. Proc. Acad. Sci. (Wash.) 65, 310-317 (1970)
70. KIRSTEN, W.H., STEFANSKI, E., PANEM, S.: An attenuated mouse leukemia virus. I. Origin and immunization. J. nat. Cancer Inst. 52, 983-985 (1974)
71. KLEMENT, V., HARTLEY, J.W., ROWE, W.P., HUEBNER, R.J.: Recovery of a hamster-specific focus-forming and sarcomagenic virus from a "noninfectious" hamster tumor induced by the Kirsten mouse sarcoma virus. J. nat. Cancer Inst. 43, 925-934 (1969)
72. KLEMENT, V., NICOLSON, M.O., HUEBNER, R.J.: Rescue of the genome of focus-forming virus from rat non-productive lines by 5'-bromodeoxyuridine. Nature New. Biol. 234, 12-14 (1971)
73. KLEMENT, V., NICOLSON, M.O., NELSON-REES, W., GILDEN, R.V., OROSZLAN, S., RONGEY, R.W., GARDNER, M.B.: Spontaneous production of a C-type RNA virus in rat tissue culture lines. Int. J. Cancer 12, 654-666 (1973)

74. LAW, L.W., MOLONEY, J.B.: Studies of congenital transmission of a leukemia virus in mice. Proc. Soc. exp. Biol. Med. 108, 715-723 (1961)
75. LEVY, J.A.: Xenotropic viruses: Murine leukemia viruses associated with NIH Swiss, NZB and other mouse strains. Science 182, 1151-1153 (1973)
76. LEVY, J.A., PINCUS, T.: Demonstration of biological activity of a murine leukemia virus of New Zealand Black mice. Science 170, 326-327 (1970)
77. LIEBERMAN, M., KAPLAN, H.S.: Leukemogenic activity of filtrates from radiation-induced lymphoid tumors of mice. Science 130, 387-388 (1959)
78. LILLY, F.: The role of genetics in Gross virus leukemogenesis. In: Comparative Leukemia Research 1969 (Ed. DUTCHER, R.M.) p. 213. Basel: Karger 1970
79. LILLY, F., DURAN-REYNALS, M.L., ROWE, W.P.: Murine leukemia virus and spontaneous leukemia in AKR mice. In: Mechanisms of Virus Disease (Eds. W.S. Robinson and C.F. Fox) p. 41, Menlo Park Calif.: W.A. Benjamin Inc. 1974
80. LIVINGSTON, D., TODARO, G.J.: Endogenous type C virus from á cat clone with properties distinct from previously described feline type C viruses. Virology 53, 142-151 (1973)
81. LWOFF, A.: Tumor viruses and the cancer problem: A summation of the Conference. Cancer Res. 20, 820-829 (1960)
82. MACMAHONE, B.: The ethnic distribution of cancer mortality in New York City, 1955. Acta Un. int. Cancer 16, 1716-1724 (1960)
83. MCALLISTER, R.M., NICOLSON, M., GARDNER, M.B., RONGEY, R.W., RASHEED, S., SARMA, P.S., HUEBNER, R.J., HATANAKA, M., OROSZLAN, S., GILDEN, R.V., KABIGTING, A., VERNON, L.: C-type virus released from cultured human rhabdomyosarcoma cells. Nature New. Biol. 235, 3-6 (1972)
83. MCALLISTER, R.M., NICOLSON, M., GARDNER, M.B., RONGEY, R.W., RASHEED, S., SARMA, P.S., HUEBNER, R.J., HATANAKA, M., OROSZLAN, S., GILDEN, R.V., KABIGTING, A., VERNON, L.: C-type virus released from cultured human rhabdomyosarcoma cells. Nature New. Biol. 235, 3-6 (1972)
84. MEIER, H., TAYLOR, B.A., CHERRY, M., HUEBNER, R.J.: Host-gene control of type C RNA tumor virus expression and tumorigenesis in inbred mice. Proc. nat. Acad. Sci. (Wash.), 1450-1455 (1973)
85. MELLORS, R. (Personal communication)
86. MELLORS, R.C., AOKI, T., HUEBNER, R.J.: Further implication of murine leukemia-like virus in the disorders of NZB mice. J. exp. Med. 129, 1045-1061 (1969)
87. MELLORS, R.C., SHIRAI, T., AOKI, T., HUEBNER, R.J., KRAWCZYNSKI, K.: Wild-type Gross leukemia virus and the pathogenesis of the glomerulonephritis of New Zealand mice. J. exp. Med. 133, 113-132 (1971)
88. MILLER, J.M., MILLER, L.D., OLSON, C., GILLETTE, K.G.: Virus-like particles in phytohemagglutinin-stimulated lymphocyte cultures with reference to bovine lymphosarcoma. J. nat. Cancer Inst. 43, 1297-1305 (1969)
89. MIRAND, E.A., GRACE, J.T., Jr., BUFFET, R.F.: Passive and active immunity to Friend virus disease. Nature 209, 696-698 (1966)
90. MOENNIG, V., FRANK, H., HUNSMANN, G., OHMS, P., SCHWARZ, H., SCHÄFER, W., STRANDSTROEM, H.: C-type particles produced by a permanent cell line from a leukemic pig. Virology 57, 179-188 (1974)
91. MOLONEY, J.L.: Biological studies on a lymphoid-leukemia virus extracted from sarcoma 37. I. Origin and introductory investigations. J. nat. Cancer Inst. 24, 933-951 (1960)
92. NEWILL, V.A.: Distribution of cancer mortality among ethnic subgroups of the white population of New York City, 1953-58. J. nat. Cancer Inst. 26, 404-417 (1961)

93. OKABE, H., GILDEN, R.V., HATANAKA, M.: Murine sarcoma virus-related nucleic acid sequences in a non-transforming virus derived from an interspecies pseudotype sarcoma virus. Cancer 15, 849-859 (1975)
94. PARKS, W.P., SCOLNICK, E.M., NOON, M.L., WATSON, C.J., KAWAKAMI, T.G.: Radioimmunoassay of mammalian type C polypeptides. IV. Characterization of woolly and gibbon viral antigens. Int. J. Cancer 12, 129-137 (1973)
95. PAYNE, L.N., CHUBB, R.C.: Studies on the nature of genetic control of an antigen in normal chick embryos which reacts in the COFAL test. J. gen. Virol. 3, 379-391 (1968)
96. PETERS, R.L., HARTLEY, J.W., RABSTEIN, L.S., WHITMIRE, C.E., SPAHN, G.J., TURNER, H.C., HUEBNER, R.J.: Prevalence of the group-specific (gs) antigen and infectious virus expressions of the murine C-type RNA viruses during the life span of BALB/cCr mice. Int. J. Cancer 10, 283-289 (1972)
97. KELLOFF, G., PETERS, R., DONOHOE, R., GHAZZOULI, I., SASS, B., NIMS, R.: An approach to type C viral immunoprevention of spontaneously occurring tumors in laboratory mice. Cancer Res. (in press) (1975).
98. PETERS, R.L., SPAHN, G.J., RABSTEIN, L.S., KELLOFF, G.J., HUEBNER R.J.: Murine C-type RNA virus from spontaneous neoplasms: in vitro host range and oncogenic potential. Science 181, 665-667 (1973)
99. RAUSCHER, F.J.: A virus-induced disease of mice characterized by erythrocytopoiesis and lymphoid leukemia. J. nat. Cancer Inst. 29, 515-543 (1962)
100. RICKARD, C.G., POST, J.E., NORONHA, F., BARR, L.M.: A transmissible virus-induced lymphocytic leukemia of the cat. J. nat. Cancer Inst. 42, 987-1014 (1969)
101. ROUS, P.: A sarcoma of the fowl transmissible by an agent separable from the tumor cells. J. exp. Med. 13, 397-411 (1911)
102. ROUS, P.: Comment - National Academy of Sciences Symposium on RNA viruses and neoplasia. Proc. Nat. Acad. Sci. (Wash.) 58, 843-845 (1967)
103. ROWE, W.P.: Studies of genetic transmission of murine leukemia virus by AKR mice. J. exp. Med. 136, 1272-1285 (1972)
104. ROWE, W.P.: Genetic factors in the natural history of murine leukemia virus infection (G.H.A. Memorial Lecture). Cancer Res. 33, 3061-3068 (1973)
105. ROWE, W.P., HARTLEY, J.W., LANDER, M.R., PUGH, W.E., TEICH, N.: Noninfectious AKR mouse embryo cell lines in which each cell has the capacity to be activated to produce infectious murine leukemia virus. Virology 46, 866-876 (1971)
106. RUBIN, H.: A virus in chick embryos which induces resistance in vitro to infection with Rous sarcoma virus. Proc. Nat. Acad. Sci. (Wash.) 46, 1105-1119 (1960)
107. RUBIN, H., CORNELIUS, A., FANSHIER, L.: The pattern of congenital transmission of an avian leukosis virus. Proc. Nat. Acad. Sci. (Wash.) 47, 1058-1060 (1961)
108. SARMA, P.S., BASKAR, J.F., HUEBNER, R.J., OLD, L.J., HARDY, W.: Feline leukemia virus: Detection of group-specific viral antigen and infectious virus by a complement-fixation test. In: Comparative Leukemia Research 1969 (Ed. R.M. DUTCHER), p. 368. Basel: Karger 1970
109. SARMA, P.S., TSENG, J., LEEN, Y.K., GILDEN, R.V.: Virus similar to RD114 virus in cat cells. Nature New. Biol. 244, 56-59 (1973)
110. SCHWARTZ, R., ANDRE-SCHWARTZ, J., ARMSTRONG, M.Y.K., BELDOTTI, L.: Neoplastic sequelae of allogenic disease. I. Theoretical consideration and experimental design. Ann. N.Y. Acad. Sci. 129, 804-821 (1966)

111. SCOLNICK, E.M., PARKS, W.P.: Harvey sarcoma virus: A second murine type C sarcoma virus with rat genetic information. J. Virol. 13, 1211-1219 (1974)
112. SHERR, C.J., TODARO, G.J.: Type C viral antigens in man. I. Antigens related to endogenous primate virus in human tumors. Proc. Nat. Acad. Sci. (Wash.) 71, 4703-4707 (1974)
113. SHOPE, R.E.: Evolutionary episodes in the concept of viral oncogenesis. Perspect. Biol. Med. 9, 258-274 (1966)
114. STEPHENSON, J.R., AARONSON, S.A.: Demonstration of a genetic factor influencing spontaneous release of a xenotropic virus of mouse cells. Proc. nat. Acad. Sci (Wash.) 71, 4925-4929 (1974)
115. STEPHENSON, J.R., AARONSON, S.A., ARNSTEIN, P., HUEBNER, R.J., TRONICK, S.R.: Demonstration of two immunologically distinct xenotropic RNA type C viruses of mouse cells. Virology 61, 56-63 (1974)
116. TENNANT, R.W., SCHLUTER, B., YANG, W.K., BROWN, A.: Reciprocal inhibition of mouse leukemia virus infection by Fv-1 allele extracts. Proc. nat. Acad. Sci (Wash.) 71, 4241-4245 (1974)
117. THEILEN, G.H., GOULD, D., FOWLER, M., DUNGWORTH, D.L.: C-type virus and tumor tissue of a woolly monkey (Lagothrix Spp.) with fibrosarcoma. J. nat. Cancer Inst. 47, 881-889 (1971)
118. THEILEN, G.H., KAWAKAMI, T.G., DUNGWORTH, D., SWITZER, J.W., MUNN, R.J., HARROLD, J.B.: Current status of transmissible agents in feline leukemia. J. Amer. vet. med. Ass. 153, 1864-1872 (1968)
119. TING, R.C.: Biological and serological properties of viral particles from a nonproducer rat neoplasm induced by murine sarcoma virus (Moloney). Virology 2, 865-868 (1968)
120. TODARO, G.J., ARNSTEIN, P., PARKS, W., LENNETTE, E.H., HUEBNER, R.J.: A type C virus in human rhabdomyosarcoma cells after inoculation into NIH Swiss mice treated with antithymocyte serum. Proc. nat. Acad. Sci. (Wash.) 70, 859-862 (1973)
121. TODARO, G.J., BENVENISTE, R.E., LIEBER, M.M., SHERR, C.J.: Characterization of a type C virus released from the porcine cell line PK(15). Virology 58, 65-74 (1974)
122. TODARO, G.J., SHERR, C.J., BENVENISTE, R.E., LIEBER, M.M., MELNICK, J.L.: Type C viruses of baboons: isolation from normal cell cultures. Cell 2, 55-61 (1974)
123. UPTON, A.C., JENKINS, V.K., WALBURG, H.E., Jr., TYNDALLY, R.L., CONKLIN, J.W., WALD, N.: Observations on viral, chemical, and radiation-induced myeloid and lymphoid leukemias in RF mice. NCI Monographs 22, 329-347 (1966)
124. VERNON, M.L., LANE, W.T., HUEBNER, R.J.: Prevalence of type C particles in visceral tissues of embryonic and newborn mice. J. nat. Cancer Inst. 51, 1171-1175 (1973)
125. WEISS, R.A.: Transmission of cellular genetic elements by RNA tumor viruses. In: Possible Episomes in Eukaryotes. (Ed. SILVESTRI, L.G.), p. 130. Amsterdam: North-Holland 1973
126. WEISS, R.A., FRIIS, R.R., KATZ, E., VOGT, P.K.: Induction of avian tumor viruses in normal cells by physical and chemical carcinogens. Virology 46, 920-938 (1971)
127. WHITMIRE, C.E.: Virus-chemical carcinogenesis: A possible viral immunological influence on 3-methylcholanthrene sarcoma induction. J. nat. Cancer Inst. 51, 473-478 (1973)
128. WHITMIRE, C.E., HUEBNER, R.J.: Inhibition of chemical carcinogenesis by viral vaccines. Science 177, 60-61 (1972)
129. WHITMIRE, C.E., SALERNO, R.A.: Influence of preinfection of C57BL/6 mice with Graffi leukemia virus on 3-methylcholanthrene-induced subcutaneous sarcoma. Proc. Soc. exp. Biol. 144, 674-679 (1973)

130. WHITMIRE, C.E., SALERNO, R.A., RABSTEIN, L.S., HUEBNER, R.J., TURNER, H.C.: RNA tumor virus antigen expressions in chemically induced tumors. Virus genome specified common antigens detected by complement fixation in mouse tumors induced by 3-methylcholanthrene. J. nat. Cancer Inst. 47, 1255-1265 (1971)
131. ZILBER, L.A., ABELEV, G.I.: The viro-genetic concept of the origin of tumors. In: The Virology and Immunology of Cancer (Ed. R. SCHACHTER), p. 150. London/New York: Pergamon 1968
132. ZIMMERMANN, E., FREEMAN, A.E., MARTIN, C.E., LANE, W.T., HUEBNER, R.J.: Slow transformation of BALB/C mouse embryo fibroblasto by a B-tropic mouse leukemia virus (in press)

Pathogenesis of Radiation and Virus-Induced Bone Tumors

M. P. FINKEL, C. A. REILLY, Jr., and B. O. BISKIS

The studies of bone cancer at Argonne National Laboratory were originally set up to evaluate the toxicity of radioactive materials involved in the development of the atomic bomb. It was learned very quickly that many of the radionuclides of special interest localized in the skeleton and that, under appropriate conditions, they caused bone cancer. In subsequent years, our efforts were directed toward delineating and understanding these "appropriate conditions," and in 1961 the studies were expanded to include a search for virus in radiation-induced osteogenic sarcomas. In this report we shall summarize what we know now, 30 years later, and what is still not known about the induction of bone cancer by radiation, and we shall describe the three bone-tumor viruses that have been isolated in the course of our investigations. The current evidence in our laboratory for a human-bone-tumor virus will also be discussed.

INDUCTION OF BONE TUMORS BY BONE-SEEKING RADIONUCLIDES

Almost all radionuclides that localize in bone and that have been extensively tested have produced bone cancer, and all mammals that have been tested with appropriate dosages of either internal or external radiation have developed osteogenic sarcomas. The route of administration is important only insofar as it influences transport of the radionuclide to osseous tissue. Thus, subcutaneous implantation or inhalation leads to bone cancer only if the material is soluble, and ingested material is oncogenic for the skeleton only if it is absorbed.

Bone cancers induced by radionuclides in experimental animals usually arise within the medullary cavity, and as they grow they invade the cortex, periosteum, and adjacent tissues. The cells that initially undergo neoplastic change seem to be located either within or not more than 10-20 μm away from the endosteum (41), where osteoblasts, preosteoblasts, and fibroblasts occur (49). An exception has been noted (37) in the case of bone tumors induced by ^{90}Sr in miniature swine. Wherever a determination was possible, it appeared that the tumors arose near to or within the periosteum.

Histologically, these experimentally induced tumors are similar to those found naturally in man. They range from densely ossified osteogenic sarcomas to osteolytic tumors with giant cells and only a small osteoid component. Fibrosarcomas and hemangiosarcomas also occur, but whether or not these tumors can be included with radiation-induced osteogenic sarcomas depends upon the specific experimental conditions. For example, in CF1 mice, the incidence of osteogenic sarcomas after the injection of bone-seekers is clearly associated with dose, whereas the incidence of fibrosarcomas and of hemangiosarcomas, which occur infrequently, is not. In addition, there is no indication that benign bone tumors are induced by radionuclides in this mouse strain, which normally has a very high incidence of osteomas (26, 16, 24). Therefore, fibrosarcomas, hemangiosarcomas, and osteomas are usually tabulated separately in mouse experiments. In dogs and cats, on the other hand, fibrosarcomas and hemangiosarcomas comprise about one-fourth of the induced bone tumors, and their incidence appears to be dose-dependent, so that for these species fibrosarcomas and hemangiosarcomas are grouped with osteogenic sarcomas for data evaluation (19, 46). In the case of ^{90}Sr in miniature swine, 10 of 14 bone tumors were found to be osteosarcomas and four were giant-cell tumors (37).

The histologic type of induced bone tumors has been reported to vary with dose level: in mice, differences in the proportion of predominantly osteoblastic and fibroblastic tumors were associated with the amount of ^{90}Sr injected (47). Histopathology may also vary with time; we observed an unusual type of bone tumor that appeared in mice 600 days or more after the injection of ^{226}Ra (5). These late radium tumors occurred in atypical fibrous bone, which formed within the marrow cavity in response to radium damage. With the exception of these late radium tumors, all bone-seeking radionuclides induce the same array of bone tumors in mice, and these tumors do not differ from those that occasionally occur spontaneously. Consequently, histopathology cannot serve as a clue to whether a particular bone cancer was induced by a specific radionuclide, or even, in fact, whether it was "induced" or "spontaneous".

Osteosarcomas can be detected roentgenographically long before they can be palpated. When young adult mice are treated with bone-seeking radionuclides, the earliest indications of bone damage occur in the metaphyses of long bones, usually in the distal femur and proximal tibia. Trabecular pattern becomes irregular, and areas of increased and/or decreased density appear. These early lesions heal, remain stable for long periods, or progress more or less rapidly to frank osteosarcoma with invasion of the cortex and extension into surrounding tissues. This sequence has been studied in detail after the injection of an equilibrium mixture of ^{90}Sr-^{90}Y (14). In spite of considerable variability among individual tumors, the growth rates of 217 osteosarcomas that were determined by measurements from serial roentgenograms could be represented reasonably well by a straight line with a slope of 2.57 on a double logarithmic plot of tumor volume against time after roentgenographic detection of tumor. Tumor doubling time was about one week, and the average time between tumor detection and death was 38.5 days. It was estimated that the smallest mass recognizable roentgenographically as a neoplasm contained 200,000 cells, but it was not possible to estimate when the neoplasm consisted of only one cell or even of 10,000 cells, because the fit of the regression line was very poor at the origin and upper end of the curve, and it was clear that an S-shaped function would provide a much better fit. Unfortunately, the data did not adequately describe that function.

It had been our impression that all osteogenic sarcomas induced in mice by radionuclides grew at about the same rate once frank osteosarcoma was present. This proved not to be the case, however, when ^{90}Y was the oncogenic agent (27). The ^{90}Y-lesions detected roentgenographically in the metaphyses of long bones often changed very little for an number of weeks, and many finally regressed. Others eventually resumed active development, after which they progressed rapidly. In contrast to ^{90}Sr-^{90}Y-tumors, which were detected radiographically about 38.5 days before the mouse died, ^{90}Y tumors were present for an average of 170 days. These differences in tumor growth are probably associated with differences in physical half-life of the two radionuclides: ^{90}Sr has a half-life of 28 years and decays with the emission of a 0.54 MeV beta particle to ^{90}Y, which has a half-life of only 64 hours and decays to stable zirconium with the emission of a 2.18 MeV beta particle. These observations suggest that the two-stage hypothesis of carcinogenesis (3) might apply to the induction of osteogenic sarcomas by radionuclides, the initiator being the intense radiation immediately following injection and the promoter being the continuing radiation from the residual body-burden. This latter factor is absent when ^{90}Y is the carcinogen because it decays so rapidly.

The Carcinogenic Dose. One very illusive goal of radionuclide studies has been the determination of the dose in rads (100 ergs absorbed/g tissue) necessary for the induction of bone cancer. This goal has not been reached for a variety of reasons, some concerned with the nature of the radionuclides themselves, some with their metabolism, and some with deficiencies in our understanding of the neoplastic progress. Three important reasons are: (1) irradiation of bone continues as long as the radionuclide is present, but irradiation is usually at a continuously decreasing rate because of physical decay and biological elimination of the material; (2) all portions of the bone are not irradiated uniformly on either a macroscopic or a microscopic scale because, under all circumstances of exposure except continuous exposure from conception to death, deposition of the radionuclide is not uniform; and (3) because the precise time when irreversible neoplastic change occurs is not known, the time span over which the dose should be evaluated is also not known.

One way to circumvent the problems of assessing oncogenic dose when bone cancer is induced by radiation is to use external instead of internal irradiation. By this means, residual radiation from a retained body-burden is eliminated, dose and dose-rate can be rigidly controlled, and the absorbed dose can be calculated in various skeletal areas with considerable accuracy. We have shown, for example, that exposure of the distal femur and proximal tibia of mice to 250 R X-ray causes osteosarcoma (27). Under the specific exposure conditions used, it was calculated that the dose to soft tissues immediately adjacent to bone was between 375 and 500 rads. This value is not inconsistent with the suggestion that 150 rads/day is close to the minimum effective dose-rate, and that 600 to 800 rads delivered within eight days is an adequate total dose for the induction of osteogenic sarcomas by ^{90}Sr. These values were based on a careful dosimetric study of ^{90}Sr deposition and retention in the mouse femur (40) and on bone-tumor data (26, 14).

Because it has not been possible to determine the true dose (in rads) responsible for tumor induction by radionuclides, it has been our practice to evaluate oncogenicity in terms of the amount of radioactivity injected per unit body weight. It was hoped that dose-response information obtained under standard conditions for a number of radionuclides with different physical and biochemical characteristics would provide a basis for estimating the smallest amount likely to cause bone cancer. In addition, since human data were already available on the oncogenicity of ^{226}Ra (42, 1), it was hoped that this radionuclide would serve as the link between animal and man for estimating the human hazard from exposure to other bone-seekers. Dose-response curves, however, have not been so useful as originally anticipated because, whatever, their shape and origin, they are always subject to criticism; more animals should have been used, or lower doses, or both. Nor have dose-response curves told us very much about the oncogenic process. They have, however, been useful in indicating relative oncogenicities of different radionuclides. For example, on the basis of amount of radioactivity injected, alpha emitters are more oncogenic that beta emitters, energetic beta particles are more oncogenic than weak particles, and radionuclides with long biologic half-times are more oncogenic than those with short half-times (9, 11, 12, 15).

Varying the exposure pattern has resulted in different tumor responses. For example, ^{90}Sr-^{90}Y given in a single injection to young adult mice produced more osteogenic sarcomas than the same total amount given in five or 20 fractional injections, and five fractions produced more tumors than 20 (27). On the other hand, ^{45}Ca produced the most tumors when divided into five fractions. MOSKALEV and STRELTSOVA (44) also reported that fractional administration of ^{90}Sr to rats was less oncogenic than a single administration, but in the case of ^{239}Pu they found fractional administration was more oncogenic than single. With ^{32}P in rats, fractional injections were found to produce more osteogenic sarcomas than a single injection of the same total amount (6, 39). The explanation for these apparently contradictory results lies in the ranges of the alpha and beta particles from these three radionuclides, their half-times, and the patterns of deposition resulting from the different injection schedules. We found that ^{90}Sr was the least oncogenic when complete uniformity of the dose in respect to both time and space was accomplished by giving the radionuclide to mice as a constant constituent of the diet (13, 27).

Differences in response to ^{90}Sr-oncogenesis also were noted between male and female mice, females being more responsive (27). Estrogen treatment can increase the incidence of bone cancer in both (47). But no differences have been noted in association with age, all indications being that very young animals are not more sensitive to the oncogenicity of radionuclides than adults when correction is made for the fact that young, growing bone retains more of a bone-seeker than adult bone (8, 13, 17. 19). Differences have been noted, however, in association with size, species with large bones being more responsive to radionuclides with energetic beta particles than species with small bones because the proportion of available energy that is absorbed increases as bone size increases (62, 51). With alpha emitters or weak beta emitters, bone size is not as important a factor in the relative oncogenic responses of different species.

The Latent Period. A well recognized but poorly understood characteristic of bone-cancer induction by radiation is that a long period of time intervenes between exposure and appearence of tumor. In our earliest experiments with bone-seeking radionuclides in mice, deaths with osteogenic sarcomas began to occur 200-250 days after injection. As a result of the increase in numbers of animals exposed, the time to first observed tumor death grew shorter. Minimum recorded periods now stand at 143 days for mice, 186 days for rats, 153 days for rabbits, 274 days for cats, and 547 days for dogs (10, 50, 61, 46). It is interesting to note that bone tumors have been reported in children in only one year after treatment with ^{224}Ra for tuberculosis and other diseases. In the animal experiments the average time to death with tumor seemed to be longer when the amount of radionuclide was smaller, but careful examination of the data showed that this apparent inverse relationship held only at the higher dosages and was merely a reflection of the fact that, as the dose increased, tumor incidence also increased, so that the probability was greater that a bone tumor would appear early. That tumor-induction time was not dependent upon dose-level became even more clear when the time of appearance of the first tumor in each dosage group was considered. A re-evaluation of many of these data, which is now in progress, supports the view that the time to tumor induction is independent of dose.

A large amount of information on the latent period has been collected after intravenous injection of radionuclides into 70-day-old female CF1 mice. For beta emitters the number of days to first death with osteogenic sarcoma was 167 for ^{90}Sr, 182 for ^{89}Sr, 190 for ^{45}Ca, and 296 for ^{90}Y; for alpha emitters it was 143 for ^{233}U, 223 for ^{239}Pu, 232 for ^{226}Ra, and 302 for ^{232}U (10). There have also been reports that in rats the period to death with osteosarcoma was shorter with the beta emitters ^{90}Sr and ^{144}Ce than with the alpha emitter ^{239}Pu; however, it was longer with beta emitters having very short biologic half-times (44, 45). These data suggest that tissue injury plays an important role in the period before a tumor appears: severe injury such as occurs with plutonium and radium may increase the time to rapid tumor growth because there must be some degree of recovery first, and minimum injury such as occurs with the very short-lived ^{90}Y may be oncogenic only if a second event eventually occurs, as noted earlier. The necessity for a second event before tumor growth progresses was also suggested by the results obtained when X-ray was the oncogenic agent. With doses that caused no externally observable injury to skin and muscle, bone tumors did not appear until 275 days after exposure.

Bone tumors may be present a long time before the animal dies. Since knowledge of the actual time when neoplastic change occurs would provide an important clue to how radiation causes cancer, we have tried various ways of detecting tumors as early as possible. In one study with retrospective examination of weekly roentgenograms of CF1 mice, positive identification of osteosarcomas was made 98 days after ^{90}Sr injection (14). In a second study, positive roentgenographic identification was made at 84 days, the same time that the average plasma alkaline phosphatase level in a group of 30 mice treated with ^{90}Sr was found to be significantly elevated above the average control level (2). With histologic examination of the distal femur and proximal tibia, identification of osteosarcoma was also made at 84 days, the earliest time so far in a study of this type. It is pertinent to note here that the presence of leukemic cells has been demonstrated as little as seven days after mice received chemical leukemogenic treatment that produced frank leukemia with an average latent period of 205 days (35).

Although the data indicate that the time to tumor induction is independent of dose, and probably also independent of isotope, the time to roentgenographic appearance of osteogenic sarcomas after the injection of ^{90}Sr was shown to be about 60 days longer in female CBA mice than in female CF1 mice (14). This difference could not be attributed to tumor incidence or growth rate once the presence of tumor had been established because total incidences, incidence rates, and growth rates were very similar in the two strains. The suggestion was made that CF1 mice provided a more favorable environment than CBA mice for the very early establishment of osteogenic sarcomas.

The term "latent period" is usually used to refer to the time between exposure to an oncogen and detection of, or death with, tumor. What processes go on before overt tumor growth are not known, but it is essential that they be discovered if we are to understand radio-oncogenesis. We prefer a more limited definition of a true latent period as the time between exposure and the occurrence of irreversible neoplastic change. When the latent period in this restricted sense is known, it will be possible to assess the dose in rads from radionuclides necessary for bone-cancer induction with some degree of accuracy. In the meantime, we can only speculate about what happens before tumors appear. Perhaps neoplastic change occurs only after sufficient tissue damage has accumulated, or after the proper number or kind of successive nuclear or cytoplasmic changes have occurred. On the other hand, neoplastic change may be an almost instantaneous event, the subsequent delay in tumor appearance being due to the necessity of one or more further events taking place. For example, the initial event may take place in an individual cell, with nothing further happening unless and until that cell is called upon to divide. Another possibility is that replication may be uninhibited, or even stimulated, until a certain cell mass is reached, after which immunosurveillance could prevent further growth until some time later when the surveillance mechanism is no longer adequate to keep the neoplasm in check.

INDUCTION OF BONE TUMORS BY VIRUSES

ROUS et al. were the first to demonstrate that bone tumors could be induced by virus, when they reported the cell-free passage of a chicken osteochondrosarcoma (57). Since then, osteosarcomas have been induced by several DNA and RNA viruses. The DNA viruses include SE Polyoma virus, which induces osteosarcomas as well as a variety of other tumors in mice (60), and SV40, which induces osteosarcoma and other neoplasms when injected to young Syrian hamsters at very high doses (7). The RNA murine sarcoma viruses produce a variety of mesenchymal tumors, including bone sarcomas. However, osteosarcoma induction with these agents usually requires that the virus be given to a species different from the species of origin, for example, the injection of Harvey or Moloney mouse sarcoma viruses to rats or hamsters (31, 36, 58). These agents that occasionally induce osteosacomas are quite different from the three bone-tumor viruses described below, which induce only bone tumors.

The Murine Bone-Tumor Viruses. FBJ osteosarcoma virus and RFB osteoma virus were obtained in CF1 mice from a spontaneous parosteal sarcoma and a spontaneous osteoma, respectively; FBR osteosarcoma virus came from a radiation-induced osteosarcoma of an X/Gf mouse (23, 28, 30, 29). All three are RNA viruses with C-type particle morphology. FBJ, the CF1 osteosarcoma virus, has been studied in several laboratories and has been found to be highly oncogenic in all strains tested except for C3H/f, C57Bl, and ICR (38, 63). In our laboratory, the two CF1 viruses are highly oncogenic in CF1, CBA and NIH Swiss mice, but they rarely induce tumors in the X/Gf strain. Conversely, the X/Gf osteosarcoma virus, which is highly oncogenic in X/Gf mice, only rarely induces tumors in the other three strains.

In spite of their strain specificities, the two osteosarcoma viruses, FBJ in CF1 mice and FBR in X/Gf mice, induce very similar tumors. Both arise on the periosteum or in adjacent muscle, and they seldom invade cortical bone. The tumors display a variety of cell types, from spindle cells to osteoblasts and osteocytes, and histopathology often varies considerably from area to area within a single tumor; however, osteoid can usually be found. Tumors are frequently multifocal and appear in 3 to 4 weeks after cell-free extracts of virus-induced osteosarcomas are injected into newborn CF1 or X/Gf mice. They grow rapidly and invasively, and quickly lead to death. Retrospective study of serial roentgenograms taken at frequent intervals after neonatal inoculation has shown tumors to be present as early as three days after treatment. Electron microscopy reveals abundant virus production in FBJ osteosarcomas (4), but only occasional particles in FBR tumors. Nevertheless, preparations of both viruses show the same extreme oncogenicity.

The RFB osteoma virus of CF1 mice induces osteomas typical of this strain, which has a relatively high incidence of this benign bone tumor in mice living 18 months or more (16, 24, 26). These well-circumscribed, noninvasive tumors consist of hard bone with osteocytes; there is very little mitotic activity. They often appear first as exostoses from the periosteum 2 to 3 months after injection of the virus into newborn mice, and as many as 36 have been counted in a single mouse. The osteomas usually grow quite rapidly for a few weeks, after which they progress very slowly and contribute to death only if they are located in a vital area, such as the spine, where they can cause paralysis, or in the mandible, where they can interfere with eating.

In an attempt to determine how these three bone-tumor viruses infect cells and bring about neoplastic change, we are conducting a series of studies in which animals receive more than one virus, one being given a day before the other, or both being given at the same time. Present data show that, in the CF1 mouse, the osteoma virus (RFB) inhibits the appearance of osteosarcomas if it is given simultaneously with or 24 hours before the osteosarcoma virus (FBJ). If FBJ precedes RFB by 24 hours, no change in tumor induction is noted. When given 24 hours earlier, the CF1 osteoma virus also interferes with the induction of osteosarcomas by the X/Gf virus (FBR) in X/Gf mice. FBJ virus has no influence on the induction of osteosarcomas by FBR virus in X/Gf mice, but FBR virus does interfere with the induction of osteosarcomas by FBJ virus in CF1 mice.

Evidence for a Human Bone-Tumor Virus. The three murine bone-tumor viruses were isolated by injecting cell-free extracts of bone tumors into newborn mice. When we embarked upon a search for a human bone-tumor virus, we injected cell-free extracts into newborn mice and Syrian hamsters. Early results indicated potential success with hamsters but not with mice (20, 21, 22). Therefore, we continued the hamster inoculations until we had processed 100 human osteosarcomas. The series also includes five chondrosarcomas and five other tumors of bone (three fibrosarcomas, one giant-cell tumor, and one reticulum-cell sarcoma). Control hamsters have received no treatment or injection of the extraction solutions, extracts of abdominal muscle from noncancer patients, or extracts of normal hamster tissues. There are about 4850 hamsters in the experimental groups and 400 in the control groups. The data are incomplete at this time; about 200 hamsters are still alive, and many more are awaiting post-mortem skeletal roentgenography and histopathology. Even with these incomplete data, however, it is evident that the hamsters inoculated with cell-free extracts of human bone tumors have a significantly higher incidence of a variety of mesenchymal tumors than do control hamsters. Sixty-one tumors of this type have been diagnosed so far, 60 in experimental animals and one in a control. The tumors in experimental animals include 20 osteosarcomas, 11 fibrosarcomas, 9 osteosarcomas, 8 schwannomas, 4 rhabdomyosarcomas, 3 leiomyosarcomas, 3 mesotheliomas, 1 liposarcoma and 1 giant-cell tumor. The tumor in the control hamster is a fibrosarcoma. At present count, the incidence of tumors of mesenchymal origin is 1.2% in experimental hamsters and 0.25% in control animals. Of the 110 patients with osteosarcoma or other tumors of bone, extracts of 32 (29%) have provided one or more of the hamster tumors. Of the 985 hamsters that lived at least 200 days and received one of the potent extracts, 60 (6%) responded with the appearance of tumor.

Further evidence that the hamster tumors were induced by a human agent was provided by the results of immunofluorescence assays (52, 55) and cytotoxicity studies (53). An indirect immunofluorescence assay showed that six of seven tested hamster sarcomas reacted with serum from patients with osteosarcoma, whereas murine osteosarcoma and hamster carcinomas, leukemia, and embryo cells did not react. One of the reactive sarcomas that has been established as a tissue-culture line was used in a cytotoxicity assay to evaluate the immunologic status of bone-cancer patients. Serum from 15 of 16 patients who had undergone amputation and had been free of diseases for six months had a high cytotoxic index, whereas serum from only 2 of 13 patients who died or had active disease within six months killed the hamster sarcoma cells.

Interaction of Radiation and Virus in the Induction of Bone Cancer. We had hoped that having two different kinds of agents oncogenic for the same mouse tissue - bone-seeking radionuclides and bone-tumor viruses - would provide a means of determining how bone cancer arises. This hope has not yet been realized, partly because of restrictions imposed by each agent. To be most effective, oncogenic virus has to be injected within a few days of birth. Radionuclides, on the other hand, should be injected after the period of rapid skeletal development in order to avoid the nononcogenic abnormalities produced by the irradiation of growing bones. When CF1 mice received FBJ virus soon after birth and ^{90}Sr at 28 days of age, ^{90}Sr-induced tumors began to appear sooner than they did without virus pretreatment, but the final incidence was only 20 percent of that observed when virus was not given (18). This effect of virus pretreatment was not noted when the mice were 70 days old at the time they received the radionuclides. The results suggest a transient immunity to ^{90}Sr-induced tumors conferred by neontal injection of FBJ virus, comparable to the immunity to radiation leukemia virus observed following neontal injection of the virus (34). FBJ-induced tumors were moderately repressed by ^{90}Sr when it was given either at 28 or after 70 days of age.

Immunization of mice against FBJ virus before they received ^{90}Sr did not alter the incidence of radiation-induced osteogenic sarcomas (25). However, treatment with ^{90}Sr one day before an intraperitoneal injection of an amount of virus known to be oncogenic in adults inhibited the appearance of FBJ osteosarcomas.

These two experiments indicated that some interaction between the two oncogenic agents did in fact occur, and they have led us to suggest that radiation produces cancer by inactivating a viral inhibitor. Evidence in support of this hypothesis has been the demonstration in neutralization tests that some ^{90}Sr-osteogenic sarcomas contain an antigen very closely related to FBJ virus (54, 29).

AREAS FOR CONTINUING RESEARCH

We have attempted to summarize our experiences relating to the induction of bone tumors by radiation and oncogenic viruses. It is somewhat discouraging that after 30 years of research so little is known about the manner in which bone-seeking radionuclides bring about neoplastic change. The answers will probably be found in the course of careful investigations of the latent period and not in further work on dose-response relationships, a type of research that is likely to be just as fruitless in the future in elucidating mechanisms of oncogenesis as it has been in the past. An important clue may be that oncogenesis by the two murine osteosarcoma viruses occurs very quickly, tumors being recognized roentgenographically as early as three days after newborn mice have been inoculated with virus. In this case the animal is overwhelmed with the oncogen. Perhaps in the case of radiation the oncogenic information present in each cell must be properly activated, then amplified, and finally produced in such abundance that the usual mechanisms for repressing neoantigens are no longer effective against the new growth. The demonstration of FBJ-antigen in some ^{90}Sr-induced osteogenic sarcomas, and the isolation of FBR virus from a ^{90}Sr-induced osteogenic sarcoma in a mouse strain that rarely develops tumors of any kind lend support to this view.

SUMMARY

Bone cancer can be induced by radionuclides that localize in the skeleton. Histologically, these experimentally induced tumors resemble those found naturally in man; they range from densely ossified osteogenic sarcomas to osteolytic tumors with giant cells and only a small osteoid component. Fibrosarcomas and hemangiosarcomas also can occur in some species. It has not been possible to determine the dose in terms of absorbed energy necessary for bone-tumor induction because radionuclides are not deposited uniformly, and they diminish in amount with time. Also, the precise time when irreversible neoplastic change occurs is not known. With X-rays, however, 500 rads delivered to the endosteal surface of a mouse femur has been shown to cause osteogenic sarcoma.

Bone tumors can be induced in mice by viruses. FBJ osteosarcoma virus and RFB osteoma virus were obtained from spontaneous tumors; FBR osteosarcoma virus came from a radiation-induced tumor. All three are RNA viruses with C-type particle morphology, and they are propagated by injecting cell-free extracts of virus-induced tumor into newborn mice. Interaction studies with bone-seeking radionuclides and these viruses have led to the hypothesis that radiation produces cancer by inactivating a viral inhibitor.

There is also evidence of a bone tumor virus in the human disease. The injection of cell-free extracts of human bone cancer into newborn Syrian hamsters has induced a variety of mesenchymal tumors at a rate significantly higher than in the control hamsters. Sixty tumors of this type, including 20 osteosarcomas, 11 fibrosarcomas, and 9 osteomas, have been diagnosed so far in experimental animals; in control hamsters there has been only one, a fibrosarcoma. Immunofluorescence assays and cytotoxicity studies indicated that these hamster tumors carried a human antigen.

Work supported by the United States Atomic Energy Commission.

REFERENCES

1. AUB, J.C., EVANS, R.D., HEMPELMANN, L.H., MARTLAND, H.: The late effects of internally-deposited radioactive materials in man. Medicine 31, 221-329 (1952)
2. BAILEY, J.M., HILL, W.D., FISCUS, A.G., REILLY, C.A., FINKEL, M.P.: Plasma alkaline phosphatase in mice with experimentally induced osteosarcomas. Laboratory Animal Science.
3. BERENBLUM, I.: A re-evaluation of the concept of cocarcinogenesis. In: Progress in Experimental Tumor Research (Ed. HOMBURGER, F.), p. 21. Basel: Karger 1969
4. BISKIS, B.O., FINKEL, M.P.: Electron microscopy of the FBJ osteosarcoma virus. In: Proc. twenty-seventh Ann. Meeting Electron Micro. Soc. Amer. (Ed. ARCENEAUX, C.J.), p. 384. Baton Rouge: Claitor's Publishing Division 1969
5. BISKIS, B.O., JINKINS, P.B., FINKEL, M.P.: The osteogenic sarcomas induced by ^{226}Ra in mice. Radiat. Res. 25, 175 (1965)

6. BLACKETT, N.M.: An effect of dose fractionation on the incidence of bone tumors using radioactive phosphorus. Nature (London) 184, 565-566 (1959)
7. DIAMANDOPOULOS, G.T.: Induction of lymphocytic leukemia, lymphosarcoma, reticulum cell sarcoma, and osteogenic sarcoma in the Syrian golden hamster by oncogenic DNA simian virus 40. J. nat. Cancer Inst. 50, 1347-1365 (1973)
8. FINKEL, M.P.: The transmission of radio-strontium and plutonium from mother to offspring in laboratory animals. Physiol. Zool. 20, 405-421 (1947)
9. FINKEL, M.P.: Relative biological effectiveness of radium and other alpha emitters in CF No. 1 female mice. Proc. Soc. exp. Biol. and Med. 494-498 (1953)
10. FINKEL, M.P.: Internal emitters and tumor induction. International Conference on the Peaceful Uses of Atomic Energy, A/CONF.8/P/80, 1955, pp. 160-164
11. FINKEL, M.P.: Relative biological effectiveness of internal emitters. Radiology 67, 665-672 (1956)
12. FINKEL, M.P.: Late effects of internally deposited radioisotopes in laboratory animals. Radiat. Res. Suppl. 1, 265-279 (1959)
13. FINKEL, M.P., BERGSTRAND, P.J., BISKIS, B.O.: The consequences of the continuous ingestion of Sr^{90} by mice. Radiology 74, 458-467 (1960)
14. FINKEL, M.P., BERGSTRAND, P.J., BISKIS, B.O.: The latent period, incidence and growth of Sr^{90}-induced osteosarcomas in CF1 and CBA mice. Radiology 77, 269-281 (1961)
15. FINKEL, M.P., BISKIS, B.O.: The induction of malignant bone tumors in mice by radioisotopes. Acta Un. int. Contre le Cancer 15, 99-106 (1959)
16. FINKEL, M.P., BISKIS, B.O.: Toxicity of plutonium in mice. Health Physics 8, 565-579 (1962)
17. FINKEL, M.P., BISKIS, B.O.: Pathologic consequences of radiostrontium administered to fetal and infant dogs. In: Radiation Biology of the Fetal and Juvenile Mammal (Eds. SIKOV, M.R., MAHLUM, D.D.), p. 535. AEC Symposium Series, No. 17 (CONF-690501) 1969a
18. FINKEL, M.P., BISKIS, B.O.: Osteosarcomas induced in mice by FBJ virus and ^{90}Strontium. In: Delayed effects of bone-seeking radionuclides (Ed. MAYS, C.W., et al.), p. 417. Salt Lake City: Univ. of Utah Press 1969b
19. FINKEL, M.P., BISKIS, B.O., GRECO, I., CAMDEN, R.W.: Strontium^{90}-toxicity in dogs: Status of Argonne study on influence of age and dosage pattern. In: Biomedical Implications of Radiostrontium Exposure (Eds. GOLDMANN, M., BUSTAD, L.), p. 285. Oak Ridge: U.S. Atomic Energy Commission (CONF-710201) 1972
20. FINKEL, M.P., BISKIS, B.O., FARRELL, C.: Pathogenic effects of extracts of human osteosarcomas. Arch. Path. 84, 425-428 (1967)
21. FINKEL, M.P., BISKIS, B.O., FARRELL, C.: Osteosarcomas appearing in Syrian hamsters after treatment with extracts of human osteosarcomas. Proc. nat. Acad. Sci. (Wash.) 60, 1223-1230 (1968)
22. FINKEL, M.P., BISKIS, B.O., FARRELL, C.: Nonmalignant and malignant changes in hamsters inoculated with extracts of human osteosarcomas. Radiology 92, 1546-1552 (1969)
23. FINKEL, M.P., BISKIS, B.O., JINKINS, P.B.: Virus induction of osteosarcomas in mice. Science 151, 698-701 (1966)
24. FINKEL, M.P., BISKIS, B.O., JINKINS, P.B.: Toxicity of radium-226 in mice. In: Radiation-induced Cancer, p. 369. Vienna: International Atomic Energy Agency (IAEA-SM-118/11) 1969
25. FINKEL, M.P., BISKIS, B.O., REILLY, C.A. Jr.: Interaction of FBJ osteosarcoma virus with ^{90}Sr and with ^{90}Sr osteosarcomas. In: Oncology, Vol. 1. Cellular and molecular mechanisms of carcinogenesis (Ed. CLARK, R.L.), p. 422. Chicago: Year Book Medical Publisher 1971

26. FINKEL, M.P., BISKIS, B.O., SCRIBNER, G.M.: The influence of strontium-90 upon life span and neoplasms of mice. In: Progress in Nuclear Energy, Series VI, Vol. 2 (Biological Sciences), p. 199. London: Pergamon Press 1959
27. FINKEL, M.P., JINKINS, P.B., BISKIS, B.O.: Parameters of radiation dosage that influences production of osteogenic sarcomas in mice. Nat. Cancer Inst. Monogr. 14, 243-270 (1964)
28. FINKEL, M.P., JINKINS, P.B., TOLLE, J., BISKIS, B.O.: Serial radiography of virus-induced osteosarcomas in mice. Radiology 87, 333-339 (1966)
29. FINKEL, M.P., REILLY, C.A. Jr.: Observations suggesting the viral etiology of radiation-induced tumors, particularly osteogenic sarcomas. In: Radionuclide Carcinogenesis, Proc. Twelfth Annual Hanford Biology Symposium (Eds. SANDERS, C.L., BUSCH, R.H., BALLOU, J.E., MAHLUM, C.C.), p. 278. U.S. Atomic Energy Commission, CONF-720505, 1973
30. FINKEL, M.P., REILLY, C.A., Jr., BISKIS, B.O., GRECO, I.L.: Bone tumor viruses. In: Proc. of the 24th Symposium of the Colston Research Soc. Vol. 24, p. 353. London: Butterworths Scientific Publications, 1973
31. FUJINAGA, S., POEL, W.E., DMOCHOWSKI, L.: Light and electron microscope studies of osteosarcomas induced in rats and hamsters by Harvey and Moloney sarcoma viruses. Cancer Res. 30, 1698-1708 (1970)
32. GOLDFEDER, A.: Studies on oncogenesis in mice of a tumor-resistant strain X/Gf. Proc. Amer. Ass. Cancer Res. 20, 20 (1972)
33. GOLDFEDER, A., KAUFFMAN, S.L., GHOSH, A.K.: Carcinogenesis in naturally tumour-resistant mice. X-irradiation versus urethane as a carcinogenic agent. Brit. J. Cancer 20, 361-374 (1966)
34. HARAN-GHERA, N.: Latent Period in leukaemia induction by the radiation leukaemia virus. Nature New Biology 238, 21-23 (1972)
35. HARAN-Ghera, N.: Relationship between tumour cell and host in chemical leukaemogenesis. Nature New Biology 246, 84-86 (1973)
36. HARVEY. J.J.: Replication of murine sarcoma virus-Harvey (MSV-H) in tissue cultures of virus-induced sarcomas. J. gen. Virol. 3, 327-336 (1968)
37. HOWARD, E.B., CLARKE, W.J., KARAGIANES, M.T., PALMER, R.F.: Strontium-90-induced bone tumors in miniature swine. Radiat. Res. 39, 594-607 (1969)
38. KELLOFF, G.J., LANE, W.T., TURNER, H.C., HUEBNER, R.J.: *In vivo* studies of the FBJ murine osteosarcoma virus. Nature 223, 1379-1380 (1969)
39. LAMERTON, L.F.: Radioisotopes in the skeleton: considerations of radiation dosage in relation to bone damage. In: A Symposium on Radioisotopes in the Biosphere (Eds- CALDECOTT, R.S., SNYDER, L.A.), p. 382. Minneapolis: Univ. of Minnesota 1960
40. MARSHALL, J.H., FINKEL, M.P.: Autoradiographic dosimetry of mouse bones containing Ca^{45}, Sr^{90}, and Ra^{226}. In: Radiological Physics Division Semi-annual Report, Argonne National Laboratory ANL-6104, 1959, pp. 48-65
41. MARSHALL, J.H., FINKEL, M.P.: Autoradiographic dosimetry of mouse bones containing Ca^{45}, Sr^{90}, and Ra^{226}. II. The sensitive region in the induction of osteogenic sarcomas. In: Radiological Physics Division Semi-annual Report, Argonne National Laboratory, ANL-6199, 1960, pp. 44-53
42. MARTLAND, H.S.: The occurrence of malignancy in radioactive persons: A general review of data gathered in the study of the radium dial painters, with special reference to the occurrence of osteogenic sarcoma and the inter-relationship of certain blood diseases. Amer. J. Cancer 15, 2435-2516 (1931)
43. MERWIN, R.M., REDMON, L.W.: Skeletal and reticular tissue disorders produced in mice by agent(s) from Sarcoma 37. J. nat. Cancer Inst. 43, 365-376 (1969)

44. MOSKALEV, U.I., STRELTSOVA, V.N.: Dependence of osteosarcomogenic activity of radionuclides on their physical properties and physiological state of the animal. In: Radionuclide Carcinogenesis, p. 307. Oak Ridge: USAEC Technical Information Center, CONF-720505, 1973
45. MOSKALEV, U.I., STRELTSOVA, V.N., BULDAKOV, L.A.: Late effects of radionuclide damage. In: Delayed effects of bone-seeking radionuclides (Eds. MAYS, JEE, LLOYD) p. 489. Salt Lake City: University of Utah Press 1969
46. NELSON, N.S., WRIGHT, J.F., LIDDLE, C.G.: Feline malignant bone tumors associated with short-term exposure to ^{89}Sr. In: Radionuclide Carcinogenesis, p. 358. AEC Symposium Series 29. Oak Ridge: USAEC Technical Information Center 1973
47. NILSSON, A.: Pathologic effects of different doses of radiostrontium in mice. Dose effect relationship in ^{90}Sr-induced bone tumors. Acta radio.: Therapy Physics Biology 9, 155-176 (1970)
48. NILSSON, A., RONNBACK, C.: Carcinogenic Effect in bone of radiostrontium and estrogenic hormones. In: Radionuclide Carcinogenesis, AEC Symposium Series 29, U.S. Atomic Energy Commission, Oak Ridge: Technical Information Center, 1973, pp. 154-158.
49. OWEN, M.: The Origin of Bone Cells. In: International Review of Cytology (Eds. G.H. BOURNE, J.F. DANIELLI), Vol. 28, p. 213. New York: Academic Press 1970
50. OWEN, M., SISSONS, H.A., VAUGHAN, J.: The effect of a single injection of high dose of ^{90}Sr (500-1000 μc/kg) in rabbits. Brit. J. Cancer 11, 229-248 (1957)
51. PARMLEY, W.W., JENSEN, J.B., MAYS, C.W.: Skeletal Self-absorption of beta-particle energy. In: Some Aspects of Internal Irradiation. (Eds. T.F. DOUGHERTY, et al.). New York: Pergamon Press 1962
52. PRITCHARD, D.J., REILLY, C.A., Jr., FINKEL, M.P.: Evidence for a human osteosarcoma virus. Nature New Biology 234, 126-127 (1971)
53. PRITCHARD, D.J., REILLY, C.A. Jr., FINKEL, M.P., IVINS, J.C.: Cytotoxocity of human osteosarcoma sera to hamster sarcoma cells. Cancer 34, 1935-1939 (1974)
54. REILLY, C.A., Jr., FINKEL, M.P.: Evidence of FBJ virus antigen in Sr-induced osteosarcomas. Radiat. Res. 47, 252-253 (1971)
55. REILLY, C.A., Jr., PRITCHARD, D.J., BISKIS, B.O., FINKEL, M.P.: Immunologic evidence suggesting a viral etiology of human osteosarcoma. Cancer 30, 603-609 (1972)
56. ROUS, P.: Transmission of a malignant new growth by means of a cell-free filtrate. J. Amer. med. Ass. 56, 198 (1911)
57. ROUS, P., MURPHY, J.B., TYTLER, W.H.: The relation between a chicken sarcoma's behavoir and the growth's filterable cause. J. Amer. med. Ass. 59, 1840-1841 (1912)
58. SOEHNER, R.L., DMOCHOWSKI, L.: Induction of bone tumours in rats and hamsters with murine sarcoma virus and their cell-free transmission. Nature 224, 191-192 (1969)
59. SPIESS, H.: ^{224}Ra-induced tumors in children and adults. In: Delayed Effects of Bone-Seeking Radionuclides. (Eds. MAYS, JEE, LLOYD), p. 227. Salt Lake City: University of Utah Press 1969
60. STEWART, S.E.: The Polyoma Virus. In: Advances in Virus Research (Eds. K.M. SMITH, M.A. LAUFFER), Vol. 7, p. 61. New York: Academic Press 1960
61. TAYLOR, G.N.: Injection Tables. In: Research in Radiobiology, Radiobiology Division of the Department of Anatomy (Ed. T.F. DOUGHERTY), p. 5. University of Utah College of Medicine 1967
62. VAUGHAN, J., OWEN, M.: The use of autoradiography in the measurement of radiation dose-rate in rabbit bones following the administration of ^{90}Sr. Lab. Invest. 8, 181-193 (1959)
63. YUMOTO, T., POEL, W.E., KODAMA, T., et al.: Studies on FBJ virus-induced bone tumors in mice. Tex. Rep. Biol. Med. 28, 145-165 (1970)

The WHO Classification of Bone Tumors

H. A. SISSONS

Both the management of individual patients and the comparison between groups of bone tumor cases can be seriously complicated by uncertainty with regard to the definition of the terms used in the pathological nomenclature and classification of these tumors, and by differences in the practical application of such definitions. Numerous attempts have been made to overcome these difficulties at both national and international levels: one of these is the classification and series of definitions proposed in a World Health Organization study (16).

The WHO scheme of classification (Fig. 1) is based on histological criteria, particularly the type of differentiation shown by the tumor cells and the type of intercellular material they produce. It simply lists the main types of primary bone tumors, according to whether they are "bone-forming", "cartilage-forming", "giant-cell tumours", etc., and implies knowledge of the histogenesis, or origin, of the tumours only for certain groups of lesions ("marrow tumours", vascular tumours," etc.) where this is regarded as established with reasonable certainty.

1 BONE-FORMING TUMOURS
- Benign
  - Osteoma
  - Osteoid osteoma and osteoblastoma (benign osteoblastoma)
- Malignant
  - Osteosarcoma (osteogenic sarcoma)
  - Juxtacortical osteosarcoma (parosteal osteosarcoma)

2 CARTILAGE-FORMING TUMOURS
- Benign
  - Chondroma
  - Osteochondroma (osteocartilaginous exostosis)
  - Chondroblastoma (benign chondroblastoma, epiphyseai chondroblastoma)
  - Chondromyxoid fibroma
- Malignant
  - Chondrosarcoma
  - Juxtacortical chondrosarcoma
  - Mesenchymal chondrosarcoma

3 GIANT-CELL TUMOUR (Osteoclastoma)

4 MARROW TUMOURS
- Ewing's sarcoma
- Reticulosarcoma of bone
- Lymphosarcoma of bone
- Myeloma

5 VASCULAR TUMOURS
- Benign
  - Haemangioma
  - Lymphangioma
  - Glomus tumour (glomangioma)

5 VASCULAR TUMOURS (Contd.)
- Intermediate or indeterminate
  - Haemangioendothelioma
  - Haemangiopericytoma
- Malignant
  - Angiosarcoma

6 OTHER CONNECTIVE TISSUE TUMOURS
- Benign
  - Desmoplastic fibroma
  - Lipoma
- Malignant
  - Fibrosarcoma
  - Liposarcoma
  - Malignant mesenchymoma
  - Undifferentiated sarcoma

7 OTHER TUMOURS
- Chordoma
- "Adamantinoma" of long bones
- Neurilemmoma (schwannoma, neurinoma)
- Neurofibroma

8 UNCLASSIFIED TUMOURS

9 TUMOUR-LIKE LESIONS
- Solitary bone cyst (simple or unicameral bone cyst)
- Aneurysmal bone cyst
- Juxta-articular bone cyst (intra-osseous ganglion)
- Metaphyseal fibrous defect (non-ossifying fibroma)
- Eosinophilic granuloma
- Fibrous dysplasia
- "Myositis ossificans"
- "Brown tumour" of hyperparathyroidism

Abb. 1. WHO classification of bone tumours (1972)

OSTEOSARCOMA AND CHONDROSARCOMA

An osteosarcoma - the recommended term for the commonest type of primary malignant tumour of bone - is defined as "malignant tumour, characterized by the direct formation of bone or osteoid tissue by the tumour cells". This does not imply that the cell of origin is a differentiated osteoblast or osteocyte, but takes account of the fact that the connective tissue of bone is able to differentiate in this direction in a tumor, as it does during normal development, or in a variety of reparative lesions such as a healing fracture.

A chondrosarcoma is defined as "a malignant tumour, characterized by the formation of cartilage, but not of bone, by the tumour cells". The distinction between osteosarcoma and chondrosarcoma is justified, of course, by the different pattern of age incidence, anatomical site, clinical presentation, radiological appearance, and response to treatment, for these groups of tumours. Only the purely cartilaginous tumours are included in the chondrosarcoma group, those containing both bone and cartilage being found to behave as osteosarcomas. Classification and nomenclature are thus based on clinical experience as well as on histological expertise, and can be expected to change as more information accumulates.

MALIGNANT MESENCHYMOMA

A problem of classification is posed by the group of rare tumours to which this term is sometimes applied. In the WHO classification it is used to describe "a malignant tumour characterized by the presence of multiple types of differentiation and structural pattern, particularly those not usually encountered in the skeleton". A special search was made for such tumours by each of the investigators concerned in the WHO exercise, but very few were found. Cases reported by two groups (14, 13) were studied, and were regarded as belonging to this group. These cases each show a combination of osteosarcomatous and liposarcomatous components. As more of these tumours are studied, the position with regard to their relative frequency and their relationship to other tumours, particularly osteosarcoma, should become clearer.

VASCULAR TUMOURS

The subdivision of primary vascular tumours of bone also poses certain problems. With the exception of haemangioma, these are all rare lesions. The WHO scheme makes provisions, in addition to haemangioma and angiosarcoma, for a group of tumours of "intermediate" malignancy, usually referred to as haemangioendothelioma (11, 20). These tumours often recur locally after excision, but rarely metastasize. Provision is also made for the occurrence of glomus tumour and haemangiopericytoma in bone, although such tumours are exceedingly rare (18, 10). The relatively common aneurysmal bone cyst is sometimes regarded as a haemangioma (7), despite equally obvious affinity with giant-cell tumour. Two other lesions which are sometimes regarded as vascular tumours are "massive osteolysis" (6) and the so-called "adamantinoma of long bones" (3), but the nature of these lesions is still debatable.

OSTEOID OSTEOMA AND OSTEOBLASTOMA

Subdivisions in tumor pathology are rarely absolute, and there is usually a delicate balance between the wish to emphasize specificity on the one hand, and broad relationships on the other: in fact, between "splitters" and "lumpers". A good example is provided, in the field of bone tumours, by the groups of cases usually referred to as osteoid osteoma and benign osteoblastoma (2, 17). It is not altogether clear whether the differences of size, site and clinical presentation between the two groups, where the histological structure of the lesions is virtually identical, are sufficient to justify their separation. But the two terms are retained in the WHO classification because of their familiarity and their clinical usefulness. Osteoid osteomas mostly occur in the shafts of long bones, particularly the tibia and femur. The lesions are generally painful; they are small (usually less than 1 cm in diameter) and do not appear to show progressive growth. Osteoblastomas usually occur in the vertebrae, ilium, ribs, and the bones of the hands and feet. They are not, as a rule, painful: they are relatively large (usually more than 1 cm in diameter at the time of clinical presentation) and in some cases they enlarge progressively while the patient is under observation.

HISTOLOGICAL DIAGNOSIS

Histological investigation is essential for the diagnosis of any case of bone tumour. It usually involves the performance of a specific biopsy, a procedure that should never be omitted when radical surgery or radiotherapy is contemplated. Open surgical biopsy is still the technique generally adopted, although needle biopsy has a definite use (15), particularly in cases where the site of the lesion, or the treatment to be adopted, make open biopsy difficult or undesirable. With open surgical biopsy, either paraffin sections or rapid frozen sections can be prepared, according to the experience of the pathologist concerned. With either open surgical biopsy or needle biopsy, imprint preparations can be prepared as well as microtome sections, and are particularly useful for cytological and histochemical studies.

In the investigation of a case of suspected bone tumor, the task of the pathologist is to provide an accurate histological diagnosis. The surgeon can help him to do this by making sure that he has access to the necessary clinical and radiological information about the case, and by providing for him an adequate and representative sample of tissue from the lesion. These aims can best be achieved if the surgeon and the pathologist, and perhaps the radiologist as well, discuss the case together before the biopsy is carried out.

POPULATION STUDIES OF BONE TUMOURS

International agreement on nomenclature and classification of bone tumours would greatly aid comparative population studies on bone tumours in different parts of the world. Until recently, little information has been available on the incidence of primary malignant bone tumours in different parts of the world, or on the relative numbers of the various types of tumour. Some idea of the incidence of primary malignant bone tumours as a whole, and of their age and sex distribution, can be obtained from the figures for bone tumour mortality for England and Wales (9, 1). Mortality - and presumably incidence - is higher in males than in females at almost all ages: it shows a peak at about 15-20 years of age, a low level in young adult life, and a steady increase after about 40 years of age. Comparable mortality figures are available from Canada (12), where the age and sex differences are similar but the total mortality appears to be less. Information for registered cases of primary bone tumours in Japan is available through the National Cancer Centre in Tokyo (1966): the Japanese figures, for both males and females, show the same adolescent peak seen in the British population, but fail to show an increase after 40 years of age. It is tempting to relate this to the absence of Paget's disease in Japan, and to its undoubted importance as a precancerous condition in relation to bone tumours in Britain (19).

Information on the relative frequencies of different types of primary malignant bone tumour in the various national series may, of course, be influenced by unrepresentative selection of cases and by the way in which diagnostic definitions are applied, as well as by any actual differences. We are, in fact, ignorant of the real position. But a comparison of series of cases from Britain (Survey of bone tumour mortality, England and Wales, 1961-63; (1), Holland (cases referred to the Netherlands Bone Tumour Registry 1953-65: Committee on Bone Tumours, 1966) the USA (cases treated at the Mayo Clinic 1909-1964;(5) and Japan (cases from Bone Tumour Registry (8) shows a rather close similarity between the different figures. Clearly, however, more information of this sort is needed.

SUMMARY

The WHO scheme of classification of bone tumors is based on histologic criteria. It simply lists the main types of primary bone tumors; knowledge of histogenesis or of tumor origin is implied only for certain groups of lesions. This international agreement on nomenclature and classification of bone tumors would greatly aid comparative population studies on bone tumors in different parts of the world.

REFERENCES

1. BOYD, J.T., DOLL, T., HILL, G.B., SISSONS, H.A.: Mortality from primary tumours of bone in England and Wales. Brit. J. prev. soc. Med. 23, 12 (1969)
2. BYERS, P.D.: Solitary benign osteoblastic lesions of bone: osteoid osteoma and benign osteoblastoma. Cancer 22, 43 (1968)
3. CHANGUS, G.W., SPEED, J.G., STEWART, F.W.: Malignant angioblastoma of bone. A reappraisal of adamantinoma bones. Cancer, 10, 540 (1957)
4. COMMITTEE ON BONE TUMOURS: Radiological Atlas of Bone Tumours. The Hague, Paris: 1966
5. DAHLIN, C.D.: Bone Tumours, 2nd ed. Springfield: Thomas 1967
6. GORHAM, L.W., STOUT, A.P.: Massive osteolysis (acute absorption of bone, phantom bone, disappearing bone): its relation to haemangiomatosis. J. Bone Jt. Surg. 37A, 985 (1955)
7. HADDERS, H.N., OTERDOOM, H.J.: The identification of aneurysmal bone cyst with haemangioma of the skeleton. J. Path. Bact. 71, 193 (1956)

8. JAPAN: NATIONAL CANCER CENTRE: The collections of the Registry of Bone Tumours in Japan. Tokyo: 1966
9. MACKENZIE, A., COURT BROWN, W.M., DOLL, R., SISSONS, H.A.: Mortality from primary tumours of bone in England and Wales. Brit. med. J. 1961 1, 1782
10. MARCIAL-ROJAS, R.A.: Primary haemangiopericytoma of bone. Review of the literature and report of the first case with metastasis. Cancer 13, 308 (1960)
11. OTIS, J., HUTTER, R.V.P., FOOTE, F.W., MARCOVE, R.C., STEWART, F.W.: Haemangioendothelioma of bone. Surg. Gynec. Obstet. 127, 295 (1968)
12. PHILLIPS, A.J.: A mortality study of primary tumours of bone in Canada. J. Canad. med. Ass. 92, 391 (1965)
13. ROSS, O.F., HADFIELD, G.: Primary osteo-liposarcoma of bone (malignant mesenchymoma). Report of a case. J. Bone Jt Surg. 50B, 639 (1968)
14. SCHAJOWICZ, F., CUEVILLAS, A.R., SILBERMAN, F.S.: Primary malignant mesenchymoma of bone. Cancer, 19, 1423 (1966)
15. SCHAJOWICZ, F., DERQUI, J.C.: Puncture biopsy in lesions of the locomotor system; review of results in 4050 cases, including 941 vertebral punctures. Cancer, 21, 531 (1968)
16. SCHAJOWICZ, F., ACKERMAN, L.V., SISSONS, H.A.: Histological typing of bone tumours. No. 6 in "International Classification of Tumours". Geneva: World Health Organization 1972
17. SCHAJOWICZ, F., LEMOS, C.: Osteoid osteoma and osteoblastoma. Closely related entities of osteoblastic derivation. Acta Orthop. scand. 41, 272 (1970)
18. SIEGEL, M.W.: Intraosseous glomus tumour. Amer. J. Orthop. 9, 68 (1967)
19. SISSONS, H.A.: Epidemiology of Paget's disease. Clin. Orthop. 45, 73 (1966)
20. UNNI, K.K., IVINS, J.C., BEABOUT, J.W., DAHLIN, D.C.: Hemangioma, hemangiopericytoma and hemangioendothelioma of bone. Cancer 27, 1403 (1971)

Primary Malignancy, Secondary Malignancy and Semimalignancy of Bone Tumors

E. UEHLINGER

At the last judgement, human beings were divided into benign and malignant Christians. However, it soon became evident that the two-class system was insufficient and it was necessary to introduce a third category. This third group was reserved for Christians who would have a chance of becoming clean in purgatory and entering Paradise later. Experience with the biologic classification of tumors was similar: between the benign and the malignant types there is an intermediate group. In English literature these intermediate bone tumors are called sarcomas of low-grade malignancy. The German language prefers the term semimalignancy. The two terms do not have quite the same meaning, but are overlapping. I shall attempt to explain what the word semimalignancy really means. It was introduced by ZOLLINGER. The semimalignant sarcomas are characterized by local invasive and destructive growth; they have a tendency to recur but do not metastasize. The intervals between recurrences vary from case to case, lasting weeks, months or years. The histologic structure can be well preserved from recurrence to recurrence in spite of the number of recurrences. The tendency to recur cannot be explained either by specific histologic details or by the structure.

The following bone tumors can be qualified as semimalignant: giant-cell tumors, chondromyxoidfibroma, large central and epiexostotic chondromas of the pelvis, and villonodular synovitis. For the parosteal osteosarcoma the term low-grade malignancy is more appropriate.

The largest group of semimalignant tumors are the giant-cell tumors. The term benign giant cell (3) seems outdated to me. Other authors have demonstrated that 10 percent of giant-cell tumors show a local invasive and destructive growth and sometimes metastasize in the lungs (13). This is true especially of giant-cell tumors in the region of the knee joint. The frequency of local recurrence is about 40 to 60 percent. In the case of giant-cell tumors a definite cure very often requires en-bloc resection, and sometimes even amputation. These facts are very well illustrated by the following case:

Case 1. semimalignant giant-cell tumor of the proximal end of the fibula:
B. Lucia, born 1952, complained of swelling and pain in the left knee joint after a fall. The X-rays showed a swelling and polycyclic destruction of the head of the fibula. The tumor was curretted. The histologic slides showed a typical giant-cell tumor with no signs of primary malignancy (mitosis and pleomorphy of the small spindle cells). The following year the giant-cell tumor recurred. One year after treatment the X-ray at check-up examination showed a ballooning of the head of the left fibula including the proximal metaphysis. Only a thin shell of bone surrounded the tumor. The changes shown on the X-rays aroused the suspicion of secondary malignancy, and amputation of the left leg was therefore performed. Seven years after amputation and eight years after

currettage of the primary tumor the patient was alive and free of local recurrence and metastases. The histologic slide of the recurrence showed the same structure and cellular details as for the primary tumor (Fig. 1).

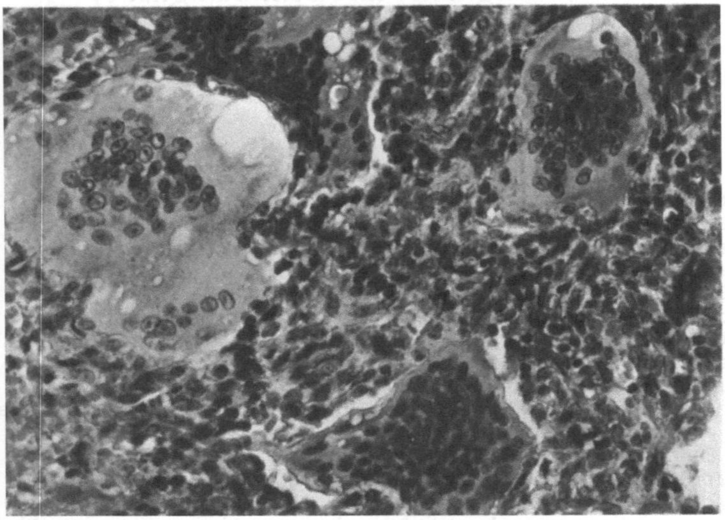

Fig. 1. Semimalignant giant-cell tumor of the proximal epimetaphysis of the fibula. First recurrence. 250 x. B. Lucia, 16 years (MB. 3134/67)

The concept of semimaligant bone tumor has to be distinguished from sarcomatous degeneration of a primarily benign bone tumor or tumor-like lesion. Two remarks are essential:

1. Present-day knowledge of bone tumors and lesions suggests that every benign bone disease can undergo a malignant sarcomatous transformation. The sarcomatous degeneration of Paget's disease was described originally by Paget himself. The literature includes many papers on sarcomatous degeneration of fibrous dysplasia, of aneurysmal bone cysts, of unicameral solitary bone cysts, of chondromas, of chronic osteomyelitis (rare) and finally of metaphyseal bone infarcts.
2. The sarcomatous degeneration of bone tumor and bone disease is enhanced by irradiation. The interval between irradiation and clinical manifestation of sarcomatous degeneration extends to ten years and more. This experience proves that the treatment of bone lesions has to be carefully evaluated, especially in young patients who are still growing. From my personal experience I would like to add that irradiation of the so-called benign giant-cell tumors tends to favor sarcomatous degeneration and should therefore be used only under special circumstances such as inoperability (6).

The following two examples will illustrate the situation:

Case 2. L.H. Marthe, born 1928, had a giant-cell tumor of the distal femoral meta-epiphysis at the age of 20 (1948) and twenty years later, after treatment by repeated currettage and irradiation, a malignant transformation of the tumor was observed so that amputation had to be performed. It should be stressed that the malignant local and invasive destructive growth did not influence the histologic picture. Both tumors, the primary tumor and the malignant recurrence twenty years later, showed the same histologic structure (Fig. 2).

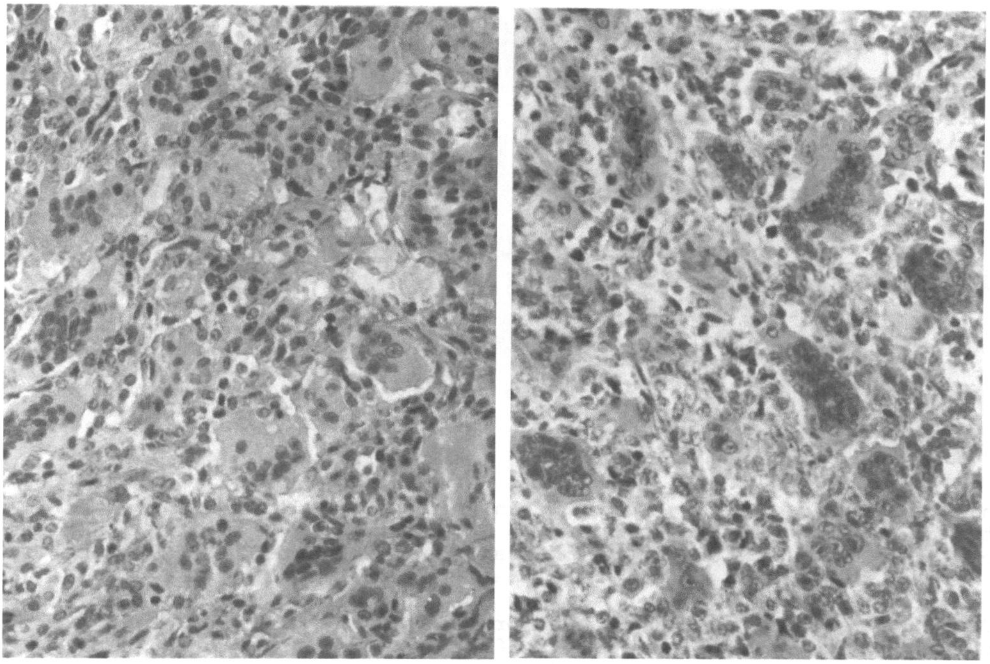

Fig. 2. Secondary malignant giant-cell tumor of the distal epimetaphysis of the femur. Left: primary tumor 1949, 250 x (MB 8777/49) Right: recurrence, 1969 (20 years later), 250 x. (MB 1662/69 Path. Inst. Zürich), L. Martha, born 1929

<u>Case 3.</u> Sarcomatous degeneration of a giant-cell tumor of the head of the humerus after currettage and irradiation:
F.G., born 1898. At the age of 43 the patient complained of rheumatoid pain in the right shoulder. X-rays of the right shoulder joint revealed polycyclic destruction of the head of the humerus. No invasion of the surrounding soft tissues was observed. Biopsy revealed the presence of a giant-cell tumor (benign). The treatment consisted in currettage followed by irradiation (up to 4200 rad). Approximately 15 weeks later, spontaneous subcapital fracture of the right humerus occurred, with lateral dislocation of the head of the humerus. The second biopsy (7 months after the first) revealed the presence of a spindle-cell sarcoma. The giant cells had completely disappeared. The right arm was amputated. To date, 31 years later, there has been no recurrence and no metastasis.

The best known example of sarcomatous degeneration of a primarily benign bone lesion is Paget's sarcoma (Fig. 3). PAGET himself mentioned five deaths from bone sarcoma in his last publication on Paget's disease. The question of how often the malignant transformation occurs

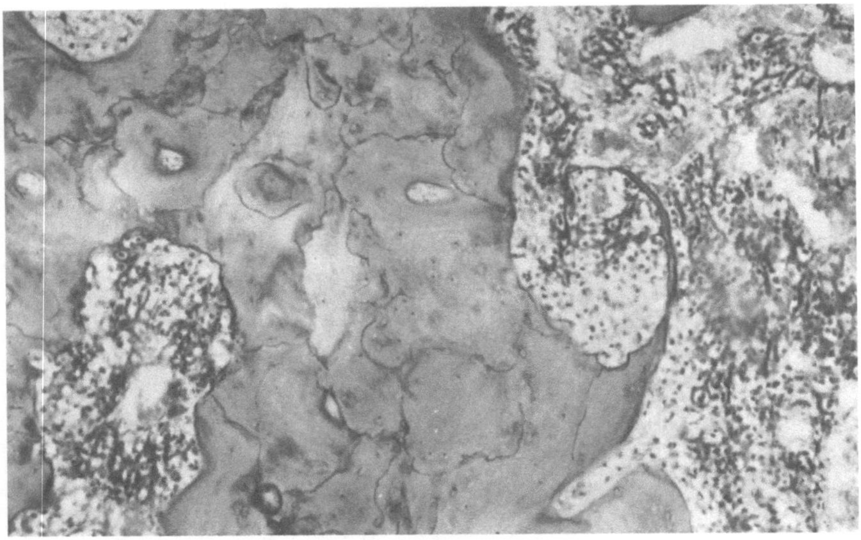

Fig. 3. Secondary osteosarcoma in Paget's disease of the vertebral column. 100x. Observation recorded by Erdheim, Vienna

has not been definitely settled. In a review the frequency was estimated at 2 percent (22). In the Mayo Clinic in Rochester, 16 of a total of 1753 patients with Paget's disease had osteosarcoma (0,9%) (before January 1965). Of a total of 121 patients with Paget's disease who were monitored over several years, only one showed secondary osteosarcoma. Thus the percentage of 1 to 2 is probably correct. The average age of patients with Paget's sarcoma is 58 years, and it is more frequent in male than in female patients. The most common symptoms of sarcomatous degeneration are pain resistent to treatment and local swelling. Life expectancy is short. The longest survival for Paget's sarcoma is 24 months. In polyostotic Paget's disease, multiple sarcomata sometimes occur. The location of Paget's sarcoma is in accordance with the location of Paget's disease. Thus, Paget's sarcoma are located preferentially in the vertebral column, the pelvis or the skull. In 16 patients at the Mayo Clinic who had Paget's sarcoma the locations were as follows: ileum 7, os ischii 8, humerus distal 3, femur 4, tibia 1.

HAUW et al. (9) collected 9 Paget's sarcomas of the vertebral column from the literature, adding 4 cases of their own. The age of the patients was over 60 years in eleven cases and under 60 in only two. The male/female ratio was 11:2. Histologic examination showed very active Paget's disease with mosaic structures and very active tumor tissue with overproduction of interstitial calcified matrix (Fig. 3). The clinical symptoms were progressive paraplegia and sphincter disturbances.

A further bone disease which predisposes for sarcomatous degeneration is the fibrous dysplasia described by JAFFE and LICHTENSTEIN. Its frequency has been estimated at 0.5 percent. Histologically the osteosarcoma is the predominant form. Secondary chondrosarcomas are extremely rare. Sarcomatous degeneration is more frequent in polyostotic than in monostotic fibrous dysplasia. The change occurs more often in males than in females. Irradiation with 3000 rads and more emhances the malignant degeneration. In a review, the age for clinical manifestation of fibrous dysplasia is calculated at 16 years, the average age for clinical manifestation of the sarcoma at 32 years, and the latent period at 13.5 years. Location of prevalence for the monostotic fibrous dysplasia with sarcomatous degeneration is the craniofacial region. The first symptoms of sarcomatous transformation are pain and inhibition of locomotion. The level of alkaline phosphatase rises at the same time.

The sarcomatous degeneration of bone infarcts is of major interest. FUREY _et al._ have published two cases of femoral bone sarcoma secondary to bone infarcts (_8_). DORFMANN observed a third case in a 64-year-old caisson worker with multiple bone infarcts in the long tubular bones. FUREY _et al_. suggest that circulatory disturbances with the change from the oxidative to the fermentative metabolism might be responsible for the bone infarcts and also for malignant transformation.

An exciting story of bone infarct with sarcomatous degeneration is reported by ARNOLD (_1_): in a pedigree of six generations, three of six siblings had developed medullary fibrosarcoma of bone. An uncle died of a metastatic bone tumor. The siblings and five of their relatives showed bone-marrow necrosis indistinguishable from bone infarcts.

With the increase of bone infarct in patients receiving long-term cortisone treatment, an increased incidence of infarct sarcoma must also be expected.

Sarcomatous degeneration of aneurysmal bone cyst is extremely rare; the American literature contains only one case. A second case of my own follows:

Case 4. Aneurysmal bone cyst of the proximal metaphysis of the humerus. Currettage irradiation, recurrences and finally myxosarcoma:
Brunhilde O., born 1952. In December 1967, at the age of 15 years, the patient suffered a traumatic fracture of the right humerus. Two months later, X-rays showed consolidation of the fracture and an expanding lesion in the proximal metaphysis, with internal erosion of the cortical bone. An aneurysmal bone cyst was recorded (Fig. 4). The treatment given was telecobalt irradiation with a total dose of 1500 rad. Six months later, the aneurysmal bone cyst recurred and increased. The lesion was again carefully curretted and the defect filled with bone chips; a second course of irradiation was also given, with a total dose of 2730 rad. Two years later there was a second recurrence with spontaneous fracture of the shaft of the humerus. Most of the bone chips were resolved. Obviously a third recurrence had developed (Fig. 5). The aggressive behavior of the bone lesion aroused the suspicion of malignancy; exarticulation was therefore performed at the shoulder. One year later, 4.5 years after detection of the aneurysmal bone cyst, a solid tumor with the typical structure of a spindle-cell myxosarcoma had developed in the fossa glenoidalis (Fig. 6).

Considering the two-fold irradiation it seems appropriate to assume that the irradiation was responsible for the sarcomatous degeneration.

A second factor which might favor sarcomatous degeneration of a benign bone lesion is the acceleration of the turnover of bone tissue.

The first clinical symptoms of secondary malignancy are local swelling and pain resistent to treatment. The X-rays show focal osteolysis and fragmentation of the cortical bone. Most secondary bone sarcomata have highly malignant behavior, local growth, and early lung metastasis.

Finally we must discuss the histologic behavior of local recurrences. The main question is whether the histological structure is identical with that of the primary lesion, or whether there are structural and cytological alterations in the sense of a lower grade of differentiation.

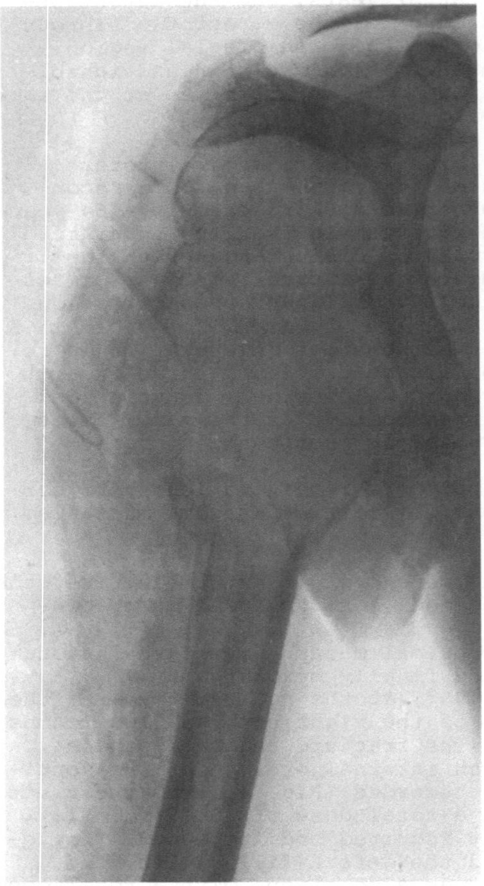

Fig. 4. Aneurysmal bone cyst with ballooning of the proximal epimetaphysis of the right humerus. Oe. Brunhilde, 16 years (U. LXXXVII/72). X-ray of 2.4.1968

As a rule, recurrences show the same structure and cellular details as the primary basic lesion (Fig. 2). In a minority of cases the recurrence shows a lower grade of differentiation. Increased differentiation is extremely rare as case 5 demonstrates:

Case 5. Higher differentiation in the first recurrence than in the primary tumor.

The patient, a young man (age 24) had a lytic bone lesion in the neck of the right femur. Biopsy showed that the lesion was a (benign) giant-cell tumor. Within a year the tumor recurred. The biopsy again revealed the structure of a giant-cell tumor, but in addition many islands of highly calcified cartilage. Thus the final diagnosis had to be changed to chondroblastoma, which is definitely a benign tumor (Fig. 6).

I wish to conclude my paper with some remarks on the expression "low grade of malignancy". The state referred to by ZOLLINGER as semimalignancy overlaps with low grade of malignancy in some aspects, but the two definitions are not identical. The clinical behavior of tumors with a low grade of malignancy is characterized by very slow growth and late metastasis (10 years or more after the beginning). Therefore the histologic structure shows the details of well-differentiated tissue, and the malignant behavior cannot be recognized from the histological structure alone. Clinical monitoring over many years and late metastasis

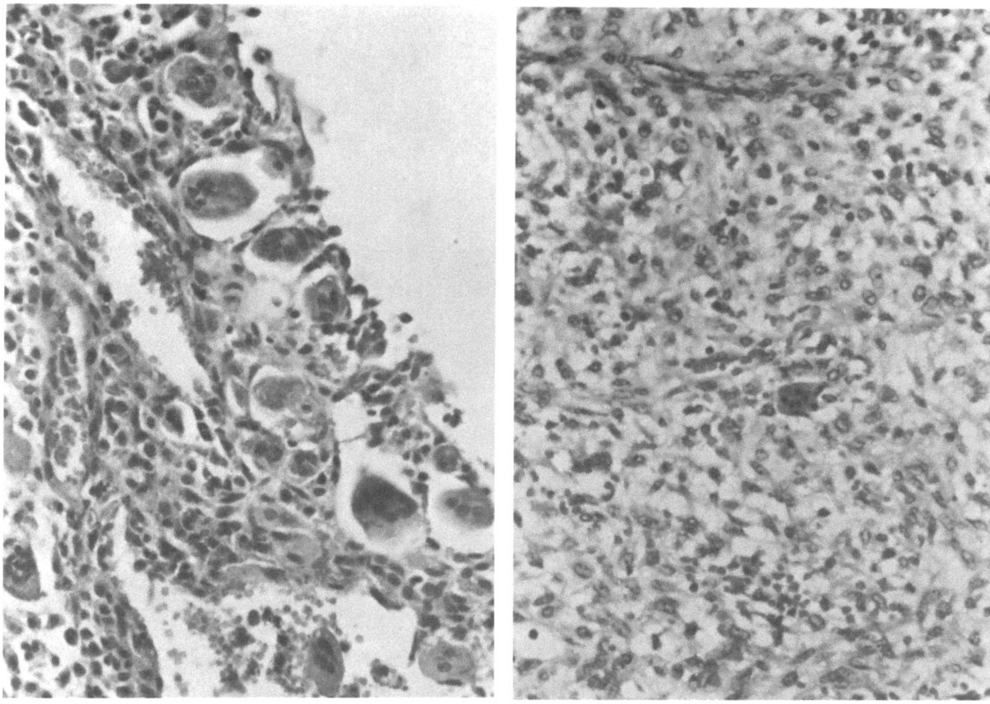

Fig. 5. Secondary malignancy in aneurysmal bone cyst of the head of the humerus. Left: primary aneurysmal bone cyst. Membrane with many giant cells (1968) Right: secondary myxomatous sarcoma in the shoulder region, 4 years later (1972). 250 x. Oe. Brunhilde, born 1952 (U. LXXXVII/72)

may prove the malignancy. Very often the qualification low-grade malignancy is misused to hide our ignorance. For the surgeon the qualification means careful resection with preservation of functual structures. By contrast the qualification semimalignancy requires wide en-bloc excision/resection/amputation. The typical example of a tumor of low-grade malignancy is the parosteal osteosarcoma of the distal femur-metaphysis.

Case 6. Parosteal sarcoma of low grade of malignancy of the distal femur metaphysis:

B. Anna, born 1914; at the age of 43 years the patient experienced some insecurity and muscle insufficiency in the right knee joint. The X-ray revealed a huge calcified tumor surrounding the distal metaphysis of the right femur. Tomograms demonstrated that the cortex in the tumor region was well preserved (Fig. 7). The tumor mass was ciseled away. Histologically the tumor tissue consisted of well-differentiated lamellar bone with no signs of malignancy (Fig. 8). In the following 15 years the tumor recurred three times without any histological changes. Finally, restriction of movement in the knee joint necessitated amputation of the leg (15 years after the initial treatment) (Fig. 7). The final histologic diagnosis was in accordance with the textbooks on bone tumors: parosteal osteosarcoma of low-grade malignancy (Fig. 8).

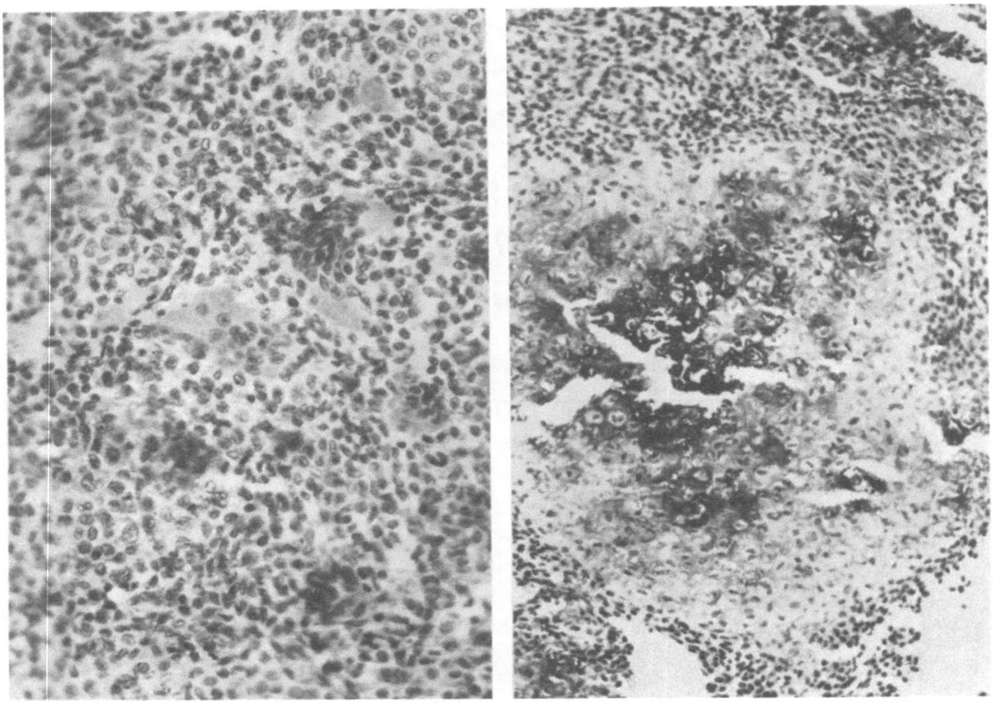

Fig. 6. First biopsy: giant-cell tumor of the trochanter. 250 x. Second biopsy: local recurrence: chondroblastoma with heavy calcified islands of cartilage. 160x. K. Josef, 24 years, (HZ. 14'124/74 Path.Inst. Zürich)

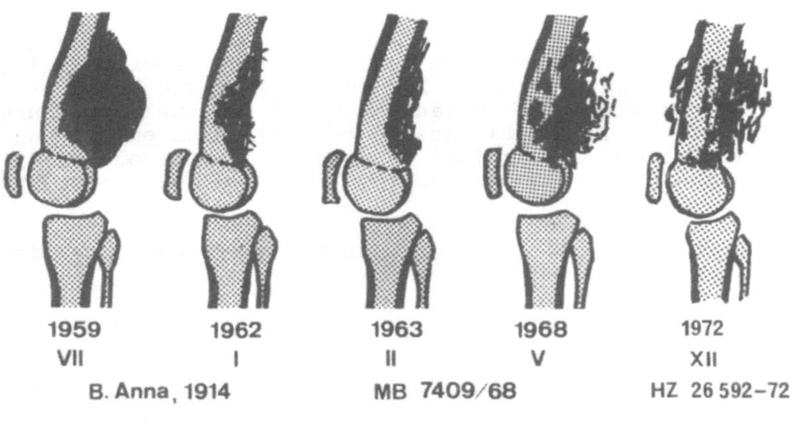

Fig. 7. Parosteal sarcoma of "low grade malignancy" of the distal femur-metaphysis. Natural case history from 1959 to 1972. B. Anna, born 1914

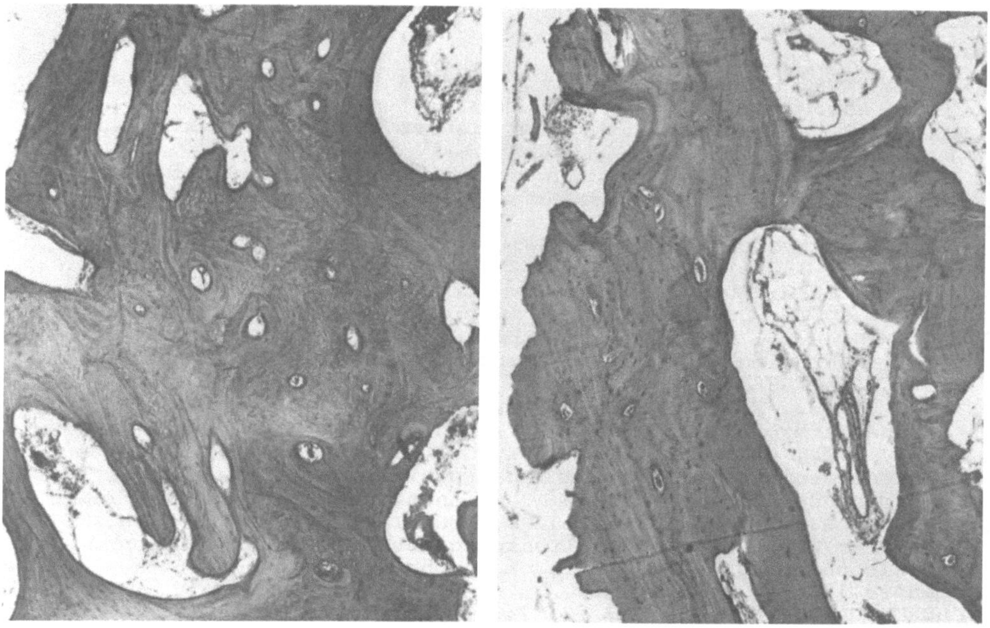

Fig. 8. Parosteal sarcoma of "low grade malignancy" of the distal femur-metaphysis. Left: specimen from 1959, 40 x (HZ. 6451/59 Histopath. Zürich) Right: specimen from 1968 (9 years later), 40 x (MB. 7409/68 Path. Inst. Zürich) Both specimens with well-differentiated lamellar bone. B. Anna, born 1914

SUMMARY

1. Bone tumors, in contrast to tumors in soft tissue, show a wide variety of clinical behavior qualified by the expressions semimalignancy, low grade of malignancy, sarcomatous degeneration and primarily benign bone tumors and bone lesions.
2. The term semimalignancy is characterized by local invasive and destructive tumor growth with a tendency to recur locally but no hematogeneous spreading. Semimalignancy requires wide en-bloc resection or amputation.
3. The term low grade malignancy is used to describe a tumor of very slow growth and with very late metastasis. Low-grade malignancy requires resection with careful preservation of functional structures.
4. The term secondary malignancy means the sarcomatous degeneration of a primarily benign lesion or bone tumor. This transformation is enhanced by irradiation and probably by acceleration of the normal turnover of bone tissue. In Paget's disease sarcomatous degeneration is to be expected in 2 percent of cases and in fibrous dysplasia in 0.5 percent of cases.
5. Sarcomatous degeneration of bone infarcts is rare, but an increase is to be expected due to an increased frequency of bone infarcts caused by long-term treatment with cortisone.
6. Primary bone tumors and recurrences show the same structure and cytology. In a minority of cases the recurrences are less differentiated; in a very few cases the recurrences are more highly differentiated and have a better prognosis than the initial lesion.

REFERENCES

1. ARNOLD, W.H.: Hereditary bone dysplasia with sarcomatous degeneration. Ann. int. Med. 78, 902 (1973)
2. BARRY, H.C.: Sarcoma in Paget's disease of bone in Australia. J. Bone Jt Surg. 34A, 1122 (1961)
3. BLOODGOOD, J.C.: Benign giant-cell tumor of bone. Its diagnosis and conservative treatment. Amer. J. Surg. 37, 105 (1923)
4. BOUTOURAS, G.D., GOODSITT, E.: Sarcoma arising in Paget's disease. Report of two cases and review of the literature. J. int. Coll. Surg, 40, 380 (1963)
5. CODMAN, E.A.: Bone sarcoma. New York: P.B. Hoeber 1925
6. DAHLIN, D.C.: Bone tumors. Springfield Ill.: Thomas 1967
7. DORFMAN, H.D., NORMAN, A., WOLFF, H.: Fibrosarcoma complicating bone infarction in a caisson worker. A case report. J. Bone Jt Surg. 48A, 528 (1966)
8. FUREY, J.G., FERRER-TORELLS, M., REAGAN, J.W.: Fibrosarcoma arising at the site of bone infarcts. J. Bone Jt Surg. 42A, 802 (1960)
9. HAUW, J.J., HENIN, D., GHOMETTE, G., ESCOUROLLE, R.: Sarcomes osseux dévélopés sur localisations rachidiennes de maladie de Paget. A propos de 4 observations. Arch. Anat. path. 21, 241 (1973)
10. HUTTER, R.V.P., WORCESTER, J.N., KENNET, C.F., FOOTE, Fr.W., STEWART, Fr.W.: Benign and malignant giant cell tumors of bone. A clinicopathological analysis of the natural history of the disease. Cancer 15, 653 (1962)
11. HUVOS, A.G., HIGINBOTHAM, N.L., MILLER, T.R.: Bone sarcomas arising in fibrous dysplasia. J. Bone Jt Surg. 54A, 1047 (1972)
12. JAFFÉ, H.L.: Tumors and tumorous conditions of the bones and joints. Philadelphia: Lea & Febiger 1958
13. JAFFÉ, H.L., LICHTENSTEIN, L., PORTIS, R.B.: Giant cell tumor of bone. 1st pathologic appearance, grading, supposed variants and treatment. Arch. Path. 30, 993 (1940)
14. JOHNSON, L.C., VETTER, H., PUTSCHAR, W.G.J.: Sarcoma arising in bone cysts. Virchows Arch. path. Anat. 335, 428 (1962)
15. LICHTENSTEIN, L.: Bone tumors. 4th ed. St. Louis: Mosby 1972
16. MCKENNA, R.J., SCHWINN, C.P., SOONG, K.Y., HIGINBOTHAM, N.L.: Osteogenic sarcoma arising in Paget's disease. Cancer 17, 42 (1964)
17. MEISTER, P., FINSTERER, H.: Der Riesenzelltumor des Knochens und seine Problematik. Münch. med. Wschr. 114, 55 (1972)
18. MIRRA, J.M., BULLOUGH, G.P., MARCOVE, R.C., JACOBS, B., HUVOS, A.G.: Malignant fibrous histiocytoma and osteosarcoma in association with bone infarcts. Report of 4 cases. Two in caisson workers. J. Bone Jt Surg. 56A, 932 (1974)
19. PORETTA, C.A., DAHLIN, D.C., JANES, J.M.: Sarcoma in Paget's disease. J. Bone Jt Surg. 39A, 1314 (1957)
20. SCHATZKI, St.F., DUDLEY, H.R.: Bone sarcoma complicating Paget's disease. A report of 3 cases with long survival. Cancer, 14, 517 (1961)
21. SCHWARTZ, D.T., MEYER, A.: The malignant transformation of fibrous dysplasia. Amer. J. med. Sci. 247, 35/1 (1964)
22. SPEISER, F.: Sarkomatöse Entartung bei Ostitis deformans Paget. Arch. klin. Chir. 149, 274 (1928)
23. SPJUT, H.J., DORFMAN, H.D., FECHNER, R.E., ACKERMAN, L.V.: Tumor Pathology. Fasc. 5: Tumors of bone and cartilage. AFIP 1971
24. TILMAN, B.P., DAHLIN, D.C., LIPSCOMB, P.R., STEWART, J.R.: Aneurysmal bone cyst: Analysis of 95 cases. Proc. Mayo Clin. 43, 478 (1968)
25. TROUP, J.B., DAHLIN, D.C., COVENTRY, M.B.: Significance of giant cells in osteogenic sarcoma: Do they indicate a relationship between osteogenic sarcoma and giant cell tumor of bone? Proc. Mayo Clin. 35, 179 (1960)

26. UEHLINGER, E.: Zur Diagnose und Differentialdiagnose der Geschwülste und geschwulstähnlichen Erkrankungen im Bereich der Gelenke. Schweiz. Rheumaliga, 5. Fortbildungskurs 1967. Bern: Huber 1968
27. UEHLINGER, E.: Die pathologische Anatomie der Knochengeschwülste. Helv. chir. Acta 26, 597 (1959)
28. UEHLINGER, E.: Pathologische Anatomie der Knochengeschwülste. Helv. chir, Acta 40, 5 (1973)
29. UEHLINGER, E.: Pathologische Anatomie der Knochengeschwülste (unter besonderer Berücksichtigung der semimalignen Formen). Chirurg 45, 62 (1974)
30. WEBER, H.G.: Semimaligne Knochengeschwülste. Tägl. Praxis 11, 607 (1970)
31. ZOLLINGER, H.U.: Geschwulstprobleme. Vjschr. naturforsch. Ges. Zürich 91, 81 (1946)

Common Errors Made by Pathologists in the Diagnosis of Bone Tumors

L. V. ACKERMAN

INTRODUCTION

Pathologists have a great deal of difficulty in diagnosing bone tumors, whether benign or malignant. The classification of bone tumors and clear definitions of the various entities have been well outlined in the World Health Monograph. It is true that bone tumors are rare. Biopsy is often improperly performed; adequate material is not obtained and, most important, the tissue is poorly processed. Before the pathologist even looks at the slides on a patient suspected of having a bone tumor, he should look at the radiographs. It must be remembered that the radiograph is merely a poor reproduction of the gross of the tumor. Its importance cannot be minimized. No pathologist should ever attempt to make a diagnosis of bone tumor before he has seen the X-rays. It is true that many pathologists are not experienced in the interpretation of roentgenograms. They should co-operate with their radiologist and look at the films with him. If a segment of bone is removed or amputation is performed, carefully prepared X-rays of the specimen should be made to allow correlation of these findings with the preoperative radiograms. Only in this fashion can the pathologist and radiologist improve their preoperative diagnosis and show the value and limitation of the method. Although strong recommendations to obtain the X-rays have been going on to pathologists for many years, it is not rare to receive slides without X-rays from pathologists working in University Centers. SCHAJOWICZ emphasizes the great value of aspiration biopsy (this volume). Errors in formal biopsy fall into several categories. Ideally, the biopsy should be performed by an orthopedic surgeon who is going to undertake further surgery if it is indicated. Biopsy specimens should be so taken that if the lesion proves to be malignant, the biospy area will be included with the definitive ablative surgery in order to avoid implantation of malignant tumor. The biopsy is so important that at one international meeting, a slide was projected which said, "Have the Professor do the biopsy - let the resident do the amputation."

INFECTION STIMULATING A BONE NEOPLASM

In the usual acute hematogenous osteomyelitis, the sequence of events (high fever and localization of the lesion) leads to an accurate diagnosis. Brodie's abscess can, of course, look exactly like an osteoid osteoma on radiographs. But again this diagnosis is usually made without difficulty. There is one other form of chronic osteomyelitis which is probably related to brodie's abscess. A patient, usually an adult in his or her thirties, develops pain in the leg. A radiograph shows a dense well-delimited area with a central area of radiolucency. This may occupy almost the entire shaft of the metaphyseal or upper diaphyseal area of the femur. At the time of operation, this lesion is made up of eburnated bone, and in the central zone there is usually a little clear fluid which is negative for culture. Undoubtedly this is an end result of an ancient infection. Difficulty arises in the case where there may be an extensive osteolytic lesion in the metaphyseal area of a long bone, such as the femur. There may be no periosteal reaction and the lesion can even cross the epiphyseal plate, The radiologist may believe it is a malignant tumor or a lesiom such as an aneurysmal bone cyst or a chondromyxoid fibroma. In the case illustrated, a young girl, aged 20, had slight hip pain without constitutional symptoms. A radiograph showed a destructive cystic lesion in the metaphyseal area of the femur (Fig. 1). It was thought to be a tumor, possibly an osteosarcoma or a benign neoplasm. Osteomyelitis was not considered. At the time of operation, material was obtained and sectioned. In some areas it had a myxoid appearance with proliferation of connective tissue. There was also proliferating fiber bone. This slide was seen by pathologists in a bone tumor seminar; most of them called it chondromyxoid fibroma. They failed to pay attention to the chronic inflammatory background, but more important, they failed to see that fiber bone was attached to dead bone and therefore the correct diagnosis was chronic osteomyelitis (Fig. 2) (5).

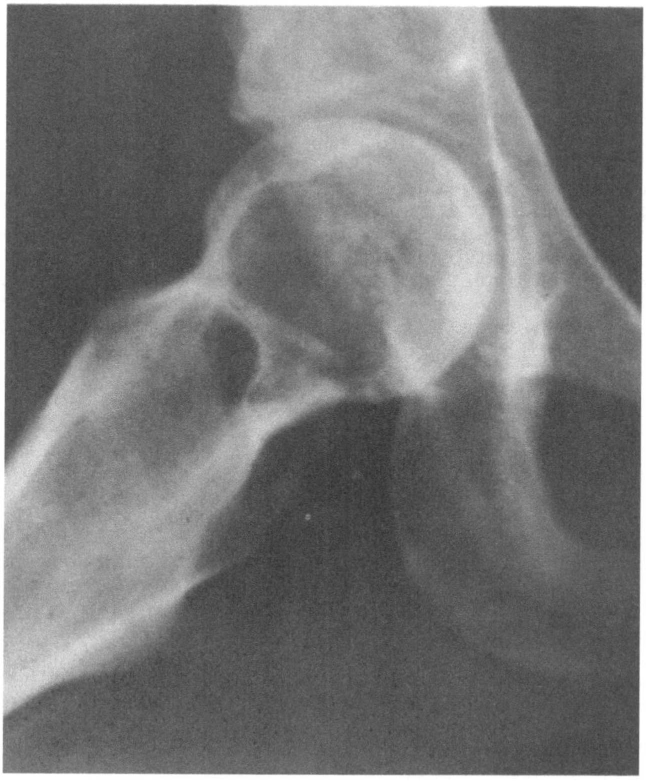

Fig. 1. Cystic, rather poorly defined radiolucent area in the metaphyseal area of the femur. No definite diagnosis could be made (VA2838K)

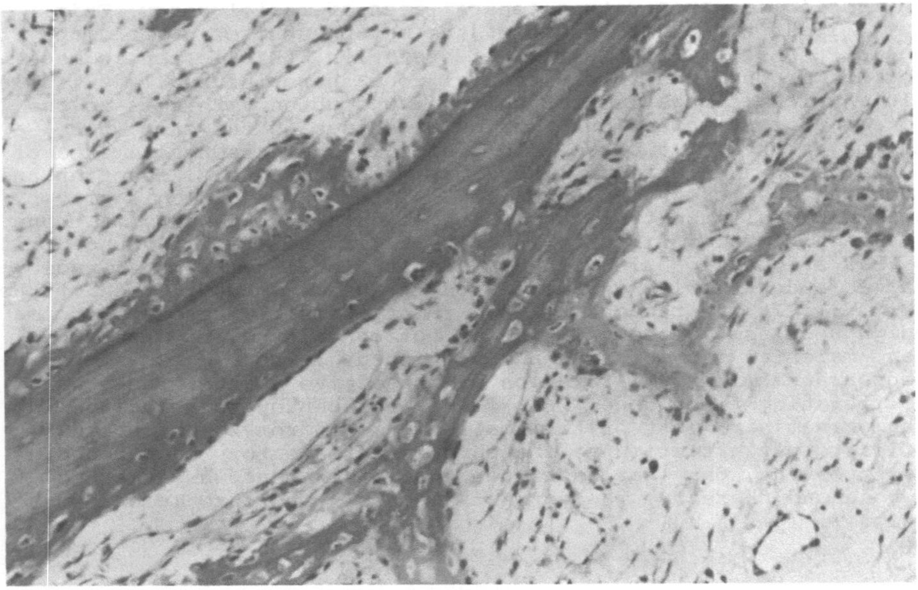

Fig. 2. Photomicrograph of material obtained by curettage. There is dead bone present with empty lacunae. Attached to this dead bone is new bone (creeping substitution). The stroma is loose with fibrous tissue and inflammatory cells (moderate enlargement). (VA2865B)

We have seen a few instances of monoarticular involvement of a vertebra with destruction without systemic symptoms. Frequently, these lesions are identified erroneously from X-rays as metastatic carcinoma or plasma-cell myeloma. There are certain examples in which periosteal bone proliferation in the shaft stimulates Ewing's sarcoma. A case of salmonella paratyphi osteomyelitis stimulating a giant-cell tumor has been reported (6). There is no way of making an accurate diagnosis except by biopsy, particularly in a patient who has no constitutional symptoms.

FRACTURE CALLUS

Fracture callus naturally has an extremely bewildering pattern, and without clinical history or radiographs it would be easy to designate such lesions as osteosarcoma. However, the patient usually has a simple fracture with callus. The clinical history and X-rays are straight-forward, and no matter how bewildering the microscopic pattern, callus is the logical diagnosis. In osteogenesis imperfecta, the X-rays might have an ominous pattern and again the amount of callus is excessive, but there is no difficulty in making the diagnosis.

It is only when fracture callus is combined with benign or malignant lesion that the pathologist makes an error. It is not at all rare for lesions such as metaphyseal fibrous defect or unicameral bone cyst to be associated with fracture. In these instances, the fracture can often be seen on the film, as well as the typical radiographic pattern of metaphyseal fibrous defect or unicameral bone cyst. The greatest difficulty occurs when the radiographic findings suggest malignant tumor or the fracture callus is difficult to visualize or is not visualized. The surgeon performs an exploratory operation and finds a mass extending out from the bone: he removes a piece which he believes to be tumor, but which is only callus. The pathologist is then informed by the radiologist that the patient may very well have a malignant bone tumor, and by the surgeon that a mass has been found extending out from the bone. The pathologist sees the bewildering pattern of callus and calls it osteosarcoma. We have seen this happen on two occasions secondary to aneurysmal bone cyst.

The following case illustrates the problem:

A 37-year-old woman had considerable hip pain. The radiograph showed an apparently cystic lesion of the upper femur. The radiologist saw no evidence of fracture (Fig. 3). The surgeon explored the lesion and found a mass extending out from the bone. He took a generous biopsy. This slide was seen by an experienced bone pathologist without the benefit of roentgenogram (Fig. 4). He diagnosed it as osteosarcoma. Later, the lesion was explored and the cystic area proved to be an aneurysmal bone cyst.

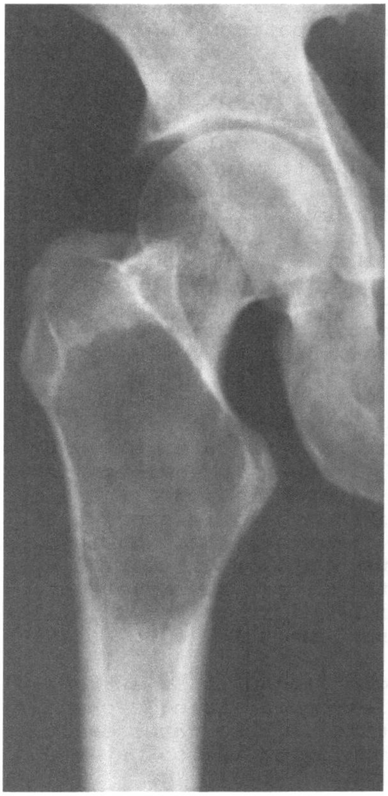

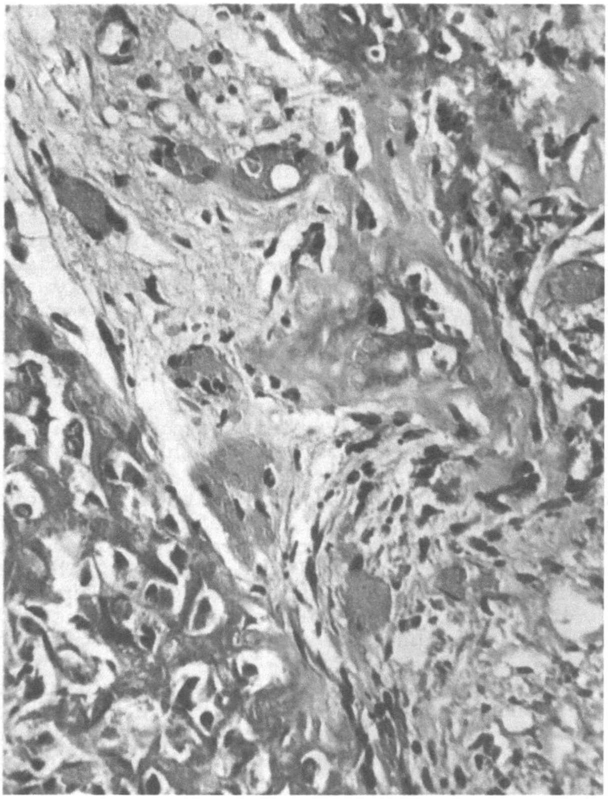

Fig. 3. Fairly well-defined radiolucent area in the metaphyseal zone of the femur. No fracture could be seen by the radiologist
Fig. 4. Biopsy of callus showing a bewildering proliferative pattern of bone formation and areas simulating sarcoma. This was erroneously diagnosed as osteosarcoma

We have also seen fracture callus in association with a metastatic carcinoma. This fracture callus was biopsied and diagnosed as a primary osteosarcoma. This was followed by disarticulation, and a correct diagnosis of secondary metastatic carcinoma with primary source in the lung was made.

This example demonstrates that fracture in association with a bone tumor or bone lesion is not always seen by the roentgenologist or recognized as callus by either the radiologist or the pathologist.

WELL-DIFFERENTIATED TUMORS

The pathologist often has considerable difficulty in evaluating well-differentiated neoplasms. This is particularly true of juxtacortical osteosarcoma and fibrosarcoma. The juxtacortical osteosarcoma has a classic radiographic pattern (Fig. 5) with a dense shadow in close apposition to the bone. It is not rare for the lesion to appear confined to the cortex, and there is some question as to whether it might arise from the periosteum. Biopsy sometimes reveals atypical bone with irregular cement lines and focal collections of well differentiated cartilage cells. (Fig. 6). The stroma is often innocuous in its pattern, i.e. the stroma does not have the obvious sarcomatous pattern which is so often seen. However, with these changes, a diagnosis is possible if the X-rays are examined. There should be no question of confusing this lesion with myositis ossificans, in which the radiographic picture is different and pathologically there is a zone phenomenon. In the past, it has been said that myositis ossificans can become malignant - this is false. Review of such cases demonstrates that they were, in reality, juxtacortical osteosarcomas from their inception. Frequently, these tumors are treated inadequately, for the surgeon tries to perform local resections. Invariably, this is impossible. Out of a total of 80 cases collected for one study, most of the patients were male, and were more than 20 years old; there was frequently a long history. After the first treatment, of whatever kind, about 80 percent survived for five years (21). However, the ten-year cure rate was poor. After local excision alone of the primary lesion a "cure" was obtained in only five of 31 patients.

Well-differentiated osteosarcomas can also give the pathologist a great deal of difficulty. However, the radiographic pattern is usually obvious (Fig. 7), but the biopsy is difficult, frequently showing disturbed trabecular bone with a rather innocuous stroma (Fig. 8). There is usually no difficulty in the diagnosis of fibrosarcoma in bone which frequently occurs in the metaphyseal of the femur or tibia and is almost completely osteolytic (Fig. 9). The usual pattern is that of undifferentiated fibrous tumor. Occasionally the biopsy shows very highly differentiated fibrous tissue and scarring, and it is very difficult to say that the change represent fibrosarcoma (Fig. 10).

In all three cases illustrated, the pathologic diagnosis is extremely difficult, and if the pathologist relies solely on histologic changes, he will make an error and call the lesion benign. These three examples illustrate vividly the necessity for the pathologist to look at and familiarize himself with radiographic patterns.

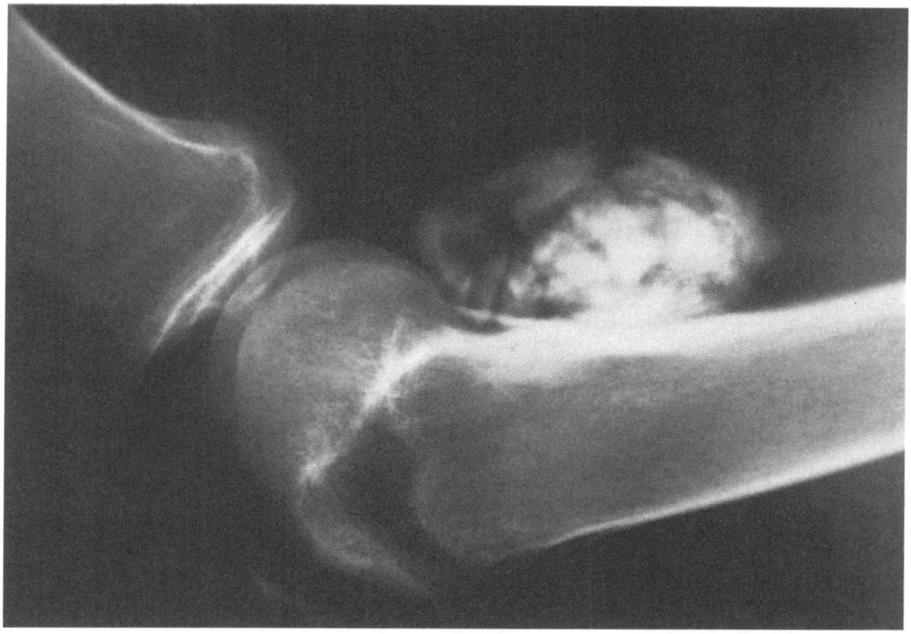

Fig. 5

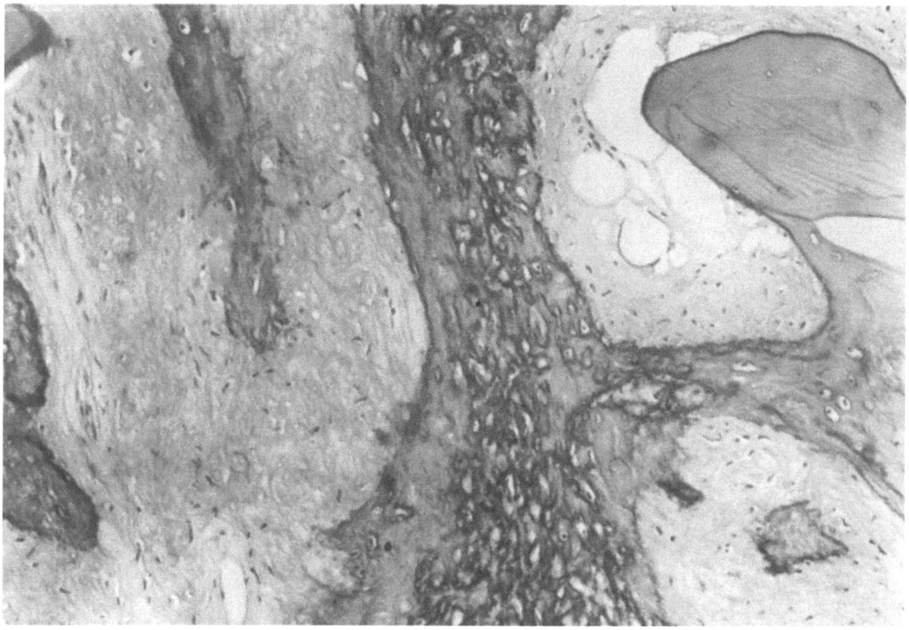

Fig. 6

Fig. 5. Roentgenogram of juxtacortical osteosarcoma of the femur. The lesion is well delimited and merges with the cortical bone and is incorporated with it. (VA2824J)
Fig. 6. Photomicrograph of tumor showing irregular cement lines and atypical bony trabeculae. The stroma appears rather innocuous. (VA2824J)

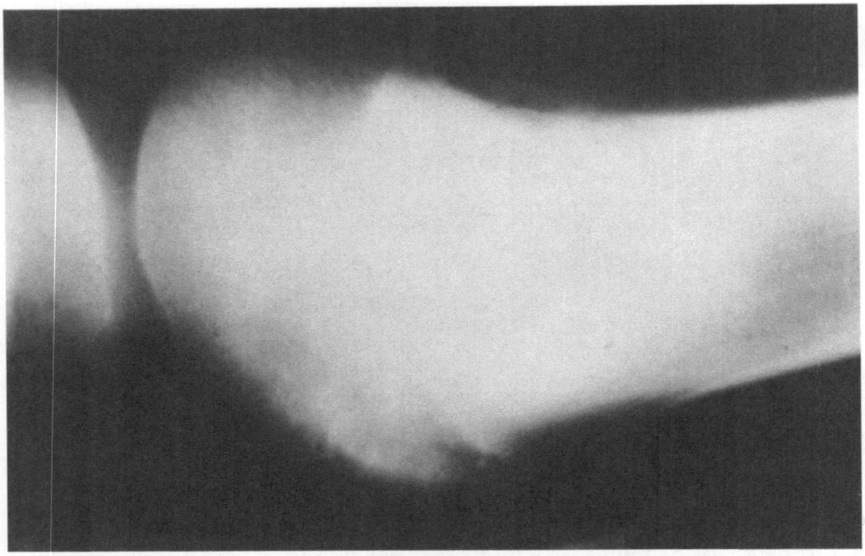

Fig. 7

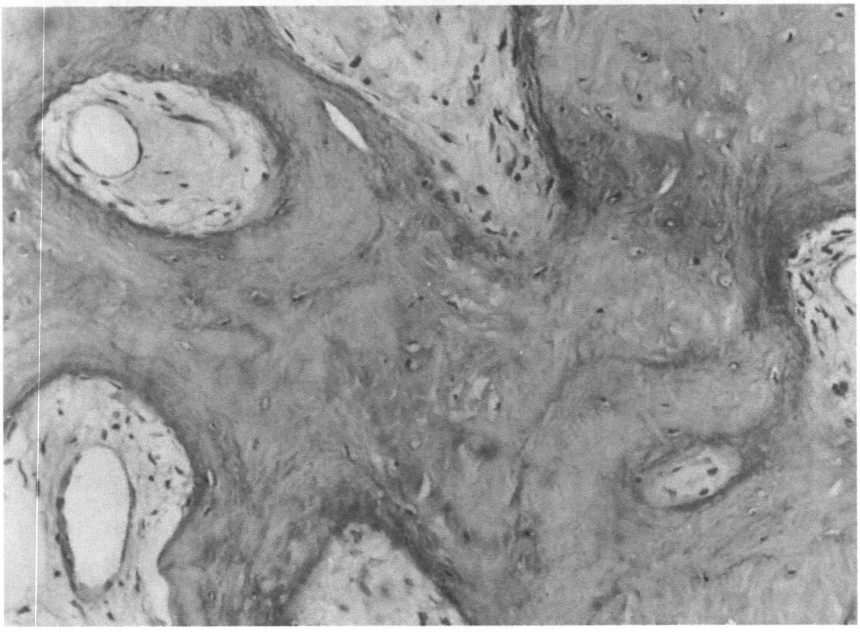

Fig. 8

Fig. 7. Extensive bone-producing lesion of the metaphyseal and of the femur in a 15-year-old female.(VA2838N)

Fig. 8. Photomicrograph of the lesion seen in Fig. 7, which demonstrates bone with abnormal appearance but has an apparently stroma. This patient developed pulmonary metastases and died. (VA2824C)

Fig. 9

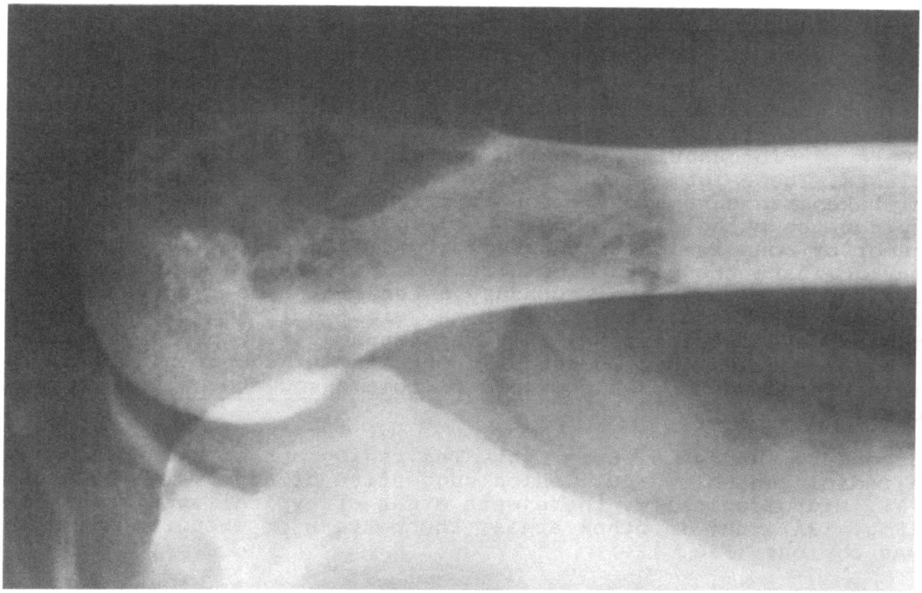

Fig. 10

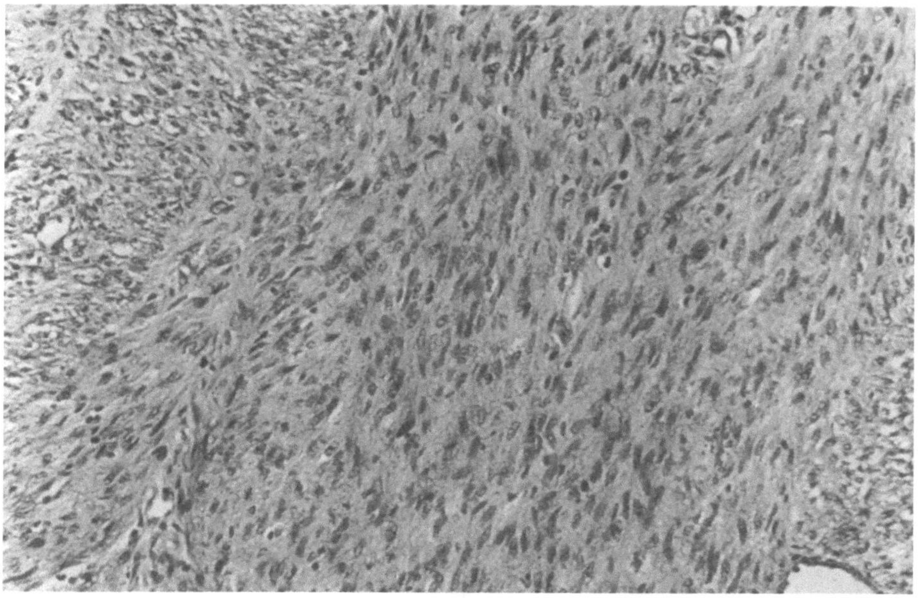

Fig. 9. Roentgenogram of extensive osteolytic lesion of the metaphysis and diaphysis of the humerus with poorly defined margins in a 19-year-old female (VY2824I)

Fig. 10. Photomicrograph of well-differentiated fibrosarcoma. The referring pathologist thought it might be a benign fibrous lesion. Operation showed this lesion to be extensive within the bone, with extension into the soft tissue. (VA2824A)

ANEURYSMAL BONE CYST

Aneurysmal bone cyst is a definite entity the pathogenesis of which is not known. The pathologic features of this lesion are clear-cut and consist of dilated vascular spaces filled with blood and crossed by septa of fibrous tissue, often containing osteoid and lined with osteoclasts. These lesions may follow trauma, may grow rapidly and may be mistaken radiographically for a malignant tumor. The greatest difficulty for the pathologist occurs when this lesion is associated with a bone tumor or bone lesion. The pathologic findings of aneurysmal bone cyst may dominate the picture both radiographically and pathologically. The lesions with which the secondary aneurysmal bone cyst can occur are fibrous dysplasia, chondroblastoma, giant-cell tumor, chondromyxoid fibroma and osteosarcoma. In some instances, the primary lesion is only a mural nodule; this occurred in one case of chondroblastoma. The case illustrated was a chondromyxoid fibroma associated with aneurysmal bone cyst.

Secondary Aneurysmal Bone Cyst. The radiograph of this case demonstrates a radiolucent blown-out lesion suggestive of aneurysmal bone cyst (Fig. 11). Microscopically, there were areas of typical aneurysmal bone cyst (Fig. 12A), but in other areas, the pattern of chondromyxoid fibroma was obvious (Fig. 12B).

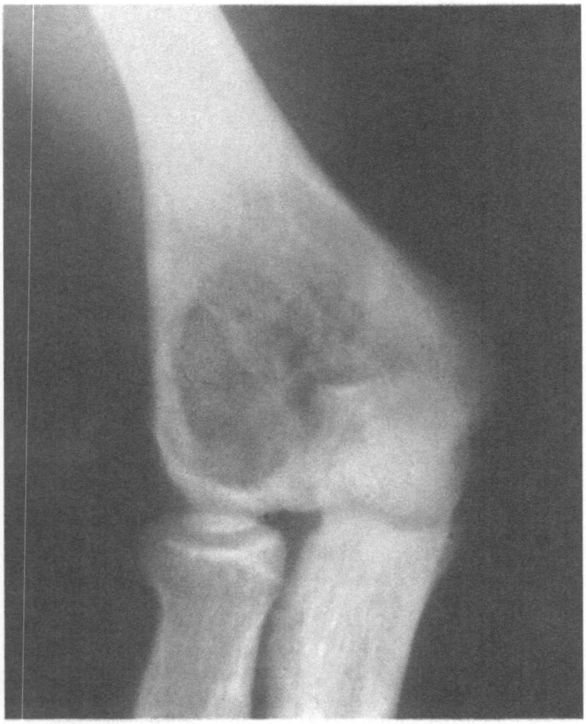

Fig. 11. Roentgenogram of a radiolucent lesion in the metaphyseal area of the right humerus. It was thought radiographically to be a giant-cell tumor

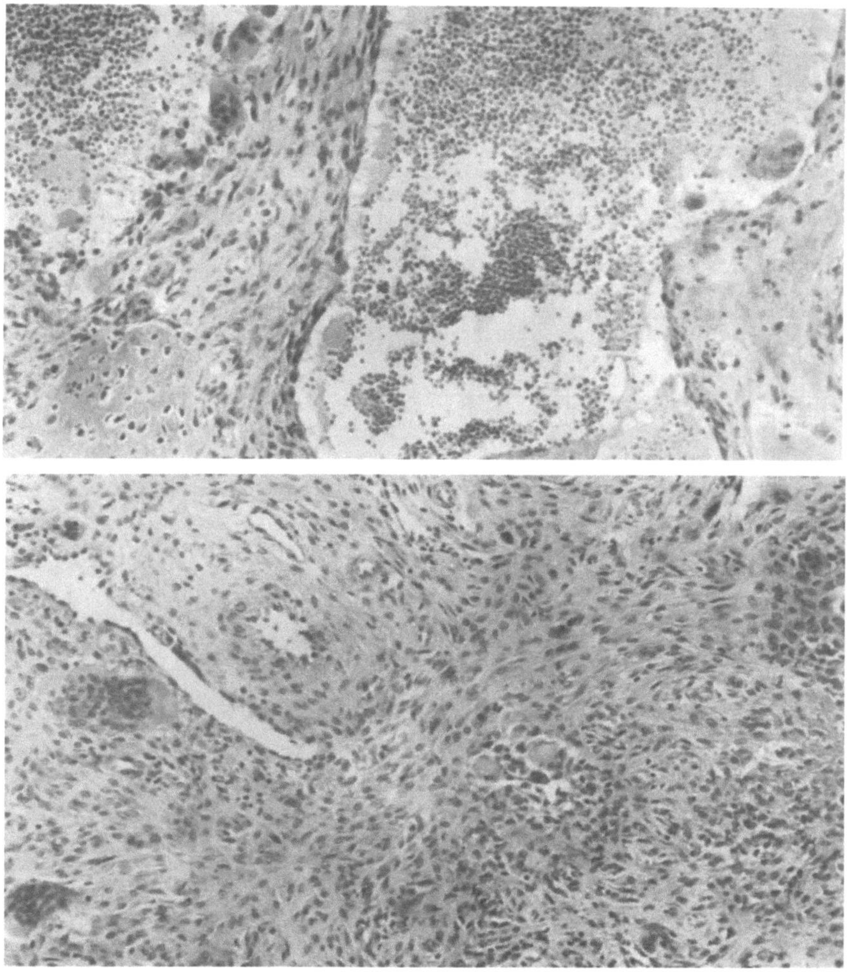

Fig. 12 (a). Photomicrograph of an area of secondary aneurysmal bone cyst demonstrating dilating spaces filled with blood and lined with fibrous-tissue septa containing osteoid, (b) photomicrograph of typical chondromyxoid fibroma, which was the primary lesion in this case

OSTEOID OSTEOMA - OSTEOBLASTOMA

Both these lesions have been well described. Microscopically, it is impossible to tell the difference between them, and the designation of either lesion may be related to size rather than to any histologic difference. It is possible that the variation of symptoms is related to the bone involvement. Osteoblastomas tend to arise in flat bone (4). The most usual osteoid osteomas, osteoblastomas, present a very classic microscopic pattern. The problem arises in extremely large or highly cellular lesions in which the pathologist has to consider whether the lesion is a malignant osteoblastoma, a well-differentiated osteosarcoma or simply a fluorid-appearing osteoblastoma.

The following cases demonstrate the problem. Examination of the lesion in the ulna of a 12-year-old girl showed a cystic lesion which was cellular; it was finally designated as benign osteoblastoma, curetted and replaced with bone chips (Fig. 13). Two-year follow-up demonstrates quiescence of the process. The second case was a large lesion in the wing of the ileum in a 15-year-old boy (Fig. 14). In this case, because of the size and the aggressive nature of the lesion, the question arose as to whether this was a malignant osteoblastoma. Miscroscopically, the decision proved very difficult because the lesion was highly cellular and there were areas which were quite disturbing (Figs. 15A and 15B). It was treated conservatively and, one year later, the child appeared to be in a stable condition. Whether this will continue is hard to say, for follow-up is still too short. The question of transition between benign osteoblastoma and malignant osteoblastoma has not been resolved and was discussed in depth at the International Skeletal Society in London in 1975.

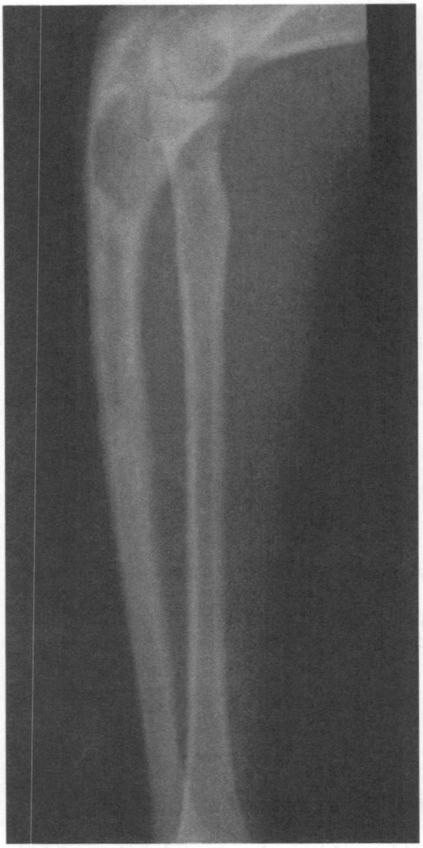

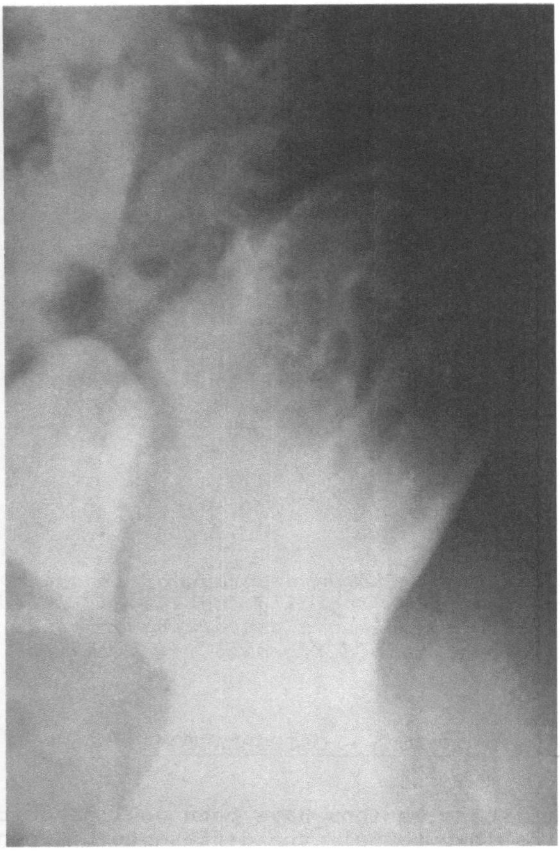

Fig. 13. Cystic lesion of the ulna in a 12-year-old female. It was well-delimited and thought to be benign, but osteoblastoma was not considered

Fig. 14. Roentgenogram shows rather poorly delimited large lesion of the ileum which was thought to be possibly malignant by the radiologist. An exact diagnosis was not made

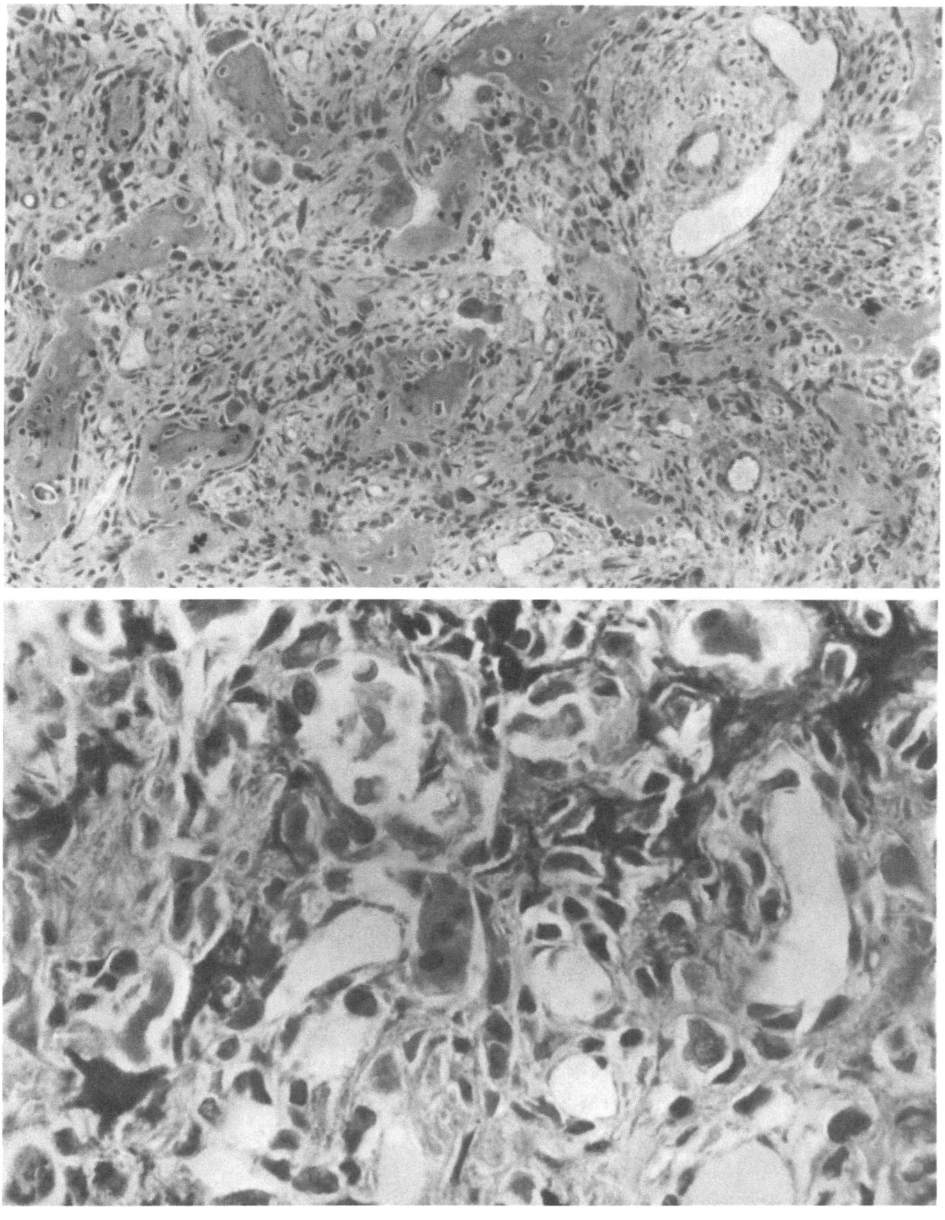

Fig. 15 (a). Photomicrograph of the lesion of the ileum shows active new bone production in a vascular background, (b) this shows areas of increased cellularity with focal calcification of immature bone. This is a disturbing histologic pattern (high power)

There is no area in tumor pathology more treacherous than the pathologic evaluation of a cartilaginous neoplasm. The diagnosis of chondroblastoma is now well established, and chondromyxoid fibroma does not usually present a problem. Both these lesions can recur locally with inadequate excision, and on rare occasions a chondroblastoma can even metastasize. There may be a poorly defined lesion in which islands of cartilage are associated with focal calcification occasionally in the long bones, particularly in the humerus in the metaphyseal area. This is a benign lesion, probably not even a neoplasm. The common enchondromata of the small bones of the hands and feet may show atypicalities which should not be interpreted as malignant, particularly if the radiographic appearance is that of a benign neoplasm. Juxtacortical chondromas may have a rather ominous radiographic pattern but they are benign (Fig. 16). Synovial chondromatosis may show extremely atypical cartilage nuclei, but only in the rarest of the circumstances is such a

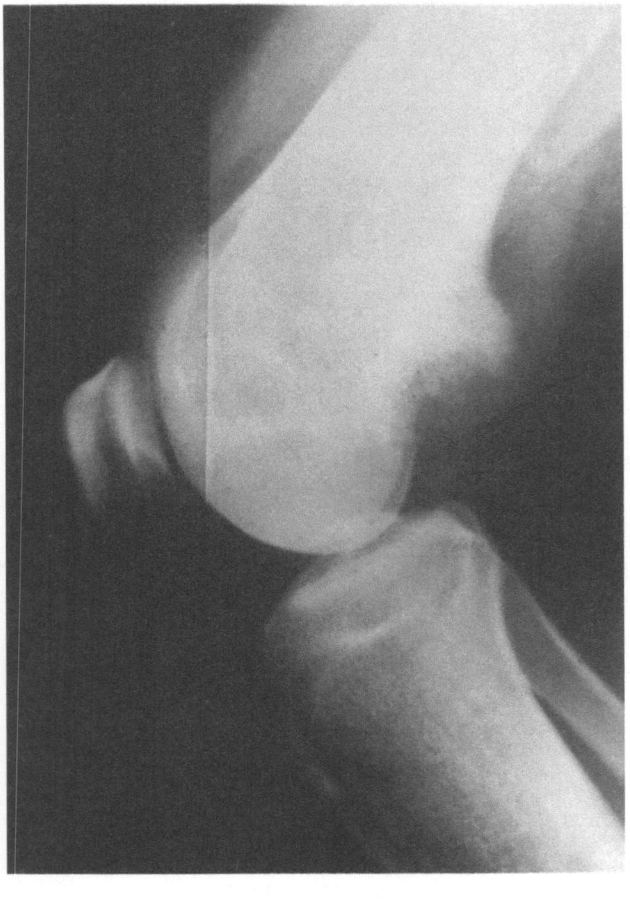

Fig. 16. Classic radiographic pattern of a juxtacortical osteochondroma of the femur in a 16-year-old female. This was successfully excised by block excision

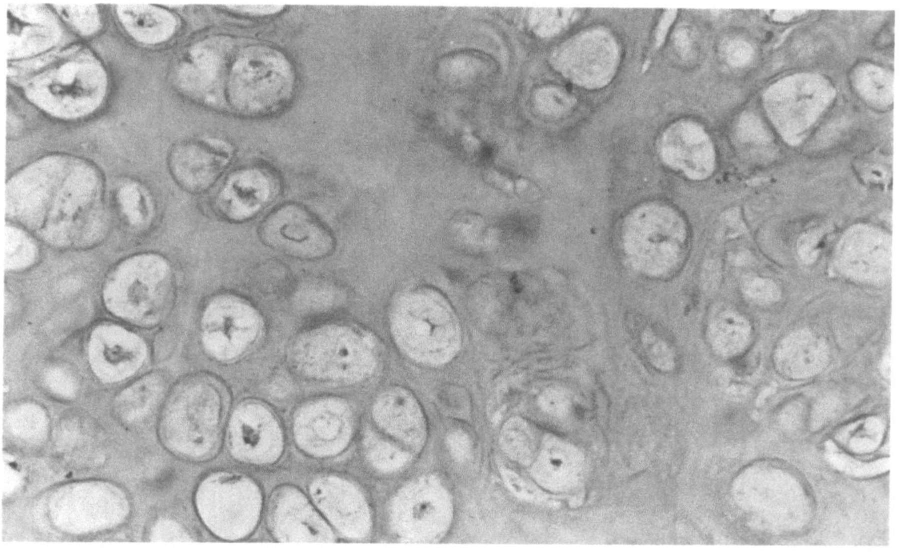

Fig. 17

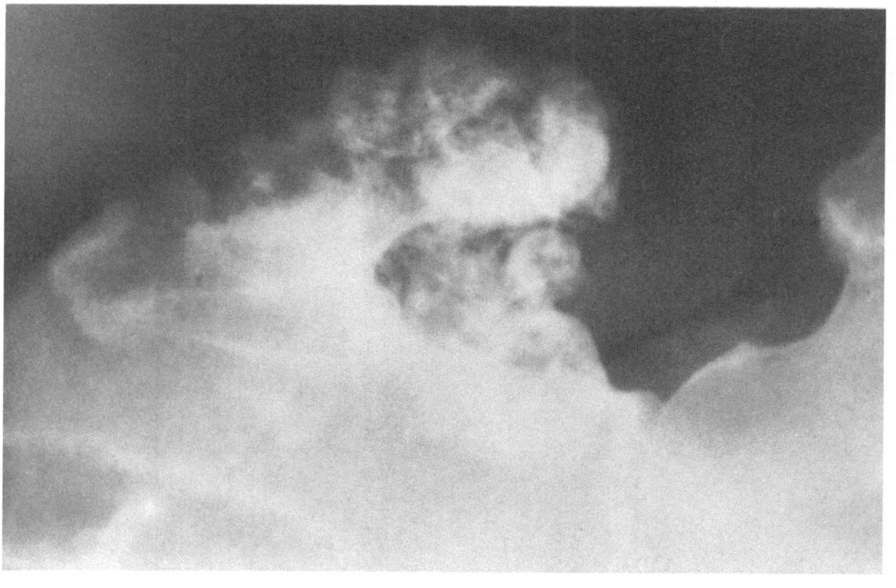

Fig. 18

Fig. 17. Photomicrograph of well-differentiated cartilage cells. It would be impossible to say this lesion was malignant on the basis of this photomicrograph.(VA2824D)

Fig. 18. Chondrosarcoma of the wing of the ileum in a 29-year-old male. The large size of the lesion and its blotchy calcifications makes its diagnosis of chondrosarcoma almost certain. (VA2824H)

lesion malignant. The extremely large cartilaginous tumors around the pelvis are often thought to be benign because of the innocuous appearance of the cartilage (Fig. 17). In the case illustrated (Fig. 18), there was a large tumor of the wing of the ileum in a 29-year-old male, which showed the typical blotchy calcification. This tumor was over 8 cm in size and had a thick cartilaginous cap. Tumors of this kind of size and with thick cartilaginous caps are malignant cartilaginous tumors almost without exception. They will inevitably recur, and through their massive recurrences (at times with metastases) they will cause the death of the patient. In the present case, it was possible to do an adequate excision.

In the next case, we have a radiographic pattern of a greatly thickened irregular cortex with focal calcification within the marrow cavitiy (Fig. 19). The patient also had pain. The best way to make a diagnosis of such a lesion is to simply do a needle biopsy (as advocated by SCHAJOWICZ). It must be emphasized that malignant cartilage can implant and grow easily, for cartilage cells require very little oxygen for their survival. If cartilage is obtained by biopsy, the only significant

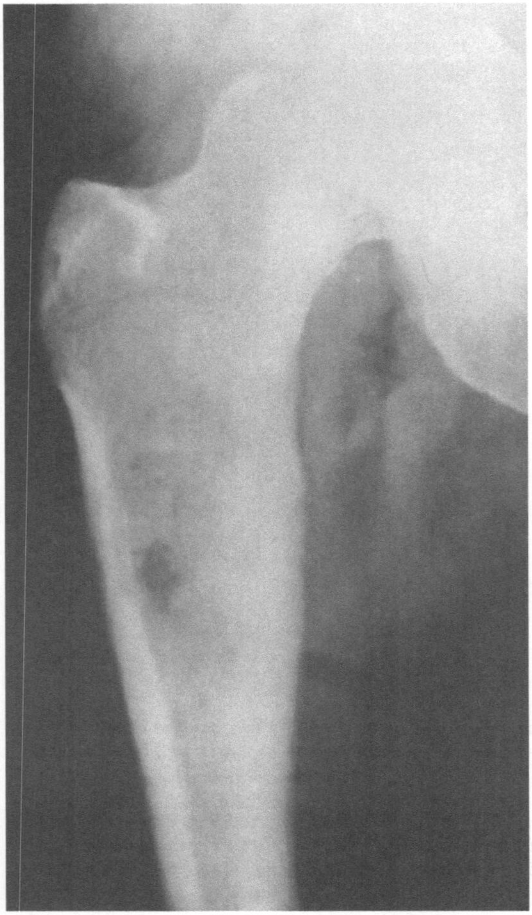

Fig. 19. Radiographic pattern of chondrosarcoma arising in the medullary canal of the femur. The cortex is irregularly thickenend, and there is a small focal area of calcification within the medullary canal. This lesion was treated by resection of the upper end of the femur, which was replaced by prosthesis

factor is that it is a cartilaginous tumor. The individual characteristics of the cells do not matter. Often this pattern is not recognized by the radiologist as indicative of a malignant tumor, and the biopsied tumor is frequently called an enchondroma by the pathologist. The lesion then recurs, frequently with metastases, and causes the death of the patient. The lesion must be treated by either disarticulation or complete excision of the lesion and replacement by a prosthesis (15). This course was successfully followed in the patient illustrated.

In conclusion, pathologists must evaluate cartilaginous tumors from the standpoint of their location in a particular bone and, most importantly, the radiographic pattern and clinical findings that accompany their presence. The microscopic pattern of the cartilage cells, although important, may be of only relative significance when evaluated with the other clinical and radiologic findings.

EWING'S SARCOMA

Ewing's sarcoma has been established clinically and pathologically as a definite entity. In the past, the overall cure rate was approximately 5 percent. With radiation therapy and appropriate chemotherapy, about 40 percent two-year survival, which is really equivalent to cure in most cases, is now recorded (14). It is essential, therefore, that an exact pathologic diagnosis be made, for there are several other pathologic conditions which have been diagnosed as Ewing's sarcoma.

Table. Errors in diagnosis -- Ewing's sarcoma

(Condensed - - Pomeroy and Johnson)	
Lymphoma	3
Soft-tissue round-cell sarcoma	2
Osteosarcoma	4
Adamantinoma	1
Histiocytosis X	2
Miscellaneous	2

This table shows a list of the incorrect diagnoses in a group of patients referred to the National Cancer Institute as Ewing's sarcoma. Speaking strictly from the pathologic standpoint, Ewing's sarcoma has uniform cells with inconspicuous cytoplasm and fine nucleoli. A positive glycogen stain helps support this diagnosis, although a negative stain does not mean that it is not Ewing's sarcoma. If the stain is positive, then with the rarest of exceptions, it cannot be reticulum-cell sarcoma or neuroblastoma (Fig. 20). Both embryonal rhabdomyosarcoma and osteosarcoma can show large amounts of glycogen (Fig. 21). Embryonal rhabdomyosarcoma may involve the bone secondarily, but if one pays attention to the location of the tumor, the radiographic pattern, and the variability of the cells, this error will not be made. Some osteosarcomas, particularly in children, are often highly undifferentiated, have a radiographic pattern similar to that of Ewing's sarcoma, and may fall within the same age group. As the photomicrograph illustrates, osteoid may be inconspicuous and seen only after many sections. However, again, the individual cells show great variability.

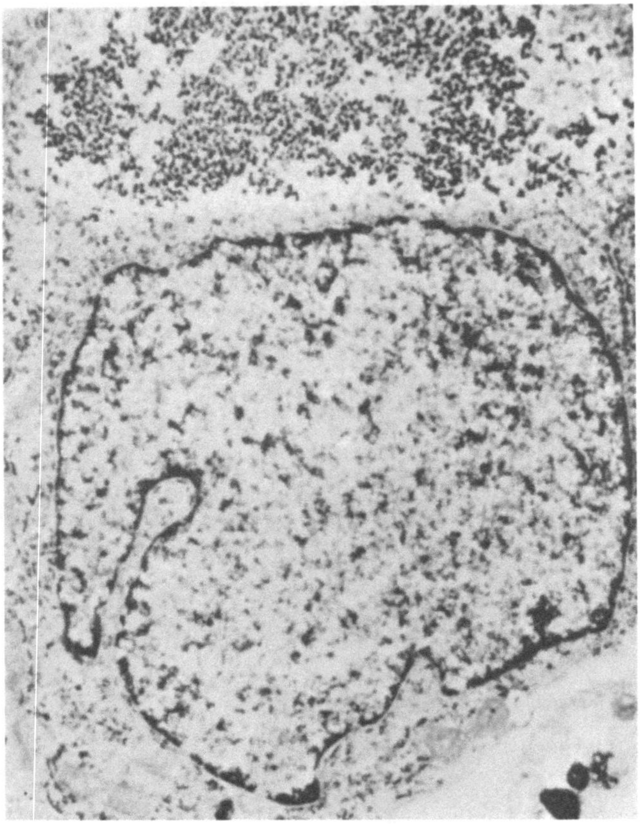

Fig. 20. Electron micrograph of a cell of Ewing's sarcoma. The upper part of the figure shows large amounts of clumped glyogen

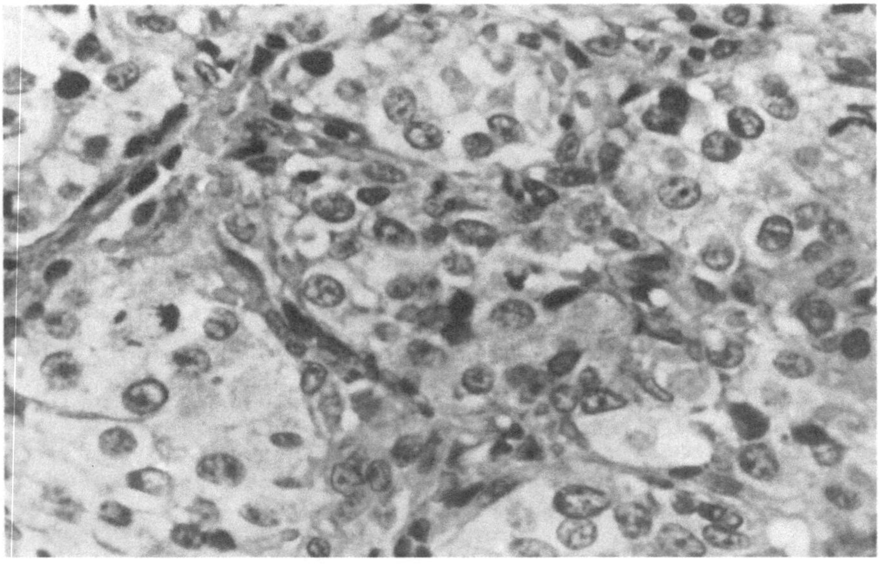

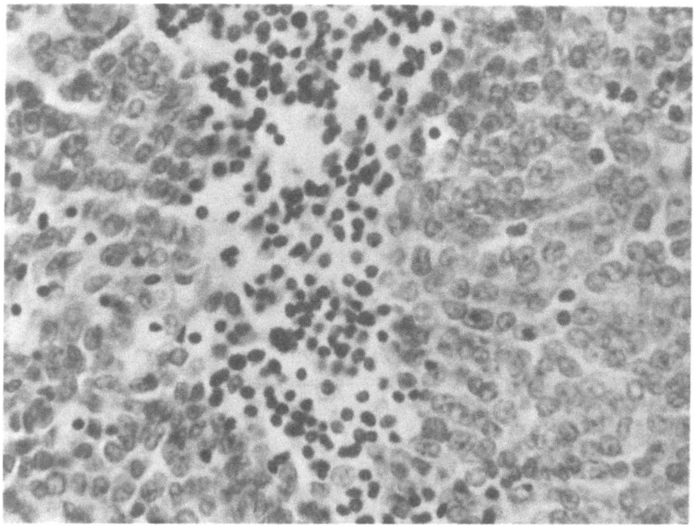

Fig. 22. This patient was erroneously thought to have Ewing's sarcoma, but glycogen stain was negative, and two different types of cells were obviously present. The patient later developed obvious disseminated lymphosarcoma

We have also observed several cases of lymphomas in children in which early in the evolution of the process, a single bone was the only one clinically involved. In such a case, the glycogen stain is negative, and there is always a variable population of cells, which rules out Ewing's sarcoma (Fig. 22).

SUMMARY

The pathologist must obtain X-rays before attempting to make a diagnosis in a bone tumor. Errors are made with both benign and malignant lesions associated with calluses. Infection may simulate a malignant bone tumor radiographically and pathologically. Secondary aneurysmal bone cyst may dominate the radiographic and pathologic findings and obscure the primary diagnosis. Osteoblastomas are becoming increasingly difficult to diagnose. The question of whether such an entity can become malignant has not been resolved. Cartilagenous tumors are often difficult to diagnose and the pathologist must not only rely on histologic findings, but in particular pay attention to the radiographic pattern which is often diagnostic. Accuracy of diagnosis in Ewing's sarcoma is essential because the treatment now can result in a cure rate of almost 40%. Certain lesions such as lymphoma or osteosarcoma can mimic this tumor. To re-emphasize the problem, the pathologist must have all the clinical information before attempting a diagnosis of a bone tumor and without the pertinent X-ray, errors are almost inevitable.

◄ *Fig. 21. Primitive highly cellular osteosarcoma in a child. This was positive for glycogen. The diagnosis was possible because in other areas osteoid was being produced, and there was a considerable variation in cell pattern. The glycogen stain was positive, resulting in an erroneous diagnosis of Ewing's sarcoma*

REFERENCES

1. ACKERMAN, L.V.: Extraosseous localized non-neoplastic bone and cartilage formation (so-called myositis ossificans). Clinical and pathological confusion with malignant neoplasms. J. Bone Surg. 40A, 279 (1958)
2. BAKER, S.L.: Hyperplastic callus simulating sarcoma in two cases of fragilitas ossium. J. Path. Bact. 58, 609-623 (1946)
3. BARNES, R., CATTO, M.: Chondrosarcoma of bone. J. Bone Surg. 48, 729-764 (1966)
4. BYERS, P.D.: Solitary benign osteoblastic lesions of bone-osteoid osteoma and benign osteoblastoma. Cancer 22, 43-57 (1968)
5. CABENELA, M.E., SIM, F.H., BEABOUT, J.W., DAHLIN, D.C.: Osteomyelitis appearing as neoplasms. Arch. Surg. 109, 68-72 (1974)
6. CHAROSKY, C.B., MARCOVE, R.C.: Salmonella paratyphi osteomyelitis. Clin. Orthop. Related Res. 99, 190-193 (1974)
7. Massachusetts General Hospital: Case records. New Engl. J. Med. 285, 166-173 (1971)
8. DABSKA, M., BURACZEWSKI, J.: Aneurysmal bone cyst; pathology, clinical course and radialogic appearances. Cancer 23, 371-389 (1969)
9. DAHLIN, D.C., IVINS, J.C.: Fibrosarcoma of bone; a study of 114 cases. Cancer 23 35-41 (1969)
10. DE SOUZA DIAZ, L., FROST, H.M.: Osteoid osteoma-osteoblastoma. Cancer 33, 1074-1081 (1974) (Extensive bibliography)
11. FALVO,K.A., ROOT,L., BULLOUGH, P.G.: Osteogenesis imperfecta: clinical evaluation and management. J. Bone Jt. Surg. 56A, 783-793 (1974)
12. HARRIS, N.H., KIRKALDY-WILLIS, W.H.: Primary subacute pyogenic osteomyelitis. J. Bone Jt. Surg. 47, 526-532 (1965)
13. KAHN, L.B., WOOD, F.W., ACKERMAN, L.V.: Fracture callus associated with benign and malignant bone lesions and mimicking osteosarcoma. Amer. J. Clin. Path. 52, 14-24 (1969)
14. POMEROY, T.C., JOHNSON, R.E., Cobined modality therapy of Ewing's sarcoma. Cancer, January 1975 (in press)
15. REITER, F.B., STAPLE, T.W., ACKERMAN, L.V.: Central chondrosarcoma of the skeleton. Radiology 105, 525-530 (1972)
16. SCHAJOWICZ, F., ACKERMAN, L.V., SISSONS, H.A., SOBIN, L.H., TORLONI, H.: Histological typing of bone tumors (International classification of Tumors) Geneva: World Health Organization, 1972
17. SCHAJOWICZ, F., CABRINI, R.L.: Histochemical studies of bone in normal and pathological conditions, with special reference to alkaline phosphatase, glycogen and mucopolysaccharides. J. Bone Jt. Surg. 36B, 474-489 (1954)
18. SCHAJOWICZ, F., DERQUI, J.C.: Puncture biopsy in lesions of the locomotor system; review of results in 4050 cases, including 941 vertebral punctures. Cancer 21, 531-548 (1968)
19. SPJUT, H.J., DORFMAN, H.D., FECHNER, R.E., ACKERMAN, L.V.: Tumors of bone and cartilage. Atlas of Tumor Pathology, Armed Forces Institute of Pathology, 2nd series, fassicle 5, 1971 (Extensive bibliography)
20. Tillman, B.P., DAHLIN, D.C., LIPSCOMB, P.R., STEWART, J.R.: Aneurysmal bone cyst: an analysis of 95 cases. Mayo Clin. Proc. 43, 478-495 (1968)
21. VAN DER HUEL, R.O., VON RONNEN, J.R.: Juxtacortical osteosarcoma. Diagnosis, differential diagnosis, treatment and an analysis of eighty cases. J. Bone Jt. Surg. 49A, 415 (1967)

Aspiration (Puncture or Needle) Biopsy in Bone Lesions

F. SCHAJOWICZ and J. HOKAMA

There is general agreement that combined clinical, radiologic and pathological study, supplemented whenever necessary by biochemical and hematologic investigations, is essential for precise diagnosis in any case of bone tumor. A biopsy should never be omitted when radical surgery of radiotherapy is contemplated, and whatever the procedure used, should be carried out by a competent surgeon under correct technical conditions and be interpreted by a pathologist who has a good basic knowledge of bone pathology. He has to be familiar with the clinical and radiographical picture and should know the exact origin of the material submitted

It is not our purpose to discuss the possible dangers and advantages of open biopsy by frozen sections or by the study of paraffin-embedded material, but to report the results of our present experience with aspiration (puncture or needle) biopsy, based on a review of more than 7000 cases, including 1900 cases of vertebral punctures, studied in our laboratory from March 15, 1941 to August 15, 1974, a 33-year period.

Aspiration biopsy of bone lesions, especially tumors, is not a new method, but we should like to mention here the outstanding importance of the work performed on this subject at the Memorial Hospital in New York by clinicians, surgeons and pathologists since 1931 (2, 5, 14, 15) and in England (3).

Like many other pathologists, we were at first sceptical about this procedure, because the pioneers of the method, the Memorial Hospital group, recommended the preferred or exclusive use of smears, a technique which requires considerable cytological experience.

However, we soon become enthusiastic about the method when we realized that it was not necessary to carry out difficult cytological interpretations, as it was possible to obtain good histological sections after embedding the more important parts of the aspirated fragments in paraffin. On our practice we use both methods whenever possible, with a preference for the histopathological interpretation of the paraffin-embedded material, which generally requires no more than 24 hours to prepare.

The technical details, and also the advantages and disadvantages of this method, have been described elsewhere (7,11). In 1968 one of us (F.S.) published the detailed results of 4050 puncture biopsies in lesions of locomotor system, comprising 3717 bon puncture, (including 941 vertebral lesions), 295 joint punctures and 38 cases of soft-tissue, with more than 70 percent positive results (11A). (Cancer 21, 531, 1968)

Our technique of vertebral puncture has been adopted at many centers with or without modifications, with various types of needle or trocars, some much larger than our original 2-mm gauge needle (13, 4, 10, 1, 12).

Although needle biopsy of the vertebrae is accepted without reservation in many important Centers, where it has replaced a difficult operation, its use in other Institutions is restricted or opposed, especially by the pathologist, one of the main objections being the relative degree of confidence inspired by a diagnosis based on very small particles of tissue.

MATERIAL AND TECHNIQUE

In this report the results of our experience with 7165 punctures of bone lesions studied in our laboratory during a 33-year period are analyzed; 1900 biopsies were taken from lesions of the spine and 5265 from other bones, including sacrum and coccyx.

In general we follow with slight modifications the technique employed at the Memorial Hospital, using a needle of 2 mm diameter with a short bevel, well sharpened, and metal syringes to which the needle can be fitted securely, but for the extraction of a specimen from the lumbar vertebrae we have designed a special set of instruments composed of a needle guide, two needles, and a lined metal plate, which makes it possible to reach this difficult site easily and with no danger. A slight modification of this technique (8), with a different length of needle (4.5 cm instead of 6.5 cm) has been used by us more recently for the approach of the second to ninth dorsal vertebrae, which we had previously considered contraindicated. For the first 3 cervical vertebrae the puncture by pharyngeal approach and from the 4th cervical to 1st dorsal vertebra the lateral approach is indicated (9).

The needle-biopsy specimen is placed in sterile physiological saline, and it is then possible to prepare smears which are air-dried and stained with methylene blue, May-Grunwald-Giemsa and hematoxylin-eosin; the residual material is embedded in paraffin for histopathological examination, and, if necessary, bacteriological examinations or inoculations of guinea pigs can be performed.

In some occasions histochemical tests (alkaline, phosphatase and glycogen stains) can be performed, and these are an important aid to diagnosis. The specimen can be kept in sterile physiological saline, even if refrigerated, for only a few hours; if it is being sent from a distant center it must first be fixed in formalin or some other fixative, in which case cytological examination by means of smears is not possible.

We consider the smear to be a supplementary method of great value for studying the fine details of cell structure, especially in conditions which involve the hematopoietic system. Moreover, it often permits a diagnosis to be made in a few minutes. The smear is generally adequate for immediate diagnosis of eosinophilic granuloma, myeloma, or metastatic carcinoma, and for differentiation of Ewing's sarcoma from osteomyelitis. In many cases, however, a smear is not sufficient for accurate classification of either benign or malignant tumors, or for differentiation between primary and metastatic malignant tumors, or between chondromas and chondrosarcomas, etc,. Moreover, in some neoplastic growths, such as fibromatous, cartilaginous or sclerosing bony tumor, or in Paget's disease, and in other lesions in which the fibrous connective tissue or bone-forming stroma predominates, it is only possible to obtain smears with little or no useful cell content; we do not, therefore, make smears in these cases.

RESULTS

We classify the results, as in previous publications, as follows:

Positive. When it was possible to establish a definite diagnosis which was confirmed by surgery or by the clinical course.

Doubtful. When the diagnosis was not definite or could not be confirmed because the outcome was unknown.

Negative. When insufficient material was obtained for diagnostic purposes or the diagnosis proved incorrect.

The total number of punctures of the skeleton was 7165, with 5276 positive results (73.65%); 1900 punctures correspond to spine lesions, excluding the sacrococcygeal region, and the remaining 5265 to other bones (Fig. 1 and 2).

The most frequent malignant primary bone tumors in which it was possible to establish a definite diagnosis were the following:

Table

Osteosarcoma (osteogenic sarcoma)	174
Chondrosarcoma	82
Ewing's sarcoma	61
Reticulum-cell sarcoma, primary and secondary (including lymphosarcoma)	65
Myeloma	254
Fibrosarcoma	39
Giant-Cell Tumor (Osteoclastoma)	96
Total	771

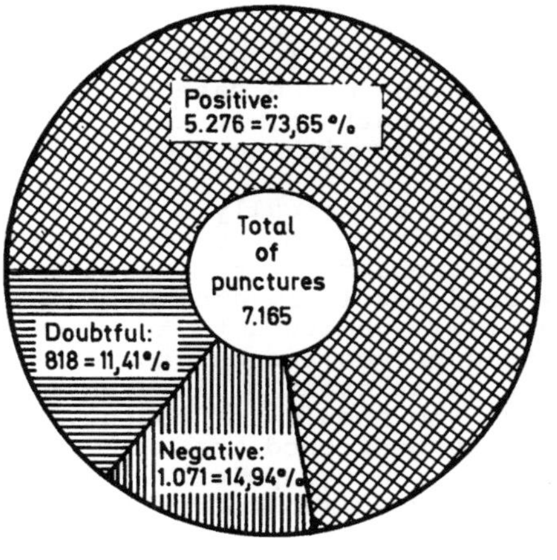

Fig. 1. Results obtained in 7165 punctures

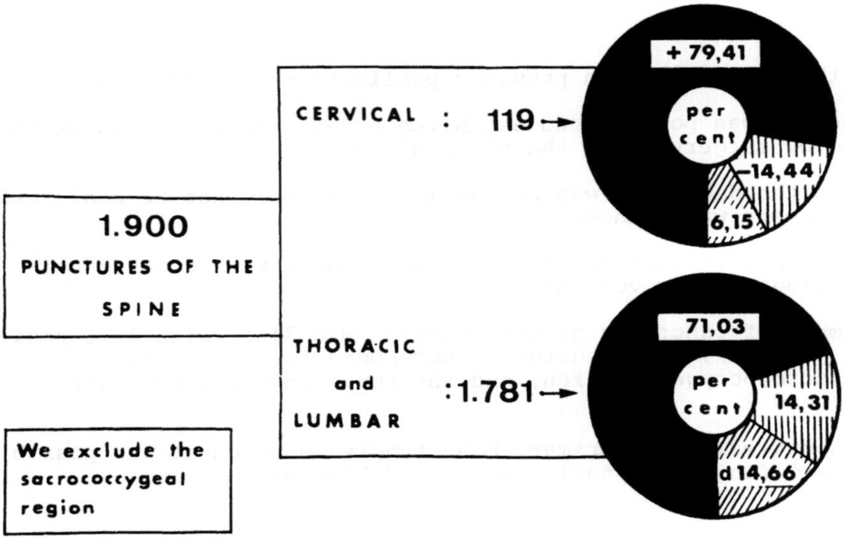

Fig. 2. Results of 1900 punctures of the spine (excluding the sarcrococygeal region); 119 cases involve the cervical spine and 1781 the thoracic and lumbar spine

DISCUSSION

Our experience justifies the recommendation of this method, which is technically simple, involves no risk to the patient, and makes it possible to extract material from a tumor at different dephts and to reach sites which are otherwise only accessible by major surgery. It saves time and money and it can be carried out in the outpatient department. When there is little material or it is insufficient for a conclusive diagnosis, the biopsy can be repeated once or twice without any ill effects. It is always possible to resort to surgical biopsy if the diagnosis remains in doubt.

It is very rarely difficult or impossible to extract sufficient material; even in the case of dense, sclerosing lesions which the needle cannot penetrate, if is often possible to extract the material after perforation with an electric or manual trephine.

Although technically a simple method, aspiration or needle biopsy nevertheless does require some experience on the part of the surgeon, and we have observed that results from medical clinics where this procedure is used regularly are much superior in the quantity and value of the material submitted to the results from clinics where lack of opportunity deprives the surgeon of the necessary experience. In our opinion, this is as great a disadvantage as lack of competence in the pathologist, who should, of course, be experienced in bone pathology. We have already mentioned that the pathologist must be familiar with the clinical and radiographical evidence if he is to interpret the histopathological specimen correctly. On this point we are in full agreement with MARTIN and ELLIS when they state with reference to the needle-biopsy technique which they introduced that "if he knows the exact site, knows what kind of tumors can originate in that region and is completely familiar with the usual sections, the pathologist is in the most favorable position to make a correct diagnosis in the great majority of cases" (5).

SUMMARY

In certain bone tumor cases bone puncture is more profitable than sample excision. Whenever necessary we are using both methods in our practice. The results of 7165 puncture biopsies are presented. A definite diagnosis by needle biopsy could be established in 771 tumors, including 254 myelomas and 174 osteogenic sarcomas. The aspiration or needle biopsy will require some experience not only on the part of the pathologist, but also of the surgeon. The pathologist must be sufficiently familiar with the clinical and radiographic evidence before interpreting the cytologic or the histopathologic specimen.

REFERENCES

1. ACKERMANN, W.: Vertebral trephine biopsy. Ann. Surg. 143, 373-385 (1956)
2. COLEY, B.L., SHARP, G.S., ELLIS, E.B.: Diagnosis of bone tumors by aspiration. Amer. J. Surg. 13, 215-224 (1931)
3. ELLIS, F.: Needle biopsy in the clinical diagnosis of tumours. Brit. J. Surg. 34, 240-261 (1947)
4. FRANKEL, C.J.: Aspiration biopsy of the spine. J. Bone J. Surg. 36A, 69-74 (1954)
5. MARTIN, H.E., ELLIS, E.B.: Aspiration biopsy. Surg. Gynec. Obstet. 59, 578-589 (1934)
6. MARTIN, H.E., STEWART, R.W.: The advantages and limitations of aspiration biopsy. Amer. J. Roentgenol. 35, 245-247 (1936)
7. OTTOLENGHI, C.E.: Diagnosis and Orthopaedic lesions by aspiration biopsy. Results of 1061 punctures. J. Bone Jt Surg. 37A, 443-464 (1955)
8. OTTOLENGHI, C.E.: Aspiration biopsy of the spine. Technique for the thoracic spine and results of twenty-eight biopsies of this region. J. Bone Jt Surg. 51A, 1531-1544 (1969)
9. OTTOLENGHI, C.E., SCHAJOWICZ, F., DE SCHANT, F.A.: Aspiration biopsy of the cervical spine. J. Bone Jt Surg. 46A, 715-733 (1964)
10. RAY, R.D.: Needle biopsy of the lumar vertebral bodies. A modification of the Valls technique. J. Bone Jt. Surg. 35A, 760-762 (1953)
11. SCHAJOWICZ, F.: Aspiration biopsy in bone lesions - cytological and histological techniques. J. Bone Jt Surg. 37A, 465-471, (1955)
11A. SCHAJOWICZ, F., DERQVICH, J.C.: Puncture biopsy in lesions of the locomotor system. Review of results in 4050 cases, including 941 vertebral punctures. Cancer 21, 531-548 (1968)
12. SICARD, A., BOUREAU, M., MARSAN, C.: La biopsie transcutanée des corps vertebraux. J. Chir. 76, 57-75 (1958)
13. SIFFERT, R.S., ARKIN, A.M.: Trephine biopsy of bone with special reference to the limbar vertebral bodies. J. Bone Jt Surg. 31A, 146-149 (1949)
14. SNYDER, R.E., COLEY, B.L.: Further studies on the diagnosis of bone tumors by aspiration biopsy. Surg. Gynec. Obstet. 80, 517-522 (1945)
15. STEWART, F.W.: The diagnosis of tumours by aspiration. Amer. J. Pathol. 9, 801-811 (1933)
16. VALLS, J., OTTOLENGHI, C.E., SCHAJOWICZ, F.: La biopsia por aspiración en el diagnóstico de las lesiones óseas. Bol. y Trab. Acad. Argentina Cir. 25, 147-180, 743-782 (1941)
17. VALLS, J., OTTOLENGHI, C.E., SCHAJOWICZ, F.: La biopsia por aspiración en el diagnóstico de las lesiones óseas. Buenos Aires: El Ateneo 1942

18. VALLS, J., OTTOLENGHI, C.E., SCHAJOWICZ, F.: Aspiration biopsy in diagnosis of lesions of vertebral bodies. J. Amer. med. Ass. 136, 376-382 (1948)
19. VALLS, J., OTTOLENGHI, C.E., SCHAJOWICZ, F.: La biopsia per aspirazione nella diagnosi delle lesioni dei corpi vertebrali. Arch. "putti" di Chir. Org. Movimento 4, 49-68 (1954)

Cytologic and Cytochemical Behavior of Primary Malignant Bone Tumors*

M. SALZER-KUNTSCHIK

Little systematic cytologic investigation has been performed on bone tumors to date (30, 31, 32). There have also been few cytochemical studies, especially of undifferentiated so called round-cell sarcoma of bone (Ewing's sarcoma etc.). Some relevant findings made in own studies carried out during the last four years will therefore be summarized here.

Material and Method. The cytologic investigations were carried out on imprints from specimens sent to the laboratory intraoperatively for frozen-section examination. The imprint preparations were air-dried briefly, then fixed with methanol (p.a. MERCK) and stained according to PAPPENHEIM[1] . The cytochemical and histochemical reactions were performed on cryostat sections and imprint preparations of the same specimens. The following histochemical and cytochemical reactions were applied: PAS and Diastase-PAS (D-PAS) reaction (26), alpha-naphthyl-acetate-esterase (15) and naphthol-AS-acetate-esterase (23) with and without sodium fluoride inhibition (8), naphthol-AS-D-chloracetate-esterase (16), peroxidase (11, 34; 15), alkaline and acid phosphatase (metal salt method; 9); peroxidase reaction for demonstration of hemoglobin (22).

The histologic examination was performed on cryostat sections, with HE staining and PAS and D-PAS reactions, and also on paraffin sections of material fixed in 5 percent neutral formalin with HE staining, PAS and D-PAS reaction, Giemsa staining and reticular-fiber staining according to GOMORI.

Cytologic, cytochemical and histochemical studies of malignant osteoplastic and chondroplastic tumors and of "undifferentiated round-cell sarcoma" of bone were carried out, with special reference to Ewing's sarcoma.

Undifferentiated Round-Cell Sarcoma of Bone. 18 cases of this tumor were available. Age and sex of the patients and localization of the tumors are shown on the table. The histologic behavior of these cases was largely similar. The tumors were characterized by high cellularity and contained no tumor-bound reticular fibers. The monotonous cells displayed round to slightly oval nuclei, often not regularly outlined.

+The Vienna Bone Tumor Registry is supported by the "Österreichen Fond zur Förderung der Wissenschaftlichen Forschung".

[1]PAPPENHEIM staining was carried out in the laboratory of the Baumgartnerhöhe, Lungenheilstätte, Wien; Director: Dr. M. FISCHNALLER.

Nucleoli could not be recognized in large sections in most of these tumors. In many tumors a small nucleolus could be found in each of a few cells. In some cases a small nucleolus was visible in some or many areas. Only in very few tumors were distinct nucleoli demonstrable in many areas. Distinct, thin, but well-defined cytoplasmic borders were recognizable in regressively altered areas only. In this areas single cells had lost their connections with the tumor formations. Elsewhere, the cytoplasm was not clearly outlined, but could be recognized as a rather indistinct reticular or granular pale eosinophilic background between the tumor cells. In areas with densely packed cells the cytoplasm was not visible at all. In several areas delicate cytoplasmic extensions were visible between the tumor cells.

Cytologic examination of these 18 cases revealed that all the cell nucleoli behaved more or less identically (Figs. 1 and 2). They were mostly round to oval, some of them flattened on one side and occasionally dented, with a delicate nuclear membrane. In one case (4620/74), deeply grooved nuclei were seen at infrequent points. The coloring ranged from light pink to dark violet. In the consistently dense, finely granular chromatin network no nucleoli could be recognized in small or large samples of tumor cells, but there were differences from tumor to tumor. In most other cells two to five nucleoli were found, occasionally six or seven small, usually not very distinct light nucleoli (Figs. 1, 2). In a few tumors, nuclei with one or two larger and more distinct nucleoli were also found. There were quantitative differences from tumor to tumor, and some of the nuclei were not surrounded by clearly defined cytoplasm (Fig. 1). They appeared to lie in a pale blue-gray reticular background, which is comparable with the indistinct cytoplasmic background in the histologic sections (Figs. 1, 2). The remaining tumor cells displayed cytoplasmic borders with different morphological behavior in the various tumors. In order to approach a possible subclassification of the nondifferentiated round-cell sarcoma of bone, the tumors examined were classified into four cytological groups according to their cytoplasmic nature

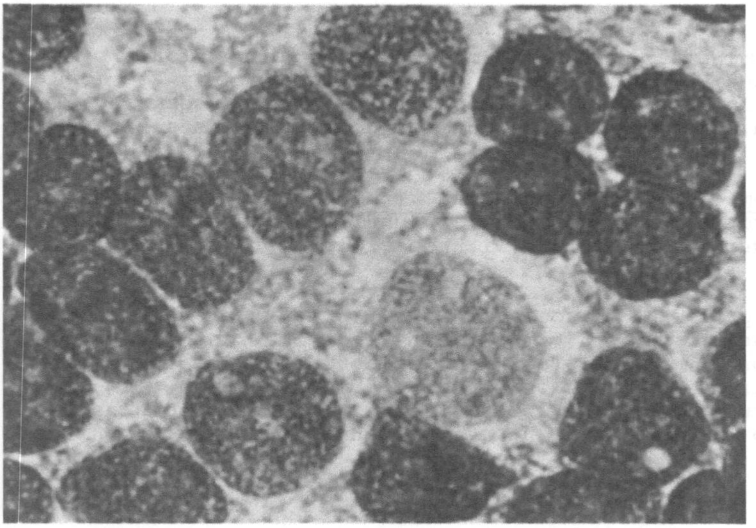

Fig. 1. K.H. ♂, 13 yrs, 13956/72. Glycogen weakly positive (+), round-cell sarcoma of scapula. Cytological group II, Pappenheim, 500 x. Light and dark nuclei; chromatin equally finely granular; no distinct cytoplasm; background of cytoplasmic frame-work; some cells with one or more nucleoli

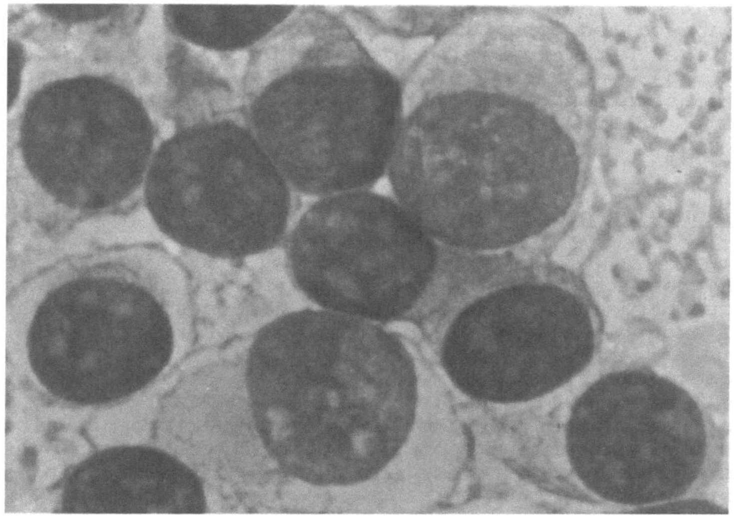

Fig. 2. T.A. ♂, 16 yrs, 4091/73. Glycogen strongly positive (+++), round-cell sarcoma of Os ilium. Cytological group I, Pappenheim, 500 x. Cytoplasmatic framework in background, and cells with varying amounts of cytoplasm, mostly well delineated, some without sharp cell borders

Group I. A large number of cells displayed pale gray-bluish cytoplasm (Fig. 2). This varied in width from case to case and also from cell to cell within a single tumor. The cytoplasmic borders appeared indistinct in parts, and were gradually lost in the surrounding similarly-stained reticular background. Many cells showed well-outlined cytoplasm. The nuclei were located either centrally or often somewhat excentrically within the cytoplasm.

Group II. Many cells displayed cytoplasmic conditions similar to those of Group I. In addition, cells were found in which the very pale cytoplasm seemed to have condensed to a very thin intensively basophilic rim in the outer parts. Occasionally there were nuclei, which were surrounded by narrow, in some cases vacuolated, strongly basophilic cytoplasm. One case in this group (4620/74) appeared particularly striking in that often deeply grooved nuclei and occasionally a very fine, azurophilic cytoplasmic granulation were visible. Such cells resembled monocytes. In one case in Group I and also in two cases in Group III, delicate azurophilic granules were also recognized in the cytoplasm.

Group III. Similar cells to those in group II were detectable in this Group: besides these, cells with a thin or somewhat more abundant cytoplasmic rim with different grades of basophilia were visible.

In all these three groups small and large cell formations were observed in addition to individually located cells. The cytoplasmic borders of the densely packed cell masses appeared indistinct in some cases and were not recognizable at all in others.

Group IV. In this Group no glycogen was demonstrable in the cells. Some cells had no visible cytoplasm, while numerous others, some of which were arranged in clusters, proved to have scanty intensively basophilic cytoplasmic rims surrounding the nuclei.

The histochemical and cytochemical behavior of the undifferentiated round-celled bone tumors investigated was not the same in all groups or even within one single group. Only with the peroxidase reaction (11, 34; see also 15-17) and the Lepehne peroxidase reaction for the demonstration of hemoglobin (22) were results in all the tumors negative. The results of the other reactions are seen in the Table.

Discussion of the Results with Round Cell Sarcomas of Bone

The results reveal no cytologically, or cyto- or histochemically uniform behavior of the round-cell sarcomas of bone, even under conditions of exceptionally similar histologic profiles.

Accordingly, there is wide-spread speculation as to whether the round-cell sarcoma of bone is a single neoplastic entity or embraces different tumor types, whether any histogenetic conclusions are possible, and whether the presence or absence of glycogen can justifiably be regarded as a decisive criterion for the diagnosis of Ewing's sarcoma as a tumor entity.

According to the presently accepted definition of Ewing's sarcoma, proof of a high glycogen content has been required (5, 6, 36, 37, 38, 40) for diagnosis of this tumor ever since this was discovered in Ewing's sarcomas (36). It is quite possible that this criterion has not yet been checked systematically for its accuracy. Only occasionally have doubts been expressed as to the diagnostic value of glycogen in classifying Ewing's sarcoma (32, 33). With an estimated graduation of the glycogen content from negative to ++++ positive (Table) wide variations were demonstrated in the four groups subjected to cytologic examination. As well as tumors with moderate to very high glycogen contents (++ to ++++), which - according to the present definition - would be freely interpreted as Ewing's sarcomas, two cases were found in Group II and one case in Group III, in which only isolated tumor cells contained scanty glycogen granules (+). These two cases, together with a glycogen-negative case in each of Groups I, III and IV, cannot be clearly attached to any category in the current bone tumor classification system. Since the glycogen content in the histologically similar cases examined exhibited quantitively pronounced variations between individual tumors and also within the same tumors, we could rather not assign an unconditionally decisive diagnostic role to the glycogen content in classifying round-cell tumors of bone. This argument is further supported by the fact that in one of our cases (Group III: 419/71 and 16703/73), the primary tumor (7035/66), which was not examined cytologically or cytochemically except for glycogen, and also two lung metastases, which were removed surgically five years later, contained glycogen, while the local recurrence seven years after irradiation of the primary tumor appeared glycogen-negative. In order to support this assumption it should be mentioned, for instance, that the glycogen content is not a reliable diagnostic criterion for the differential diagnosis of neoplasms of the erythro- and myelopoetic or the lymphatic system. Acute lymphatic leukemia and acute erythremia, for example, normally exhibit a high glycogen content, but there are wide quantitative variations (12, 17, 25, 42). In contrast to the earlier opinion, we now know that monocytic and myelocytic leukoses can give a coarsely lumpy glycogen reaction (12, 17, 18). In contrast to the cells of the normal erythromyelopoetic system, polysaccharides can appear in large amounts in very immature cells of malignant hemoblastoses as well as in cells in which it is not demonstrable at all under physiological conditions (42). The value of the glycogen reaction in the differentiation of leukoses has,

Table

Histological number	NN	sex	age	localization primary tumour	cytolog. groups	PAS	αN	NAS	ASDCL	alk.P.	acid P.
11366/71	W.E.	♀	1 1/2	femur	I	+++	-	-	-	o	o
11926/73	L.H.	♂	16	os ilium	I	++++	+	-	-	-	+++
4091/73	T.A.	♂	16	os ilium	I	+++	-	-	-	-	++
7865/73	-"-		-"-	(meta lungs)							
13336/73	-"-		-"-	(meta lungs)							
6274/73	K.C.	♀	13	femur	I	+++	++	-	-	-	++
5279/74	H.C.	♀	25	tibia	I	-	-	-	-	-	+++
6009/74	H.R.	♀	14	femur	I	+++	++	++	-	++	-
3578/70	H.C.	♀	17	costa	II	+++	-	-	-	o	o
3812/71	B.A.	♂	10	tibia	II	++++	++	-	-	o	o
8921/72	F.W.	♂	21	humerus	II	++	+++	++	-	++	-
13956/72	K.H.	♂	13	scapula	II	+	++	-	-	o	o
3951/74	G.E.	♀	12	rib	II	+++	++	++-+++	++	-	-
9269/74	K.H.	♂	28	femur	II	+	→+++	→+++	-	-	-
4620/74	Sch.P.	♀	11	os ilium	II	++	+++	++++	++	++	-
419/71	R.H.	♂	12	meta lungs	III	++	-	-	-	o	o
16703/73	-"-			humerus (recurrence)	III	-	-	-	-	++	-
6201/71	Sch.S.	♂	23	femur	III	++++	-	-	-	o	o
2953/72	K.E.	♀	28	fibula	III	+++	++	++	-	++	+++
9605/73	Sch.R.	♀	13	os ilium	III	+	-	-	-	++	-
5969/72	W.G.	♀	9	scapula	IV	-	-	-	-	-	-
12624/72	-"-		-"-	(recurrence)	IV	-	++-+++	-	-	-	-

αN = α-naphthylacetate esterase; NAS = Naphthol-AS-acetate esterase; ASDCL = ASD-chloracetate esterase; alk.P. = alkaline phosphatase; acidP. = acid Phosphatase.
o means no reaction was done. - means reaction was negative.
+, ++, +++, ++++ means the quantitative estimated reaction: + a few fine positive granula in some cells.
++ some fine granules in many or most cells; or a weak diffuse colouring in ASDCL.
+++ many fine granules in the whole cytoplasm of most cells;
PAS +++ clumps in addition in some cells, PAS ++++ clumps in many cells.

contrary to previous opinions, proved to be limited. The same may be true for differentiation of the round-cell sarcomas of bone.

Cytologic behavior in Group I was uniform except for variations in the amount of cytoplasm. In all cases examined except one, a positive acid phosphatase reaction was seen after incubation for 60 minutes. The high glycogen content of most cases of this group together with the positive acid phosphatase reaction suggest that a tumor of lymphocytic origin as well as one of monocytic origin has to be considered. With respect to the very different opinions concerning the morphologic and cytochemical behavior (unspecific esterases and acid phosphatase) of the reticulum cells and the reticulum-cell sarcomas (4, 7, 17, 19, 20, 21, 27, 41, etc.), the inference of conclusions concerning a tumor of this type is not easy. It should be kept in mind that the positive acid phosphatase reaction suggests reticulo-sarcomas. The acid phosphatase-negative case in this group (6009/74) could also be accomodated under this heading. The positive alkaline phosphatase reaction in this and a second case (5279/74) in this group defies interpretation at present. A positive alkaline phosphatase reaction with reticulum cells is reported occasionally (27); this is denied by other authors (17, 19).

The cytologic behavior of tumors in Group II was also largely similar. One case (4620/74) differed from the others in that it displayed cells with strongly grooved nuclei and a fine azurophilic granulation in the cytoplasm, identical to monocytes as well as cells similar to those found in the other tumors. The strongly positive naphthol-AS-acetate-esterase reaction inhibited by sodium fluoride in this case and in a second one (9269/74), the cells of which were cytologically not differentiated and were unmistakably monocytes, makes it believable that these two tumors were sarcomas of the monocytic series. The weakly positive ASD-chloracetate-esterase reaction in one of the two cases is also suggestive of this.

The acid phosphatase reaction was negative. The possibility that leukoses might develop from both these tumors cannot yet be excluded, due to the short follow-up period (3 and 6 months) of the patients, who are under constant observation. The positive alkaline phosphatase reaction in these cases and in one more in this group (8921/72) cannot be interpreted with certainty at present.

With respect to the largely similar cytologic behavior of all cases in this group, it should be remembered that in spite of the negative and only weakly positive naphtol-AS-acetate-esterase reaction in some cases, tumors of the monocytic system may also be present. It is known that during increasing dedifferentiation in monoblastic leukemia, the naphthol-AS-acetate-esterase reaction declines first (17). One case (3951/74) in this group was the only round-cell sarcoma of bone that displayed analogous tumor cells in the peripheral blood (13%) and within the sternal marrow (3%) before cytostatic therapy. The ASD-chloracetate-esterase reaction was weakly positive in this case, as was the naphthol-AS-acetate-esterase reaction, which was not completely inhibitable by sodium fluoride. The possibility of a tumor-forming leukosis of the myelocytic or monocytic series must be considered in this case.

Cytologic behavior was least uniform in Group III, varying in the amount of cytoplasm present and the stages of basophilia. One case (2953/72) demonstrated a distinctly positive alkaline phosphatase reaction as well as a weakly positive alpha-naphthyl-acetate-esterase reaction and naphthol-AS-acetate-esterase reaction which was inhibitable by sodium fluoride, along with a strongly positive acid phosphatase reaction. This tumor could perhaps also be assigned to the monoblastic series. In view of the positive acid and alkaline phosphatase reactions, a tumor of the erythroblastic series must be considered. A tumor of lymphocytic origin can not be excluded completely, as recent examinations have revealed that, in contrast to earlier views, alkaline phosphatase-positive lymphocytes can appear in humans as well as in many animal species (13, 35). In one case (419/71 and 16703/73), holes and cleft structures lined by tumor cells were demonstrated histologically in many sections of the primary tumor (7035/66), which had not been subjected to any further cytological or cytochemical examination, in two surgically removed lung metastases (419/71). On the basis of these findings and the distinctly positive alkaline phosphatase reaction, the existence of a primitive tumor was considered, which could be traced back to endothelial cells. According to the suggestion for classification of the cells of the monocytic series (14), again, there may be some connection with the monocytic sarcomas. In the opinion of these authors the endothelial cells of the sinus of the bone marrow are derived from monocytes.

The case in Group IV displayed no sort of cytologic similarity to the cases in Groups I-III. This tumor is thought to be a stem-cell tumor or undifferentiated blast tumor, on the basis of the negative behavior of all cytochemical reactions of the tumor cells, many of which had a narrow, intensively basophilic cytoplasmic rim. In the recurrence following this tumor the alpha-naphthyl-acetate-esterase reaction appeared strongly positive, in contrast to that of the primary tumor, a feature which could be interpreted as indicative of differentiation of the tumor.

OSTEOSARCOMA

When imprint preparations of osteoplastic parts of the tumor were used, cytologic examination of 23 osteosarcomas revealed a high degree of polymorphism; cells were round, oval, triangular or polygonal, often with eccentrically located nucleis (Fig. 3). The cytoplasm showed a changing basophilia, and in some cases a recognizable but often not

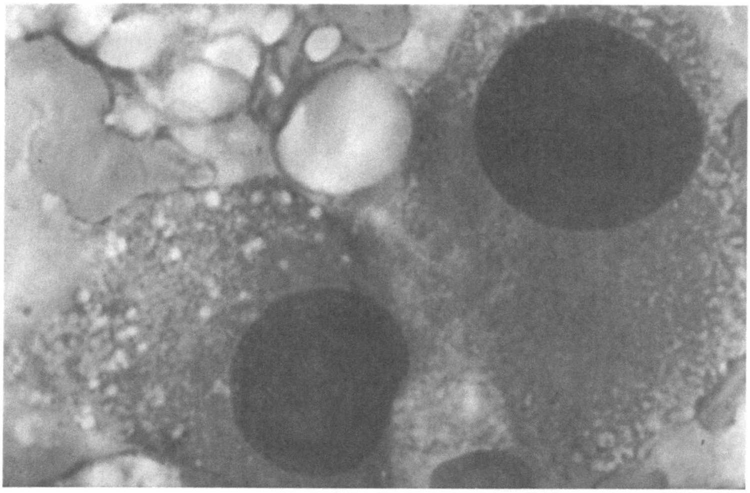

Fig. 3. G.M. ♂, 6 yrs, 12914/72. Osteosarcoma of femur. Pappenheim, 500 x. 2 malignant osteoblasts, nucleus eccentrically located

really distinct delineation. The cells were repeatedly seen in small clusters. The nuclei were dark violet. These cells have a malignant counterpart in osteoblasts. In comparison, nonmalignant osteoblasts from osteoblastoma, osteoid osteoma, Paget's osteodystrophia fibrosa, myositis ossificans and reactive bone neoformation show no polymorphism; they are smaller; the cytoplasm is developed more abundantly in comparison to the nucleus. The nucleus is located eccentrically and, in contrast to the malignant osteoblasts of the osteosarcoma, there is perinuclear cytoplasmic clearing (archoplasma). In addition, characteristic malignant osteoblasts were often found in the undifferentiated parts of osteosarcomas, in which only abortive bone neoformation or none at all was demonstrable histologically. The alkaline phosphatase reaction was positive in these cells. In imprints from fibroplastic parts of osteosarcomas there were polymorphic spindle cells like those found in fibrosarcomas, and in imprints of chondroplastic areas there were cells like those that can be found in chondrosarcomas.

The eight chondrosarcomas examined also revealed an extremely variable appearance cytologically, which corresponds histologically to the signs of malignancy. Chondrosarcoma cells are roundish and of different sizes (Fig. 4a - c). Their cytoplasm (Fig. 4a - c) sometimes reacts amphoterically. However, in most of our cases there was basophilia of varying degrees, ranging from pale blue to intensive dark blue. The amount of cytoplasm varied according to the dedifferentiation of the tumor. The roundish nuclei appeared to be light and loosely structured or very dark and dense; their sizes varied (Fig. 4a - c). The frequency of binuclear and multinuclear cells and cells with giant nuclei rose with increasing anaplasticity of the tumor. Nucleoli were not recognizable in most cases; sometimes there were two, occasionally several, and they varied in size. The cytoplasm is outlined with varying degrees of clarity, and often vacuolized. In imprints from myxomatous parts the cytoplasm has drawn-out tips. The nuclei of most cases are located centrally in the cell.

In comparison, a chondromyxoid fibroma contained smaller cells than the chondrosarcoma. The cytoplasm exhibited moderately pronounced basophilia and often had irregularly drawn-out tips, but it was distinctly outlined. Some nuclei were pale while others were hyperchromatic,

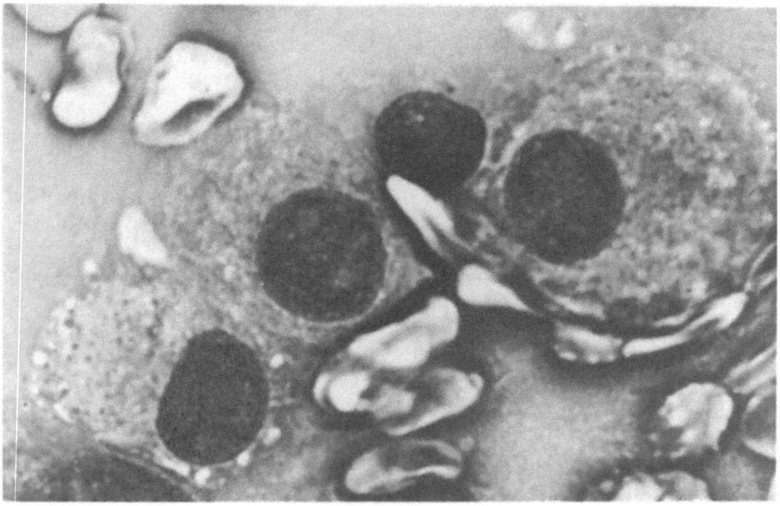

a

b

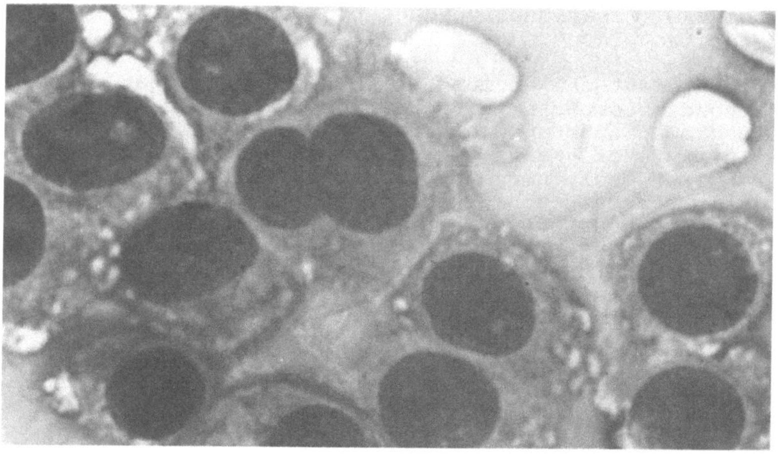

c

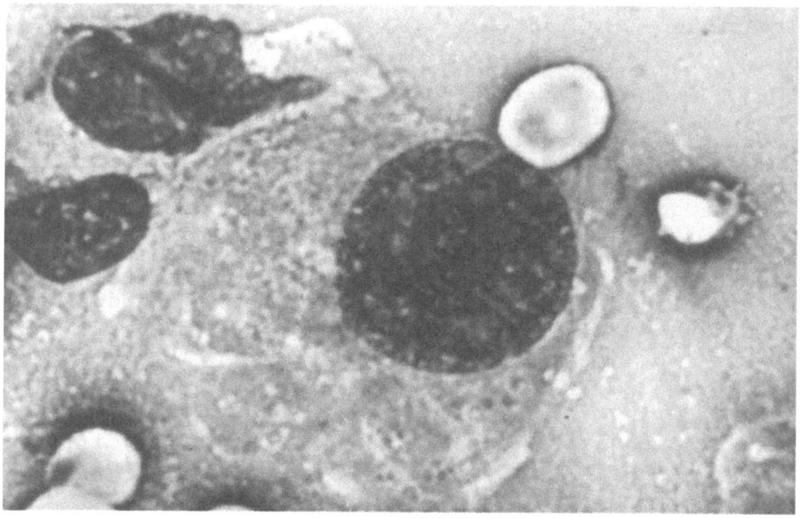

Fig. 4a - c. St.D. ♀, 42 yrs. Chondrosarcoma of sacrum; Pappenheim, 500 x. (a) cells of a tumor section with low histologic malignancy; relatively large amount of palely stained cytoplasm; (b) cells of a histologically more anaplastic section of the tumor; less and more basophilic cytoplasm than in 4a; (c) tumor cell with a giant-nucleus

and they also varied in size; occasional binuclear cells were also detected.

The cells of a chondroblastoma, which is rich in giant cells and has sparsely developed ground substance, were relatively uniform, including mononuclear as well as multinucleoled cells. The round nuclei stained dark violet without distinct structure, and were surrounded by an intensively basophilic, in most cases sharply defined, narrow, round cytoplasm. Occasionally the cytoplasm had slightly drawn-out tails in one or two places.

Since a giant-cell tumor has to be ruled out at differential diagnosis of chondroblastomas that are rich in giant cells and devoid of chondroid ground substance or develop only small amounts of it, the cytologic picture of giant-cell tumors should also be mentioned: the cells of a giant-cell tumor have roundish, although sometimes more oval nuclei, in contrast to the chondroblastoma. Their cytoplasm varies in width but never shows such intensive basophilia as that present in chondroblastoma. The alpha-naphtyl-acetate-esterase reaction is strongly positive with both tumors; however, the chondroblastoma has a high glycogen content in its tumor cells, while the glycogen reaction is negative in the giant-cell tumor.

Sometimes the differentiation between chondrosarcoma and chordoma in the sacral region presents difficulties. One chordoma was investigated cytologically. An absolutely characteristic cytologic picture was revealed; the cells were rich in cytoplasm; the nuclei, most of which were centrally located, were round and displayed a moderate coloration. The cytoplasm varied from faintly basophilic to colorless and cloudy. There was multiple indenting of the outer contour of the cell boundary, of a type that was never found in the chondrosarcomas examined. The borders of the cells, which were arranged in clusters in some parts, were often indistinct.

The use of cytologic and cytochemical technics in the investigation of round-cell sarcoma of bone thus allows us to draw substantially more conclusions than does histologic examination only. A cytologically and cytochemically nonuniform tumor pool seems to be involved in this group. It seems entirely possible that the positive glycogen reaction is not a conclusive criterion for the classification of such tumors as a uniform Ewing's sarcoma group. Conclusions concerning the histogenesis lead to the opinion that these neoplasms include tumors of the monocytic series and probably also tumors of lymphocytic origin and reticulum-cell sarcomas, and occasionally tumors of the myelocytic and erythroplastic series, as well as tumors of endothalial origin and stem-cell tumors. Cytologic investigations and cytochemical reactions, especially those now used for the differentiation of leukoses, seem to be necessary for the classification of these tumors.

In instances of osteosarcomas and chondrosarcomas there are characteristic cytologic pictures with possibilities for differential diagnosis, in connection with the application of histochemical reactions, and for comparison of benign tumors of the osteoplastic and chondroplastic series with giant-cell tumors and chordoma.

SUMMARY

Cytologic and cytochemical examination of eighteen cases of round-cell sarcoma of bone allowed classification of these tumors into four cytologic groups. Additional cytochemical examinations based on the PAS and D-PAS reactions, and the demonstration of the activity of peroxidase, naphtol-ASD-Chloracetate esterase, alpha-naphthylacetate esterase, naphthol-AS-acetate esterase with and without sodium fluoride inhibition, acid and alkaline phosphatases yielded no evidence of uniform behavior among the individual groups or within any single group. The studies showed that a positive glycogen reaction cannot be used as a basic criterion for the classification of such tumors as Ewing's sarcoma and for regarding them as a uniform tumor group. It is possible that a pool of tumors is involved, including tumors of monocytic and probably of lymphocytic origin, reticulum-cell sarcoma, tumors of myelocytic and erythroplastic origin, stem-cell tumors, and endothelial-cell tumors. Histologic examination alone is not sufficient for the classification of round-cell sarcomas of bone, and it should be supplemented by cytologic and cytochemical or histochemical methods.

Osteosarcomas (23 cases) and chondrosarcomas (8 cases) display cells which are characteristic for these tumors and which could be correlated with their benign counterparts, osteoblasts and chondroid cells. The histologically recognizable degree of malignancy of chondrosarcoma can be evaluated better with the cytologic than with the histologic technic. Indications of the possibilities of differential diagnosis based on the cytologic pictures of benign and malignant osteoplastic and chondroplastic tumors, giant-cell tumors and chordoma are discussed.

REFERENCES

1. ARNOLD, M.: Histochemie. Berlin Heidelberg New York: Springer 1968
2. BARKA, T., ANDERSON, P.J.: Histochemistry. New York, Evanston, London: Harper & Row 1968
3. BEGEMANN, H., RASTETTER, J.: Atlas der klinischen Hämatologie. Heidelberg, New York: Springer 1972
4. BEGEMANN, H., RASTETTER, J., KABOTH, W.: Klinische Hämatologie. Stuttgart: Thieme 1970
5. DAHLIN, D.C.: Bone tumors, 2nd ed. Springfield, Ill.: Thomas 1967
6. DOMINOK, G.W., KNOCH, H.G.: Knochengeschwülste und geschwulstähnliche Knochenerkrankungen. Jena: Fischer 1971
7. DORFMAN, R.F.: Enzyme Histochemistry of Normal Hyperplastic and Neoplastic lymphoreticular Tissues. Symp. Lymph. Tumors in Africa-Paris 1963. Basel, New York: Karger 1964
8. FISCHER, R., SCHMALZL, F.: Über die Hemmbarkeit der Esteraseaktivität in Blutmonozyten durch Natriumflorid. Klin. Wschr. 42, 751 (1964)
9. GOMORI, cit.: BARKA, T., ANDERSON, P.J.: Histochemistry
10. GOMORY, TAKAMATSU: cit.: BARKA, T., ANDERSON, P.J.: Histochemistry
11. GRAHAM, KNOLL: cit.: Undritz, 1972
12. KAHN, P.: Zytochemische Befunde während Therapie von Leukosen. In: Chemo- u. Immunotherapie der Leukosen und malignen Lymphome. International Workshop, Vienna 1969 (Ed. A. Stacher). Vienna: Bohmann 1969
13. KAPLOW, L.S.: Alkaline phosphatase activity in peripheral blood lymphocytes. Arch. Path. 88, 69 (1969)
14. LANGEVOOT, H.L., COHN, Z.A., HIRSCH, J.G., HUMPHREY, J.H., SPECTOR, W.G., VAN FURTH, R.: cit.: Meuret
15. LEDER, L.D.: Über die selektive fermentzytochemische Darstellung von neutrophilen myeloischen Zellen und Gewebsmastzellen im Paraffinschnitt. Klin. Wschr. 42, 553 (1964)
16. LEDER, L.D.: Zur Praxis der bioptischen Hämoblastosediagnostik mit zytochemischen Methoden. Beitr. Path. 141, 396 (1970)
17. LEDER, L.D.: Zytochemische Differenzierung normaler mononukleärer Blut- und Knochenmarkszellen. Acta histochem. Suppl. 9, 141 (1971)
18. LEINONEN, E.A.: Cytochemical Studies of Acute Leukemias. Acta Haematol. 43, 219 (1970)
19. LENNERT, K.: Handbuch d. spez. path. anat- Hist. Bd- 1/3: Lymphknoten. Berlin, Göttingen, Heidelberg: Springer 1961
20. LENNERT, K.: Pathologie der Halslymphknoten. Berlin, Göttingen, Heidelberg: Springer 1964

21. LENNERT, K., LEDER, L.D., LÖFFLER, H.: Fermenthistochemische Untersuchungen des Lymphknotens. Virchows Archiv path. Anat. 338, 285 (1965)
22. LEPEHNE: cit.: Undritz, 1972
23. LÖFFLER, H.: Zytochemischer Nachweis von unspezifischer Esterase in Ausstrichen. Beiträge zur Technik und Ergebnisse im Blutausstrich des Menschen. Klin. Wschr. 39, 1220 (1961)
24. LÖFFLER, H.: Zytochemische Klassifizierung der akuten Leukosen. In: Chemo- und Immunotherapie der Leukosen und malignen Lymphome. International Workshop, Vienna 1969 (Ed. A. Stacher). Vienna: Bohmann 1969
25. LORBACHER, P.: Zytochemischer β-Glukuronidasenachweis, ein Beitrag zur Differenzierung lymphatischer Leukosen. In: Chemo- und Immunotherapie der Leukosen und malignen Lymphome. International Workshop, Vienna 1969 (Ed. A. Stacher). Vienna: Bohmann 1969
26. MCMANUS: cit.: Arnold
27. MERKER, H.: Zytochemie der Blutzellen. In: Handb. d. inneren Medizin, Vol. II/1. Berlin, Heidelberg, New York: Springer 1968
28. MEURET, G.: Monozytopoese beim Menschen (Vol. 13 of Hämatologie und Bluttransfusion). Munich: Lehmann 1974
29. PIETSCHMANN, H.: Der Lymphozyt. 1. Tagungsbericht der österreichischen Gesellschaft für Hämatologie. Vienna: Wiener Medizin. Akademie 1972
30. RAJCIC, V.: Zytodiagnostik der Knochenkrankheiten, Bilt. transf. 21, 133 (1966)
31. RAJCIC, V.: Zytodiagnostik der Knochentumoren. Libri oncol. I, Suppl. 1, 1435 (1972)
32. SALZER-KUNTSCHIK, M.: Zytologisches Verhalten primärer maligner Knochentumoren. Verh. Dtsch. Ges. Path. 57, 280 (1973)
33. SALZER-KUNTSCHIK, M.: Zur Beurteilung von Probeentnahmen bei Knochentumoren. Verh. Dtsch. Ges. Path. 58 (1974) (in press)
34. SCHÄFER, H.E., FISCHER, R.: Der Peroxydasenachweis an Ausstrichpräparaten sowie an Gewebsschnitten nach Entkalkung und Paraffineinbettung. Klin. Wschr. 46, 1228 (1968)
35. SCHÄFER, H.E., NIEDERALT, G., FISCHER, R.: Alkalische Phosphatase in Lymphozyten. In: H. Pietschmann, Der lymphozyt. Tagungsbericht d. Österr. Ges. f. Hämatologie. Vienna: Wiener Medizin. Akademie 1972
36. SCHAJOWICZ, F.: Ewing's sarcoma and reticulum-cell sarcoma of bone with special reference to the histochemical demonstration of glycogen as an aid to differential diagnosis. J. Bone Jt Surg. 41A, 349 (1959)
37. SCHAJOWICZ, F., ACKERMAN, L.V., SISSONS, H.A.: Histological Typing of Bone Tumours. Internat. Histological Classification of Tumours. Geneva: WHO 1972
38. SPJUT, H.J., DORFMAN, H.D., FECHNER, R.E., ACKERMAN, L.V.: Tumors of Bone and Cartilage. Atlas of Tumor Pathology. Armed Forces Inst. Washington: 1971
39. STACHER, A. (Ed.): Chemo- u. Immunotherapie der Leukosen und Malignen Lymphome. International Workshop, Vienna 1969. Vienna: Bohmann 1969
40. UEHLINGER, E.: Geschwülste des retikuloendothelialen Systems. In: Hdb. d. Ges. Hämatol. Bd. V/1. Munich: Urban & Schwarzenberg 1964
41. UNDRITZ, E.: Die Differentialdiagnose der malignen Hämoblastosen. In: Chemo- und Immunotherapie der Leukosen und malignen Lymphome. International Workshop, Vienna, 1969 (Ed. A. Stacher). Vienna: Bohmann 1969
42. UNDRITZ, E.: Hämatolog. Tafeln. Bask: Sandoz 1972
43. WHO: Burkitt's Tumor. Bulletin. Geneva: WHO 1969

Histochemical and Electron-Microscopic Aspects of Bone Tumor Diagnosis

W. REMAGEN, F. GUDAT, and P. HEITZ

In recent years, special methods have been increasingly introduced into the investigation of bone tumors, namely, electron microscopy, histochemistry, and organ culture. Examples of cartilage- and bone-forming tumors are used in this paper to illustrate the contributions that can be made by histochemistry and electron microscopy, and their limitations, in differential diagnosis.

Histochemical and, in particular, enzyme-histochemical, investigations of bone tumors have hitherto been relatively rare, except in the case of Ewing's sarcoma: According to SCHAJOWICZ the demonstration of glycogen is essential for diagnosis of this tumor (19, 20). Recent findings, however, should encourage us to adopt a more flexible approach to this problem (18).

It is quite interesting to compare matrix production observed in different cartilage-forming tumors by histochemical methods. At acid pH values, the glycosaminoglycans display a qualitatively quite uniform pattern in a number of histologically rather different cartilaginous tumors. On differentiation of the different components by means of alcian blue (22), all of them are shown to contain weakly acid sulfomucins in fairly large quantities. In cartilaginous callus tissue, strongly acid sulfomucins are also found in large quantities. In callus tissue and in sarcomas, hyaluronic acid and sialomucin are found in significant quantities, whereas the reaction is weak in osteochondroma. In enchondroma and in the parts of chondroblastoma with cartilaginous differentiation, the findings are like those in osteochondroma. The rich concentration of hyaluronic acid and sialomucins in the fast-growing cartilaginous tissues, namely callus and sarcomas, appears to be quite characteristic. In this property they differ from chondroblastoma. On the other hand, these findings are further evidence for the view that chondroblastoma is a tumor derived from cartilaginous tissue (29). Up to now, enzyme histochemistry of tumorous conditions has not yielded more than scattered findings. It is already possible, however, to draw certain conclusions from the enzymatic pattern. If acid and alkaline phosphatases are considered as key enzymes of formation and destruction of mesenchymal matrix, the extraordinarily low concentration of these enzymes in chondrosarcomas is conspicuous. In this respect, these tumors differ clearly from epiphyseal growth cartilage, which shows considerable activity of alkaline and acid phophatase. Similarly, chondroblastoma which contains parts with cartilaginous differentiation and completely cellular parts, shows no activity of alkaline phosphatase in the cartilaginous parts and only scanty activity in the cellular parts, again behaving like a cartilaginous tumor rather than one derived from reticulohistiocytic elements (26). A brief recapitulation of the meaning of this phosphatase activity might be appropriate. In the literature, the interpretation of findings has changed. It was originally felt that enzyme activity was connected with the formation of organic matrix (2, 11, 24). Later on, the hypothesis was put forward that these enzymes regulated the deposition and the dissolution of mineral in the matrix. Pyrophosphates are thought to block the precipitation of calcium phosphate in the tissue. When the cells of this tissue produce phosphatase, the pyrophosphates are dissociated, and thus the conditions for the precipitation of calcium salts are created. Apparently, at least in vitro, phosphatases are capable of pyrophosphate dissolution. On the other hand, the apatite crystals in the tissue are thought to be covered by pyrophosphate, which blocks their dissolution. If the cells of those tissues produce phosphatase, the pyrophosphate cover is destroyed and the apatite crystal is thus rendered more soluble (5). There are experimental and clinical findings that support this hypothesis (25, 17). Within this framework it is interesting to compare the pattern of phosphatases in benign and malignant tumorous bone conditions. The activity pattern of alkaline phosphatase in fibrous dysplasia is a good example of a benign condition; the cells of the connective-tissue stroma show a certain amount of activity, which is considerably increased in regions of bone formation (Fig. 1). The enzyme appears to have a rôle in the formation of organic bone matrix, since, if the primitive fiber bone trabeculae mineralize at all, they do so with considerable retardation. However, the young osteocytes in these fiber bone trabeculae also show alkaline phosphatase activity. This seems to indicate that mineralization is also influenced by this enzyme. Apparently, with the same histochemical method, multiple kinds of enzymes with alkaline pH optima are demonstrated, which are active in the formation of matrix as well as in mineralization. Activity of acid phosphatase is almost exclusively restricted to the very few osteoclasts. This pattern is very similar to that seen in nonossifying fibroma (12). Comparison of these findings with those made in a malignant bone-forming tumor, i.e. osteosarcoma, reveals a completely different pattern. There is a rather pronounced activity of

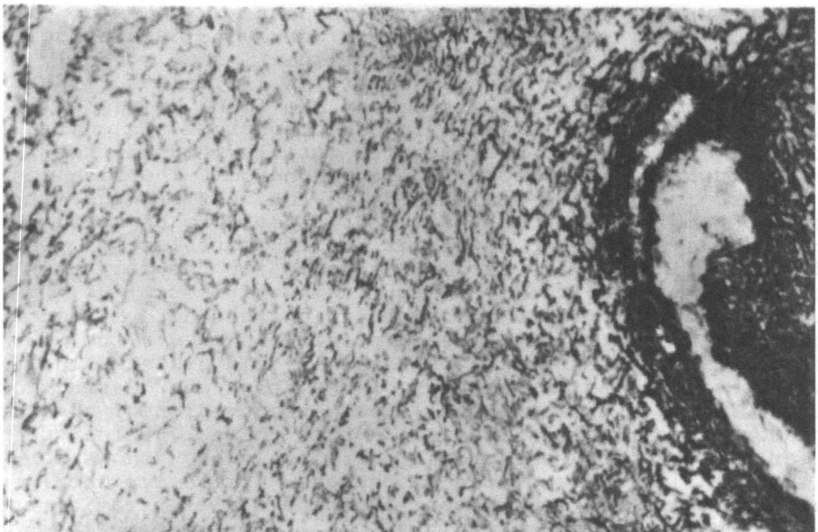

Fig. 1. Fibrous dysplasia, alkaline phosphatase: moderate activity in the stroma cells, considerably increasing around metaplastically formed bone trabecula (right). α-naphthyl phosphate, Echt blau BB, 126 x

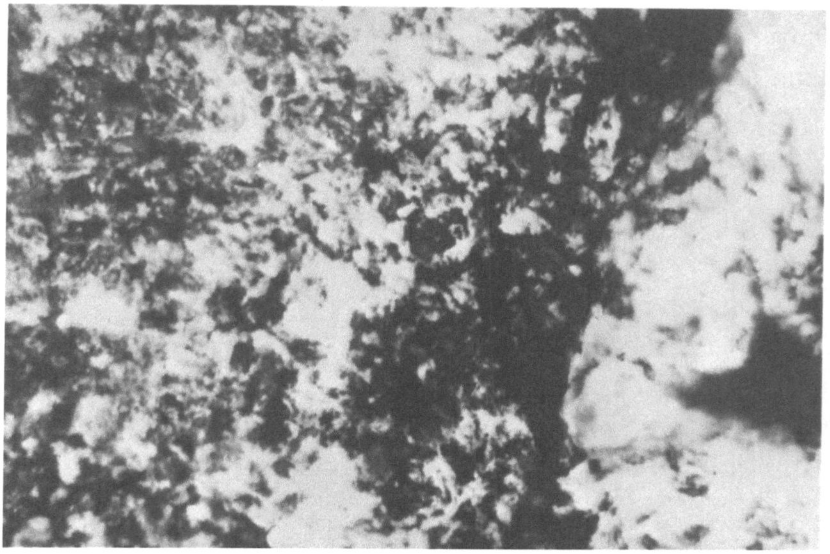

Fig. 2. Osteosarcoma, alkaline phosphatase: marked activity in the regions without and with (right) bone formation. α-naphthyl phosphate, Echt blau BB, 252 x

alkaline phosphatase in the tumor cells, which do not display any distinctive differences between the regions with or without bone formation (Fig. 2). This enzymatic activity must be regarded as associated with the production of matrix. In contrast to the situation in fibrous dysplasia, all the tumor cells also show extremely significant activity of acid phosphatase (Fig. 3). As this enzyme is considered to be the key enzyme of the lysosomes, it indicates pronounced cyto- and histolytic activity. After comparing this activity with the low activity found in chondrosarcoma, we should like to put forward the following speculative explanation: in contrast to chondrosarcoma, there is a very strong infiltrative and destructive growth potency to be found in osteosarcoma. It could therefore be supposed that the lytic enzymes, the key enzyme of which is acid phosphatase, play a rôle in the breakdown of the host tissue infiltrated by the tumor. The low enzyme activity in fibrous dysplasia is quite consistent with this concept. Apparently this enzyme production is an integrated part of malignant transformation of cells. The example of an osteosarcoma which has formed metaplastically from thyroid carcinoma clearly demonstrates this factor: the tumor shows an activity pattern of alkaline and acid phosphatases that corresponds very closely to that of a genuine osteosarcoma.

Electron-microscope investigation of the matrix of cartilaginous and bony tumorous conditions has brought out some interesting findings: when we measured the periodicity of the collagen fibrils, we found no difference between benign and malignant bone-forming entities. We measured a mean value of 640 Å for the width of the crossbanding periodicity, which corresponds to that of regular collagen. The thickness of the fibrils varied, of course, according to the growth potency of the different tumorous conditions.

Furthermore, besides normal fibrils, we were able to show a different kind of fibrils in fibrous dysplasia (Fig. 4); these were observed

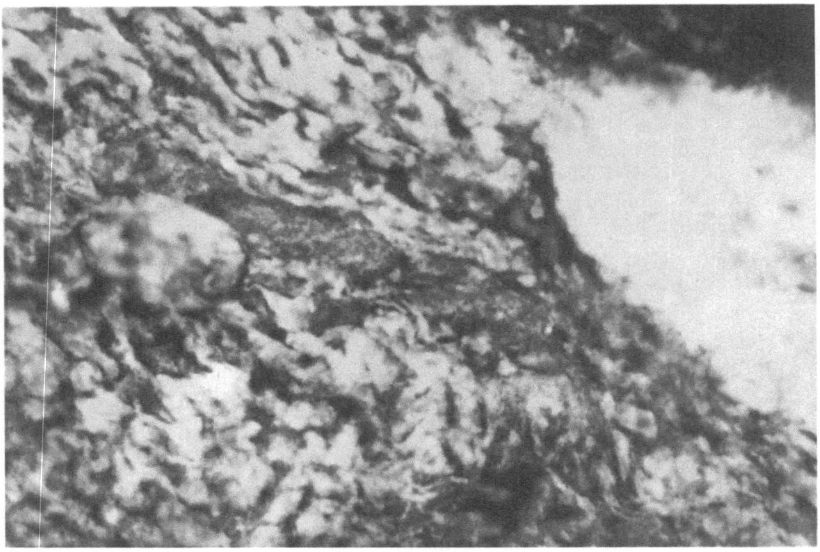

Fig. 3. Osteosarcoma, acid phosphatase: marked activity in all the tumor cells (grey). Osteoid formation on the right. Naphthol-AS-BI-phosphate, pararosaniline, 252 x

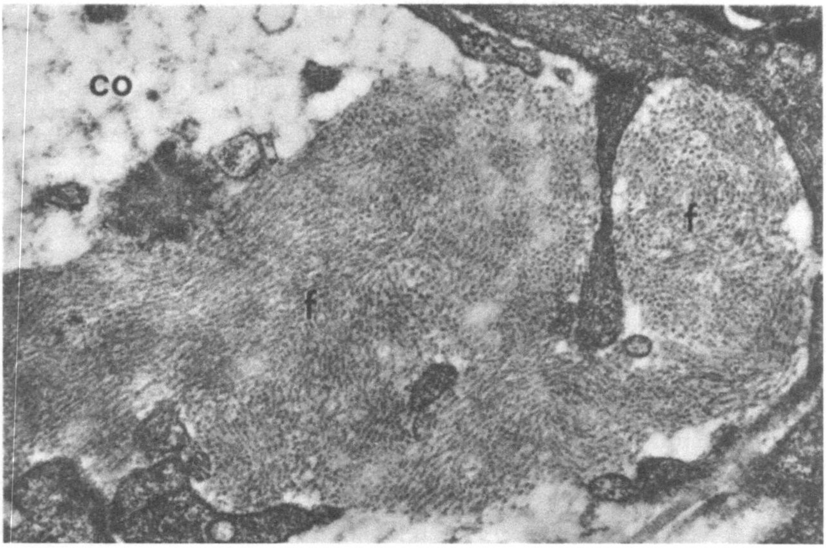

Fig. 4. Fibrous dysplasia, electron microscopy of matrix: besides normal collagen fibrils (co), there are densely packed fine fibrils without clear-cut periodicity (f), especially in contact with cell extensions 31,700 x

especially in close contact with the cell extensions of the fibroblast-like stroma cells, and consisted of densely packed, very fine fibrillar structures without clear-cut periodical crossbanding. They are different from other fine fibrils which have been found in metaplastically formed cartilage tissue and which have been considered as an early aggregation phase of tropocollagen macromolecules (1) in that the fibrils observed by us are more densely packed; it is possible, however, that we are dealing with a similar phase of collagen fibril maturation or with a retardation of this maturation. Up to now, we have not been able to detect variants of collagen fibril formation of this kind in other tumors or tumor-like conditions of the skeletal system, and in particular not in matrix of cartilaginous tumors. Furthermore, these fibrils are not like the fine filaments which have been found in the superficial layer of articular cartilage (27). Further collection of data in this field will help us to classify and to interpret this finding.

Electron-microscopic comparison of cells of different benign and malignant bone tumors reveals very few qualitative differences between them (Fig. 5). They all possess sets of organelles corresponding to those of active fibroblasts. They all have a large nucleus with varying degrees of indentation. A particularly conspicuous finding in the cartilaginous tumors is that the cytoplasm is densely packed with bundles of fine filaments arranged in parallel fashion; these microfilaments apparently connect different regions of the cell membrane. It may well be that these organelles are involved in cell motility. The indentations of the nucleus could perhaps be similarly interpreted (6).

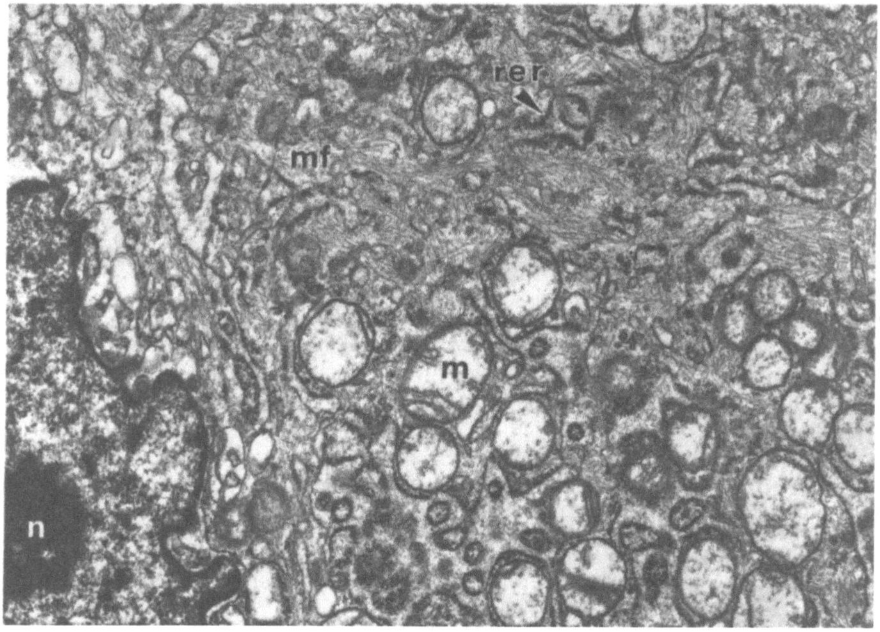

Fig. 5. EM of part of an osteosarcoma cell: the indented nucleus with prominent nucleolus (n), rough endoplasmatic reticulum (rer), mitochondriae (m), and other vesicles and further microfilaments (mf), are visible. 4,100 x

We have observed a nuclear structure that is peculiar to osteosarcoma: the nuclear membrane is extensively folded, forming very narrow channel-like invaginations in places. The significance of this tremendous increase in the nuclear surface cannot be unaequivocally interpreted as yet. This, as well as groups of tiny roundish particles near to the membrane, which are considered as perichromatin granules and are thought to be involved in nuclear RNA synthesis, strongly suggest increased nuclear activity. Furthermore, the large nucleoli are conspicuous, and they are sometimes increased in number. In all these conditions, parts of the endoplasmatic reticulum (ER) are generally found to be densely occupied by ribosomes. Quite often, the ER is enlarged, forming cysternae that contain fine granular or amorphous substances. Furthermore, mitochondriae and membranes of the Golgi apparatus are numerous. The number of lysosomes, in contrast, is small, despite the histochemical demonstration of intense acid phosphatase activity, which leads one to postulate a large number of lysosomes. This dilemma may be resolved by the finding that other cell organelles, in particular the Golgi apparatus and cytoplasmatic vesicles near to the Golgi apparatus, may also contain this enzyme in large amounts; this has been shown to be the case by histochemical investigations on fracture callus at the electron-microscopic level (8). Fairly large agglomerations of glycogen in cartilaginous tumors have already been found by other authors (29, 28, 23, 21) (Fig. 6). We were not able to establish any parallel between the grade of malignancy determined clinically and by light microscopy and the density of cell organelles in the cytoplasm. Furthermore, we did not find any correlation between the quantity of glycogen and the grade of malignancy. This is in contrast to the fingings of other authors, who have stated a parallel between increasing malignancy and decreasing number of cell organelles (21). In a highly differentiated chondrosarcoma arising in rib cartilage, we observed a pronounced paucity of organelles but abundant glycogen as well as some lipid droplets. Another sarcoma of moderate differentiation, arising from the thyroid cartilage of the larynx, was clearly richer in organelles, and glycogen and lipid droplets were found in addition. Furthermore, the cells of a cartilaginous callus, which also shows a marked growth potency and thus parallels fast-growing malignant tumors, contain abundant organelles, particularly rough endoplasmatic reticulum. A point of importance which should be mentioned here is the presence of dense granules in the matrix of all of the cartilaginous tumors as well as in that of cartilaginous callus. There is evidence that these granules represent protein polysaccharide within the matrix and that they change in size prior to calcification (13).

There is increasing evidence from experimental investigations in recent years, in particular from those involving inoculation of cell-free tumor extracts from human osteosarcomas to golden hamsters (3, 4) and from experiments applying immunofluorescence (15) that human osteosarcomas may contain virus-like particles. In most papers dealing with electron microscopy of human osteosarcomas, however, they have not been mentioned or - as in our observations - habe been reported as absent (9, 16, 7, 14, 10). Thus, FINKEL's inhasitating assertion that C-type virus particles should be found in every human osteosarcoma if studies are sufficiently careful must be questioned. Furthermore, even these inoculation experiments cannot be considered absolute evidence for an etiological rôle of these virus particles in the genesis of osteosarcomas.

In conclusion, we can say that histochemistry and electron microscopy of bone tumors are still in the early stage of material gathering. The histochemical findings available up to now can already be used as a diagnostic tool, e.g., in the case of Ewing's sarcoma. It is possible that in the fairly near future the demonstration of phosphatase activity will allow diagnostic guidelines concerning benignancy or malignancy of bone

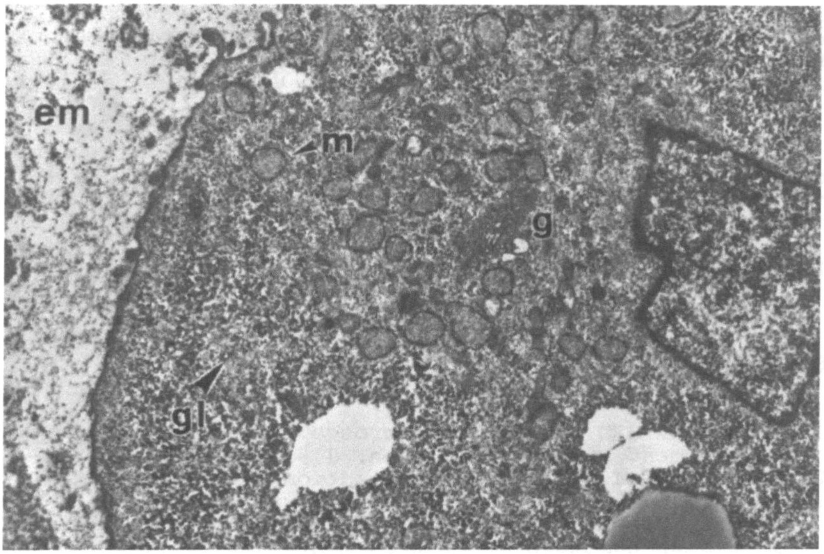

Fig. 6. EM of part of a chondrosarcoma cell: the nucleus, some mitochondriae (m), parts of the Golgi apparatus (g), lipid droplet (lower right), and abundant glycogen (gl) are visible. The cell membrane with some extensions borders the extracellular matrix (em), which contains scarce collagen fibrils and finely granular material. 3,100 x

tumors to be drawn up. At present, electron-microscope findings are contradictory: No criteria that could be useful in differential diagnosis have yet been formulated in the field of cartilage-forming tumors or that of bone-forming tumors.

SUMMARY

In recent years, histochemistry and electron microscopy have been applied more and more to the investigation of bone tumors. The contributions and limitations of these methods in differential diagnosis are discussed. The levels of glycosaminoglycans in cartilaginous tumors display distinct differences between slow- and fast-growing types. All cartilaginous tumors are poor in phosphatase activity. Demonstration of these enzymes at acid and alkaline pH in bone-forming conditions reveals differences between benign and malignant tumors. Osteosarcomas display a rich activity of both phosphatases in bone-forming and in bone-free regions. Acid phosphatase may play a rôle in the breakdown of the host tissue infiltrated by the tumor.

Electron microscopy of bone tumors has brought out some interesting findings. In fibrous dysplasia a particular kind of very fine fibrillar structures was observed besides the regular collagen fibrils. This may indicate retardation of collagen maturation. Cell organelles in benign and malignant bone tumors usually differ quantitatively. They resemble active fibroblasts. In bone- and in cartilage-forming tumors we observed large quantities of microfilaments in the cytoplasm. Nuclear indentations and invaginations probably indicate increased nuclear activity. The intense acid phosphatase activity demonstrated histochemically seems inconsistent with the low number of lysosomes in the cytoplasm of osteosarcoma cells, but other organelles (Golgi apparatus and vesicles) may also contain the enzyme. Virus-like particles have not been observed in human osteosarcomas up to now.

Other authors have observed a correlation between the number of cell organelles and the grade of differentiation, but this was not detected in our sample of benign and malignant cartilaginous tumors. Histochemistry and electron microscopy of bone tumors are still in the early stage of material gathering. Some histochemical findings, however, can already be used as diagnostic tools.

REFERENCES

1. ANDERSON, H.C.: Electron microscopic studies of induced cartilage development and calcification. J. Cell. Biol. 35, 81-101 (1967)
2. BRADFIELD, J.G.R.: The localization of enzymes in cells. Biol. Rev. 25, 113-157 (1950)
3. FINKEL, M.P., BISKIS, B.O., FARRELL, C.: Osteosarcomas appearing in Syrian hamsters after treatment with extracts of human osteosarcomas. Proc. nat. Acad. Sci. (Wash.) 60, 1223-1230 (1968)
4. FINKEL, M.P., REILLY, jr. C.A., BISKIS, B.O., GRECO, J.L.: Bone tumor viruses. Bone - certain aspects of neoplasia. Proc. 24th Symp. Colston Res. Soc. (Eds. C.H.G. Price, F.G. Ross), p. 353. London: Butterworths 1973
5. FLEISCH, H.: Physiologie und Biochemie der Knochenbildung. Klin. Wschr. 44, 360-363 (1966)
6. GABBIANI, G., HIRSCHEL, B.J., RYAN, G.B., STATKOV, P.R., MAJNO, G.: Granulation tissue as a contractile organ. A study of structure and function. J. exp. Med. 135, 719-734 (1972)
7. GHADIALLY, F.N., MEHTA, P.N.: Ultrastructure of osteogenic sarcoma. Cancer 25, 1457-1467 (1970)
8. GOETHLIN, G., ERICSSON, J.L.E.: Fine structural localization of acid phosphomonoesterase in the osteoblasts and osteocytes of fracture callus. Histochemie 35, 81-91 (1973)
9. GONZALEZ-LICEA, A., YARDLEY, J.H., HARTMANN, W.H.: Malignant tumor of the breast with bone formation. Cancer 20, 1234-1247 (1967)
10. HIROHATA, K., MORIMOTO, K.: Ultrastructure of Bone and Joint Diseases. Amsterdam: Excerpta Medica 1971
11. KROON, D.B.: Phosphatase and the formation of protein-carbohydrate complexes. Acta anat. (Basel) 15, 317-328 (1952)
12. LLOMBART-BOSCH, A., PEYDRO-OLAYA, A., LOPEZ-FERNANDEZ, A.: Non-ossifying fibroma of bone. A histochemical and ultrastructural characterization. Virchows Arch. path. Anat. A 362, 13-21 (1974)
13. MATUKAS, V.J., KRIKOS, G.A.: Evidence for changes in protein polysaccharide associated with the onset of calcification in cartilage. J. Cell.Biol. 39, 43-48 (1968)
14. MCALLISTER, R.M., GARDNER, M.B., GREENE, A.E., BRADT, C., NICHOLS, W.W., LANDING, B.H.: Cultivation in vitro of cells derived from a human osteosarcoma. Cancer 27, 397-402 (1971)
15. MORTON, D.L., MALMGREN, R.A.: Human Osteosarcomas: Immunologic evidence suggesting an associated infectious agent. Science 162, 1279-1281 (1968)
16. PEYDRO-OLAYA, A., LLOMBART-BOSCH, A., LOPEZ-FERNANDEZ, A.: Estudio histoquimico y microscopico electronico de un osteosarcoma de femur. Patologia 5, 231-244 (1972)

17. RUSSELL, R.G.G., FLEISCH, H.: Pyrophosphate, phosphonates and pyrophosphatases in the regulation of calcification and calcium homeostasis. Proc. roy. Soc. Med. 63, 876 (1970)
18. SALZER-KUNTSCHIK, M.: Zur Beurteilung von Probeentnahmen bei Knochentumoren. Verh. Dtsch. Ges. Path. 58, 235-248 (1974)
19. SCHAJOWICZ, F.: Ewing's sarcoma and reticulum cell sarcoma of bone; with special reference to the histochemical demonstration of glycogen as an aid to differential diagnosis. J. Bone Jt Surg. 41A, 349-356 (1959)
20. SCHAJOWICZ, F.: Differential diagnosis of Ewing's sarcoma. Bone - certain aspects of neoplasia. Proc. 24th Symp. Colston Res. Soc. (Eds. C.H.G. Price, F.G.M. Ross) p. 189. London: Butterworths 1973
21. SCHAJOWICZ, F., CABRINI, R.L., SIMES, J.R., KLEIN-SZANTO, A.J.P.: Ultrastructure of chondrosarcoma. Clin. Orthop. 100, 378-386 (1974)
22. SCHULTZ-HAUDT, S.D.: Histochemistry of connective tissue ground substances. Progr. Histochem. Cytochem. 5/2. Stuttgart: Fischer 1973
23. STEINER, G.C., MIRRA, J.M., BULLOUGH, P.G.: Mesenchymal chondrosarcoma. Cancer 32, 926-939 (1973)
24. TEN CATE, A.R.: The histochemistry of human tooth development. Proc. Nutr. Soc. 18, 65-70 (1959)
25. VAES, G.: Hydrolytic enzymes and lysosomes in bone cells. Proc. 2nd Europ. Symp. Calc. Tiss. Liège, 1964, p. 51-62
26. VALLS, J., OTTOLENGHI, C.E., SCHAJOWICZ, F.: Epiphyseal chondroblastoma of bone. J. Bone Jt Surg. 33A, 997-1009 (1951)
27. WEISS, C., ROSENBERG, L., HELFET, A.J.: An ultrastructural study of normal young adult human articular cartilage. J. Bone Jt Surg. 50A, 663-674 (1968)
28. WELLMANN, K.F.: Chondroblastoma of the scapula. Cancer 24, 408-416 (1969)
29. WELSH, R.A., MEYER, A.T.: A histogenetic study of chondroblastoma. Cancer 17, 578-589 (1964)

Morphological, Biological, Immunological and Biochemical Studies on Bone Tumors of Animals and Man

L. DMOCHOWSKI

INTRODUCTION

In a discussion on bone tumors in animals and man, the thoughts of a clinician and of a practicing physician may well turn first to their importance in terms of occurrence, death, survival, and estimated appearance of new cases within the general statistics of cancer of all sites and organs in humans of both sexes. Even a brief glance at the available statistics may give the impression of that this neoplasia is relatively rare within the general framework of incidence of cancer of various sites in man, and lead to the conclusion that this type of neoplasia is of relatively little importance in the overall incidence of cancer of other sites of man. In a utilitarian approach, it may be argued that this type of neoplasia does not deserve as much attention and, another important point, as much financial support as do other types of neoplasia in man. However, when even a single case of a bone tumor in a child is diagnosed and referred for treatment, its importance and its challenge to the clinician are equal to if not greater than those in any other type of neoplasia.

The occurrence of primary cancer of the bone in humans, like the incidence of a similar type of cancer in animals, accounts for a small proportion of all malignancies. The incidence of this type of cancer in animal species extending from mice to monkeys cannot be given with any accuracy.

According to the Third National Cancer Survey (22), primary cancer of the bone accounts for a small proportion (0.5 percent) of all malignancies. The age-adjusted incidence rate is about 1 per 100,000 (1.1 for males and 0.8 for females). During the period 1955-1964, 40 percent of bone cancer patients were under 25 years of age, and a little over 20 percent of patients were 65 years or older. Prognosis is poor, although as far as a 10-year relative survival rate is concerned it is not the worst of all cancers, the rate for stomach cancer, for example, being lower (30 percent compared with 10 percent). The poorest survival was observed for patients under 25 years of age and those over 65 years. For comparison (22), leukemia accounted for 4.1 percent of all malignant neoplasms in males and 3.1 percent in females during the period 1955-1964. There has been an increase in the 1-year survival rate from 39 to 44 percent for all leukemia patients for 1955-1969 (1). However, the 3-year rate has remained at 20 percent (1), in spite of the dramatic increase in the 3-year survival rate for children. Among the estimated new cases of cancer in 1974, totalling 655,000 (in USA), there will be 2,000 cases of bone cancer and 21,000 cases of leukemia (47).

On the assumption that viruses may be involved in human neoplasia, it is not known to what extent, if any, such viruses are involved in the origin of human bone tumors and of human leukemia, or, if they exist, how they are interrelated in these two types of human neoplasia. There is, of course, a considerable literature on the interrelationship of leukemia and sarcoma viruses in a number of animal species (56). Interest in a similar relationship between viruses causing bone tumors in animals and those causing leukemia has only recently started to develop as a result of reports on the implication of viruses in bone tumors of mice and their induction by known leukemia viruses.

The RNA viruses associated with leukemia, lymphoma, and sarcoma of various species of animals have a number of important morphological, biological, antigenic and biochemical properties in common. All are of the so-called type-C morphology, induce similar cellular changes in their respective host cells, have common as well as distinct antigens, and possess characteristic genomic RNA. These viruses also contain unique enzyme complexes including the RNA-dependent DNA polymerase (reverse transcriptase (13).

Some time ago we demonstrated the presence of virus particles of the C type in diseases of some patients with leukemia, lymphoma, lymphosarcoma, and osteosarcoma (8, 9, 11, 16). These virus particles were morphologically similar to the virus particles responsible for leukemia of mice and animals of other species. As isolation of oncogenic viruses from human tumor tissues has been difficult, it has been necessary to apply information obtained from studies of known animal viruses to the problem of human neoplasia.

Animal sarcoma viruses have been shown to induce transformation *in vitro* of cells from homologous and heterologous host species. These viruses are known to be frequently defective in their ability to replicate and produce infectious progeny. However, the transformed cells contain the genetic material of the virus in a covert form (32, 37).

Animal leukemia viruses produce infectious virus when inoculated into cells grown *in vitro*, and generally do not produce cell transformation. They can, however, act as so-called helper viruses in the replication of the defective sarcoma viruses. When cells transformed by sarcoma virus are infected with leukemia virus they produce both leukemia and sarcoma virus. This phenomenon is called retrieval or rescue of sarcoma virus (14, 55).

As already mentioned, type-C virus particles have been demonstrated in human tumors including bone tumors, although infrequently and in small numbers. These virus particles have been found even less frequently in cells grown in tissue culture (10). In spite of the presence of small numbers of type-C virus particles in human osteosarcoma biopsy specimens, the virus may be present in tumor cells in a hidden form resembling that of animal sarcoma viruses. Attempts were therefore carried out to rescue any viral information present in human sarcoma by the use of human leukemia material, as a possible source of a human leukemia helper virus. Before the results of these studies are described, the results of various animal bone tumor studies will be presented.

STUDIES ON ANIMAL BONE TUMORS

Spontaneous bone tumors in mice are rare (17). However, the occurrence of these tumors in mice of a number of strains has been recorded with a frequency of under 1 percent (1, 2, 29, 46, 57). However, mice of a subline of the Simpson strain have been reported to have a high incidence of bone tumors (51). Unfortunately this Pybus-Miller subline of Simpson mice was lost. Renewed interest in the bone tumors of mice resulted from the report of FINKEL and her associates (27) on the isolation of a virus described as FBJ from a spontaneous osteosarcoma observed in a CF1/Anl mouse. Further biological and morphological studies demonstrated that the virus was inducing mainly osteosarcomas in mice and was the so-called type-C particle (4, 24). The successful isolation of an oncogenic virus from a spontaneous malignant bone tumor of a mouse led to a search for a virus in human bone tumors. These studies led to a suggestive but not conclusive demonstration of the induction of osteosarcomas in hamsters inoculated with extracts of human osteosarcomas (25, 26). Type-C virus particles were found in the induced tumors and in some extracts of the human osteosarcomas examined (26).

Studies of the FBJ osteosarcoma virus in tissue culture (44) have demonstrated that the murine leukemia virus is associated with it, thus producing a complex similar to other murine RNA oncogenic viruses with typical morphology, group-specific antigen and characteristic density. This virus also induced characteristic foci in mouse and rat embryo cells (44).

Since the isolation of a murine sarcoma virus (MSV) by HARVEY (33, 34), and by MONOLEY (45) numerous studies have been carried out on the behavior of these two viruses. In our own studies on these two virus isolates, we have observed induction of bone tumors and their cell-free transmission in New Zealand black rats and in Syrian hamsters (53). Characteristic type-C murine leukemia virus particles have been observed in these bone tumors induced by the SD-MSV-M virus in specimens grown both in vivo and in vitro (30, 53, 54). These tumors have been found transmissible by cell-free material from rats to rats, from rats to hamsters, and from hamsters to hamsters (54). Further studies have also demonstrated that the FBJ bone tumor-inducing virus is capable of inducing bone tumors in mice of all strains examined (58). Similarly, the SD-MSV-M virus was found to induce bone tumors in rats of all strains tested (14) (Fig. 1).

There have been further biological studies on the SD-MSV-M virus in mice, rats, and hamsters following passage in tissue cultures of mouse, rat, and hamster embryo cells (14). Tumorigenicity of the virus for hamsters was lost after passage in mouse and rat embryo cells (14). However, the tumor-inducing property of the hamster-adapted SD-MSV-M virus for hamsters was retained after tissue-culture passage in rat and hamster embryo cells and in mouse 3T3 cells. Passage of this virus in GP and ICR mouse embryo cells led to the loss of tumor-inducing property in hamsters and acquisition of tumorigenicity for mice (14). Both budding and typical type-C virus particles have been observed in both tumors and in transformed tissue culture cells of animals of all species examined (14). Cell-free material from 3T3 cells transformed by rat-adapted SD-MSV-M induced bone tumors and in some cases effusions in mice and hamsters and bone tumors in rats (14). This material also had focus-forming ability in mouse and rat embryo cell cultures, but not in hamster embryo cell cultures. Virus from hamster bone tumor cultures was tumorigenic only in hamsters, but induced foci in hamster, rat and mouse embryo cultures. Virus from these transformed cultures, except for mouse embryo cultures, induced bone tumors in hamsters and in mice but not in rats (14). Virus from the transformed mouse embryo cultures induced bone tumors only in mice and foci in mouse embryo cultures. Thus, successful transmission of hamster-adapted rat bone tumor virus to species other than hamster has been achieved, as demonstrated by focus formation in mouse, rat, and hamster embryo cell cultures and tumor induction in mice as well as in hamsters (14) (Figs. 2-3).

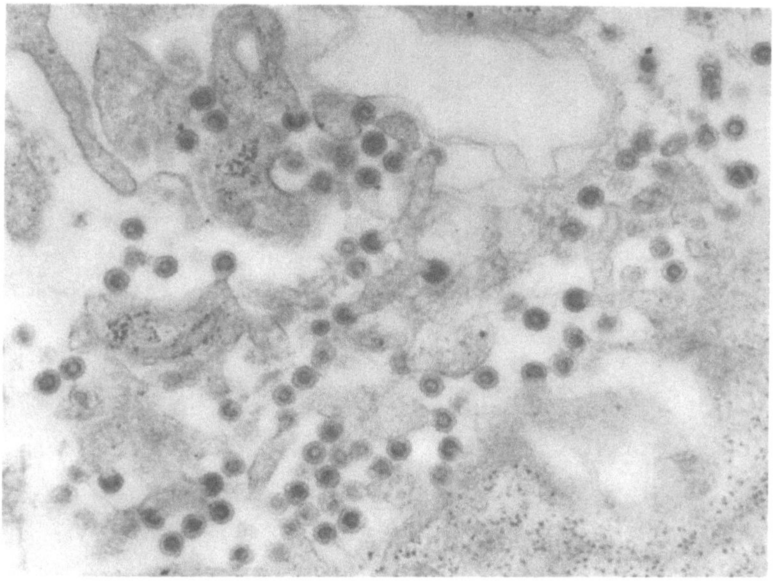

Fig. 1. Tumor cells grown in tissue culture from a CF-1 strain mouse tumor induced by FBJ virus, showing budding, immature, and mature type-C virus particles. X 33,500

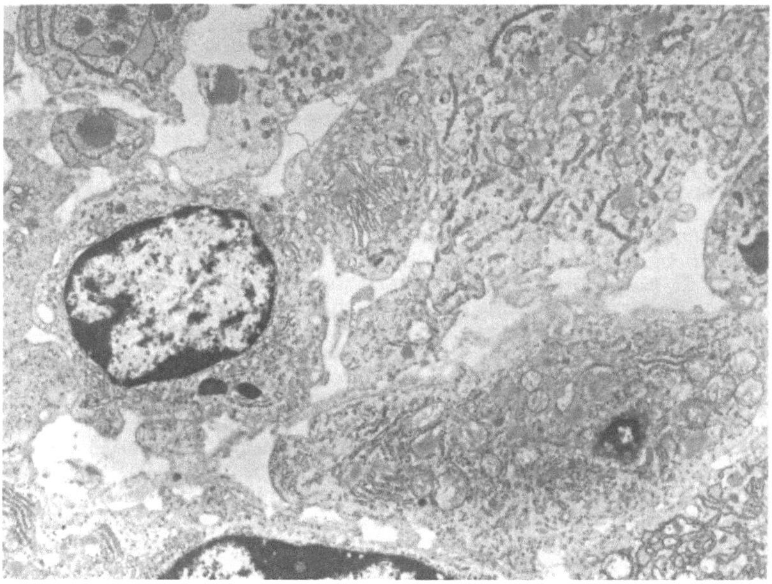

Fig. 2. General view of a hamster bone tumor induced by MSV-SD. X 4,000

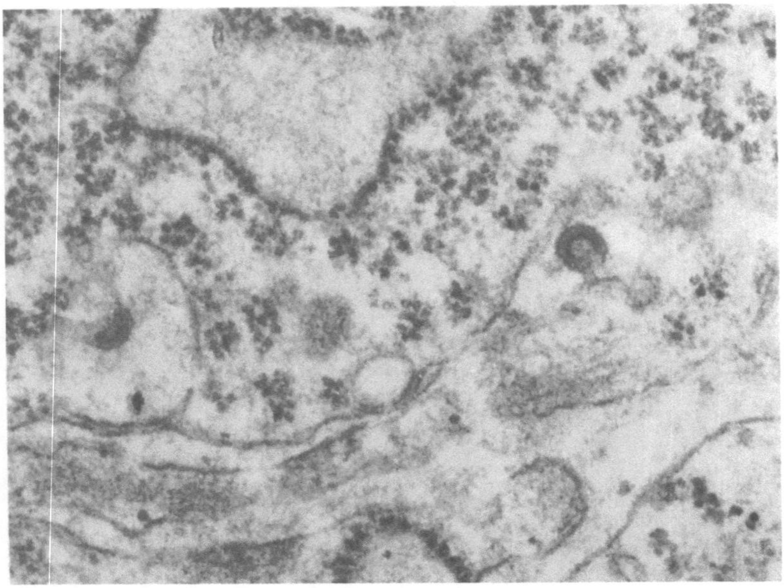

Fig. 3. Higher-magnification view of two budding type-C virus particles in the same tumor as is shown in Fig. 15. X 60,000

The results of immunoelectron-microscope studies (36) using immunoferritin and immunoperoxidase demonstrated that the envelope antigens of MSV-SD virus in rat bone tumor cells were distinct from those of MSV-SD virus recovered from the hamster bone tumor cells. This may explain the hamster tropism of the virus recovered from hamster bone tumor culture cells (36).

Isolation of hamster-specific sarcoma virus from hamster tumors induced by murine sarcoma viruses has been reported by a number of investigators (3, 42, 43, 49, 52). Some of these authors consider that the hamster-specific sarcoma virus represents the murine sarcoma virus genome encapsidated in the envelope of an indigenous hamster-tropic helper virus (42). The results of our studies (36) based on the finding that hamster bone-tumor cells contain a rescuable murine sarcoma virus genome and that the hamster-derived virus induces similar bone tumors also favor the notion that the hamster virus or MSV-SD (HBT) is the product of encapsidation of the parental MSV-SD genome in a hamster-specific envelope. In our opinion, final proof will come from molecular hybridization studies on nucleic acid sequences between the rat or MSV-SD (RBT) or hamster tumor derived viral genomes.

The induction of osteosarcomas in rats and also in mice has recently been reported from Japan (38, 39, 40). Osteosarcomas were produced predominantly in rats and myosarcomas predominantly in mice (40). Typical type-C virus particles were again found in the induced tumors of mice and rats (40). The viruses with similar properties for rats and mice could also be retrieved from tumor cells grown in vitro (39). In these experiments (40), as in our own experience (54), the coexistence of both sarcomas and leukemia virus has been demonstrated by development of lymphomas in rats (54). Multiple oncogenic potentiality is a phenomenon observed in other tumor-inducing viruses such as Rous sarcoma virus, which was first shown by DURAN-REYNALS (18) to induce bone tumors in ducks, turkeys and guinea-fowls (19). This may be due to modification of multivalent potentials of the viruses involved or to alterations in a mixed population of virus particles.

Establishment of a culture from an osteosarcoma induced in a rat (39) led to the observation of morphological alterations of some cells into refractile fusiform cells and finally into small rounded cells, some of which produced the bone tumor-inducing virus (39). This phenomenon has been observed by us in rat and hamster bone tumor cultures (14) and also in some human sarcoma cultures (50).

In our tissue-culture studies of MSV-SD rat bone tumors, two separate cell cultures have been established (7). One of them releases both MSV and MuLV and contains, therefore, sarcoma-positive and leukemia-positive transformed cells. The other culture, which also forms colonies on soft agar and also has an increased 2-deoxy-D-glucose-^{5} H, uptake produces only MuL virus. Cocultivation with MulV-producing mouse cells or addition of MuLV exogenous helper virus has not resulted in rescue of MSV activity (7). However, the MuLV in this cell line has helper activity, as shown by the rescue of MSV genome from bone-tumor cells transformed by MSV-SD (7).

These findings support the notion that this culture contains sarcoma-negative and leukemia-positive (S-L+) transformed cells (7). Several explanations could be put forward for the S-L+ rat bone tumor culture. One of them is that the MSV genome is still present but under suppression (Except for genes responsible for transformation). Partial expression of MSV or MuLV genome has previously been reported (28). Revertant cells have been isolated from the S+L- transformed cells; these contained no rescuable MSV genome but did contain some MuLV gs antigens (48). Some spontaneously transformed revertants which regained neoplastic properties contained no rescuable MSV and had lost MuLV gs antigens (48). These findings appear to support the existence of separate control mechanisms for partial expression of genes responsible for neoplastic properties, virus replication and synthesis of gs antigens (7). However, further experiments are obviously needed to clarify this problem.

In our studies on the development of immunological response in rats in relation to tumorigenesis of MSV-SD, several pathological parameters were observed which influenced the humoral and cell-mediated responses (23). New Zealand black rats inoculated at 7 days of age with MSV-SD developed erythroblastosis which progressed concomitantly with tumor growth, while rats inoculated at 21 days of age developed osteosarcomas but not erythroblastosis or anemia (23). The animals inoculated at 7 days showed depression of humoral response to sheep red blood cells as well as reduction in secondary antibody response. Animals inoculated at 21 days showed no depression of primary humoral response to sheep red blood cells, and only after tumor development was a lower level of antibody titer recorded (23). Serum-blocking factors were found in rats with progressively growing bone tumors, as demonstrated by colony inhibition tests (23). Non-tumor-bearing animals showed no detectable serum-blocking factors, which may indicate that these factors have some role in the growth of MSV-SD-induced tumors (23). Animals with progressively growing tumors exhibited a growth-enhancing factor like one described for murine sarcoma system (35). Thus, in MSV-SD induced infection in rats there is a complex virus interaction with both specific and nonspecific physiological parameters.

Biochemical studies were carried out by us on structural rearrangement and subunit composition of RNA released from MSV-SD virus (20). The results of these studies demonstrated that two forms of native genome

RNA exist in the released virus particles, depending on the age of the particles examined (20). These two forms differ in their sedimentation coefficients and in their subunit composition (20). The major subunit of both forms is a 28S component (20). Studies are now in progress to correlate the different forms of RNA in released virions with infectivity and physical structure.

STUDIES ON HUMAN OSTEOSARCOMA

If a human sarcoma virus exists, at least in a covert form, it may be present in the tumor cells in a form similar to that of defective sarcoma viruses in animal tumors. An attempt was made to study possible activation of either type-C virus particles or virus-controlled information by using human leukemic material as a source of a potential human helper virus. These studies were based on a correlative application of tissue culture, morphological, immunological and biochemical methods (11, 15) (Fig. 4).

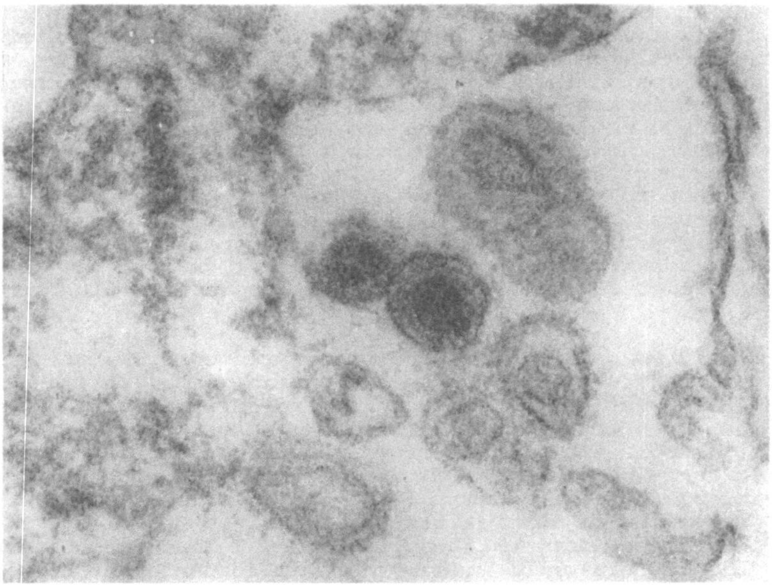

Fig. 4. High magnification view of two type-C virus-like paticles in human osteosarcoma tissue culture. X 100,000

In the attempts at a retrieval of virus-directed information, 49 cocultures derived from human osteosarcoma were established with cells from bone marrow or peripheral blood of patients with different types of leukemia, especially acute lymphocytic and granulocytic leukemia. The cocultures were examined in short- and long-term cultures. Changes in cellular morphology and pattern of growth were observed in 7 of 13 long-term cocultures. The observed morphological changes resembled the morphologic changes induced in animal cells by RNA tumor viruses (15) (Fig. 5).

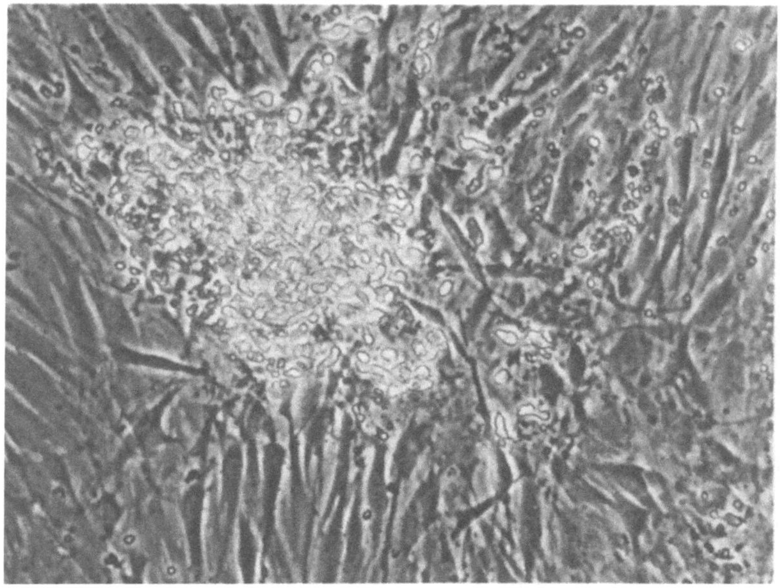

Fig. 5. Appearance of morphological changes in cells after 23 days in coculture of human osteosarcoma cells and white blood cells from a patient with acute leukemia. X 200

The morphologic changes were accompanied by the appearance of a cytoplasmic antigen as demonstrated by fixed immunofluorescence test with sera of patients with osteosarcoma, leukemia and of some normal donors. A total of 165 sera (including 49 from apparently normal donors) were tested against cells of one of the osteosarcoma-leukemia cocultures. A total of 44.9 percent of sera gave cytoplasmic fluorescence in the fixed immunofluorescence test (15). Fourteen of 49 normal sera (28.5 percent) were positive; 18 of 28 osteosarcoma sera, 24 of 48 sera of patients with sarcoma of different types; 10 of 20 sera of leukemic patients; and 8 of 20 sera of patients with other solid tumors were possible in these tests (15). Absorption of the positive sera with coculture cells removed the reactivity but not absorption with sheep red cells, guinea-pig kidney-cell powder or mycoplasma. Furthermore, absorption with WISH, HeLa, Wilm's tumor, and Hep 2 cells also failed to remove the cytoplasmic reaction. It is of interest and as yet unexplained that the reaction was also removed by absorption with KB cells (Figs. 6, 7).

In the fixed immunofluorescence tests, only one of ten of the parental osteosarcoma cultures was positive, while all three of the cocultures available were positive. It is of interest that cells of all six cultures grown from leukemic bone-marrow aspirates gave a positive cytoplasmic reaction with the sera tested (15) and that cells of some cocultures were negative for the cytoplasmic antigen in early tissue-culture passages but became positive in later passages.

The distribution of antibodies to the cytoplasmic antigen in cells of the cocultures showing changes in morphology and growth pattern was found similar to that in human embryonic cultures transformed by fluid from different osteosarcoma-leukemia cocultures (12).

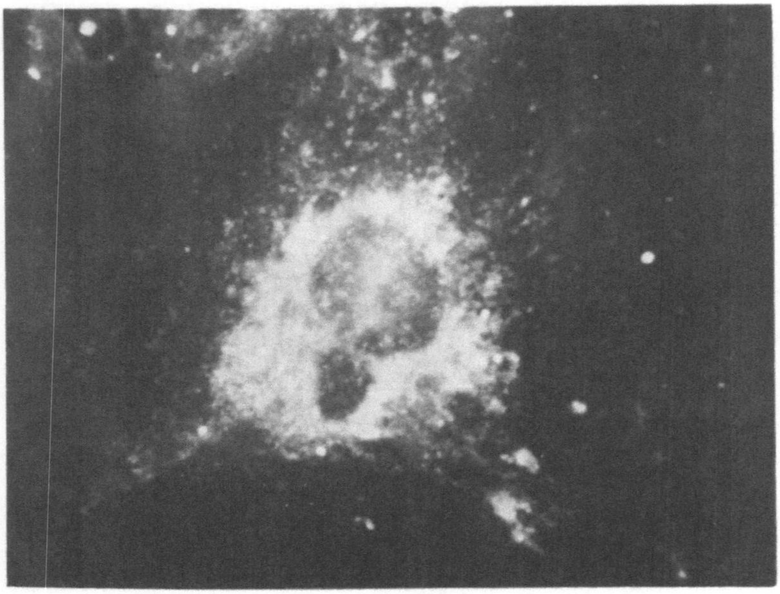

Fig. 6. Fluorescence photomicrograph of coculture of human osteosarcoma and white blood cells from a leukemic patient. The culture was treated with serum of a patient with osteosarcoma, then with fluorescein conjugated human IgG antiserum. X 1,000

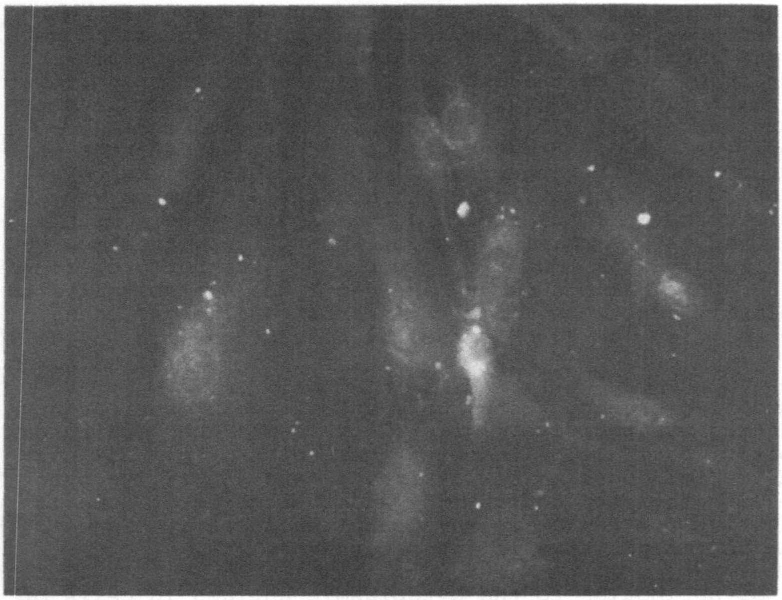

Fig. 7. Control fluorescence photomicrograph of the same coculture as in Fig. 6. The cells were treated with PBS then with fluorescein conjugated human IgG anti serum. X 630

It was possible to induce production of the cytoplasmic antigen in negative osteosarcoma cells by cocultivation with antigen-positive leukemic bone-marrow cells. It is not known whether this reflects transmission of antigen-producing activity or activation of its synthesis by osteosarcoma cells.

The cytoplasmic antigen was detected in cells of a few tumors other than leukemia and osteosarcoma, including KB cells, a cell line derived from human oropharyngeal carcinoma. The antigen could not be detected on the plasma membrane of viable KB cells, and an allotypic reaction can, therefore, be ruled out, but this finding requires further study.

Attempts were made to study the possible viral nature of the observed morphological and immunological changes by their transmission to appropriate target cells (15, 12). Cell-free supernatants from long-term cocultures (3 months or longer) induced foci of cells of altered morphology in some of the recipient human embryo cultures. A total of 23 of 24 cocultures tested induced morphological alterations in the recipient human embryo cells (15). Whole human embryo cultures whether untreated or treated with supernatant fluid from bone-marrow cultures, showed 10 morphological changes (15). It is of interest that whole human embryo cells treated with fluid from leukemic bone-marrow cultures (but not from parental cultures) showed the presence of the cytoplasmic antigen when tested with positive sera but they showed no morphological changes (15) (Figs. 8-9).
Absorption of the positive sera with sheep red blood cells, guinea-pig kidney powder, Hep-2, HeLa, WISH, or Wilm's tumor cell suspension did not remove the cytoplasmic reaction in whole human embryo cells treated with fluid from osteosarcoma-leukemia cocultures. Cell-free fluid from leukemic bone marrow cultures did not induce morphological alterations but gave cytoplasmic fluorescence in the recipient whole human embryo cells (15) (Fig. 10).

These observations are similar to those reported by GIRALDO and his associates (31). They described foci of morphologically altered cells and a cytoplasmic antigen in long-term cultures of human osteosarcomas. They also observed the induction of foci of altered cells in human embryonic lung and skin cells by cell-free tissue-culture medium of osteosarcoma cultures.

In connection with these observations, a recent report on transformation of human fibroblasts with DNA of cultured human rhabdomyosarcoma cells (41) may be mentioned. Morphological changes and abnormal karyotypes were observed after 8 months in human embryo skin fibroblasts treated with DNA extracted from cultured human rhabdomyosarcoma cells which showed an abnormal growth pattern, pleomorphic cytology, and distorted karyotypes. This report may indicate transmission of viral coded information from human malignant cells (41).

Biochemical studies on osteosarcoma leukemia cocultures and on the human embryonic cells transformed by coculture fluid demonstrated that some of the cultures released a fast-sedimenting RNA and less frequently particulate components associated with an RNA-dependent-DNA polymerase. However, the appearance of this oncorna virus-like biochemical activity was variable and could not be consistently demonstrated. These results suggest that the transforming factor or agent may be present in the examined material in low concentration or that it may be defective (15). However, the biological and immunological observations indicate the existence of a human leukemia-sarcoma complementation system resembling that of animal leukemia-sarcoma system.

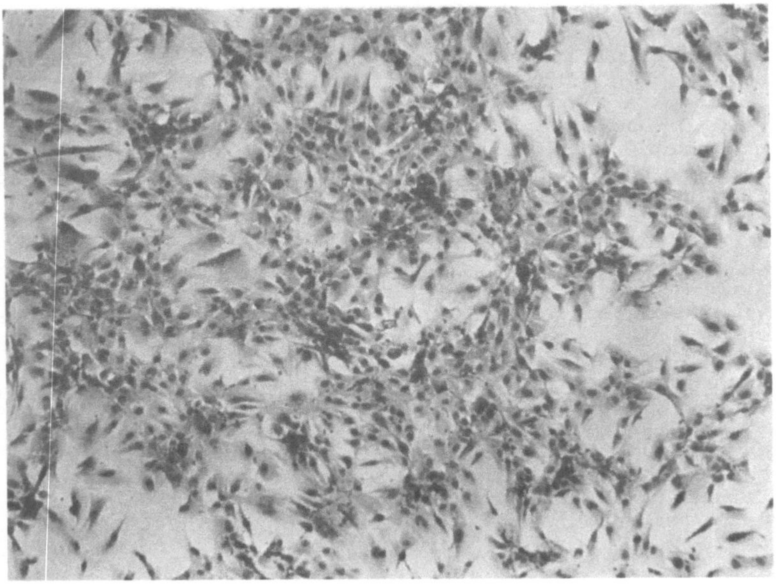

Fig. 8. Appearance of whole human embryo cell culture treated with cell-free fluid of a long-term coculture of human osteosarcoma and peripheral white blood cells of a patient with acute lymphocytic leukemia. Stained with Giemsa. Characteristic appearance of cells. Photomicrograph. X 40

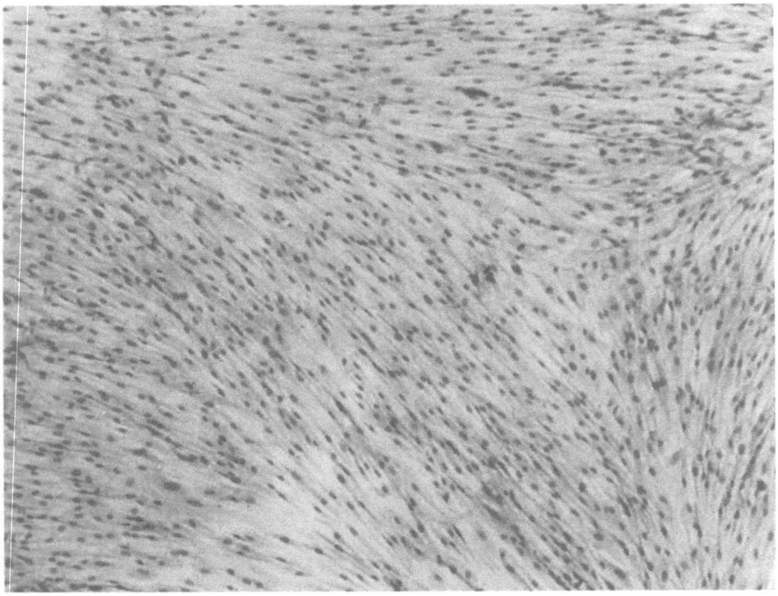

Fig. 9. Appearance of untreated control whole human embryo cell culture. Stained with Giemsa. Photomicrograph. X 40

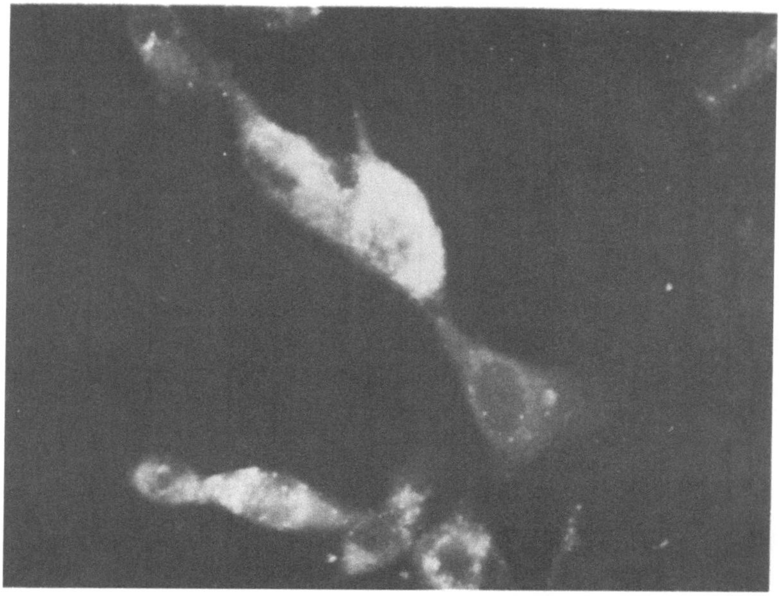

Fig. 10. Fluorescence photomicrograph of whole human embryo cell culture transformed by cell-free fluid from human osteosarcoma-leukemia coculture. Cells treated with serum of an osteosarcoma patient and then with fluorescein conjugated anti-human IgG serum. Diffuse cytoplasmic reaction may be seen. X 600

In our biochemical studies we have also applied molecular hybridization techniques in search of virus-related nucleotide sequences in human osteosarcoma cells. Recently, we have examined human sarcoma tissue-culture cell lines for the release of high-molecular-weight RNA species associated with particulate components. In several instances, such RNA species have been detected (5, 6).

A typical sedimentation profile of high-molecular-weight RNA from concentrated fluid medium of a human osteosarcoma cell cultures (designated OS-392) is illustrated in Figure 11a. The sedimentation coefficient of this RNA species was estimated to be 68S. For comparison, the sedimentation pattern of MSV-SD genomic RNA from virions released by a virus-producing rat tumor cell culture is presented in Figure 11b. The MSV-SD genomic RNA species had a sedimentation coefficient of 58S (20).

Sufficient quantities of radioactive high-molecular-weight RNA species are being obtained in many instances from human sarcoma-cell cultures so that their biochemical characteristics can be further analyzed. After measurement of their sedimentation coefficients, the high-molecular-weight RNA species are treated with pancreactic ribonuclease in high salt to determine their strandedness and with alkali to ascertain whether they are contaminated with DNA.

As shown in Table 1, the high-molecular-weight RNA species released by four human sarcoma-cell cultures had sedimentation coefficients ranging from 62S to 68S.

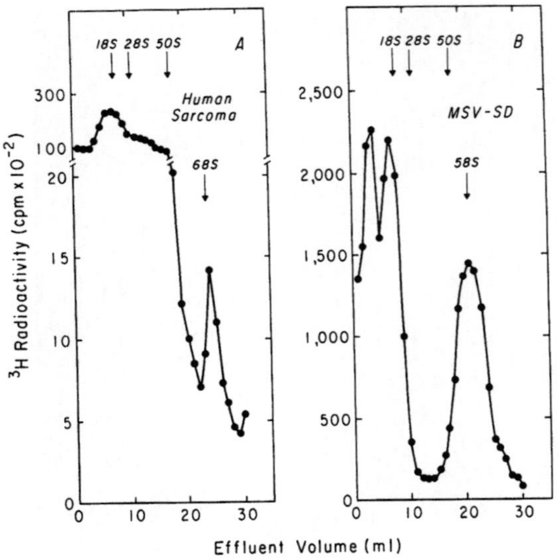

Fig. 11

Table 1

RNA	Radioactivity (CPM/ml)	Sedimentation constant	Percent resistance RNase A	NaOH
FS-B	12,220	68S	4	3
FS-437	9,400	62S	5	3
OS-392	109,300	68S	5	2
OS-7197	7,700	64S	22	9

[a]Abbreviations: FS, fibrosarcoma; OS, osteosarcoma.

Three of the four high-molecular-weight RNA species exhibited low ribonuclease-resistant values of 4 to 5 percent and low alkali-resistant values of 2 to 3 percent. In the case of the high-molecular-weight RNA species from the osteosarcoma-cell culture OS-7197, the ribonuclease-resistant value of 22 percent was excessively high, suggesting that a considerable portion of the molecules was double-stranded. For this reason, that particular RNA was not examined further.

The three high-molecular-weight RNA species exhibiting low ribonuclease-resistant values and alkali-resistant values were tested for sequence homology with known murine RNA tumor viruses. The design of the molecular hybridization tests was such that two distinct but related questions could be asked, i.e. (1). Do these high-molecular-weight RNA species share nucleotide sequences with viral RNA genomes? And (2) if so, to what extent are these sequences shared? This was accomplished by annealing the radioactive high-molecular-weight RNA species with saturating amounts of unlabeled, viral complementary DNA products synthesized in endogenous reverse transcriptase reactions. Pancreatic ribonuclease was used to measure hybrid formation annealing in 0.24 M sodium phosphate buffer at pH 6.7, for 3 hours at 70°C.

The results of these hybridization tests are presented in Table 2. The hybridization values shown for the viral systems are the values observed after annealing of a given radioactive viral genomic RNA with a saturating amount of its homologous, unlabeled complementary DNA product. Hybridization values ranged from a minimum of 51 percent for the homologous Kirsten sarcoma virus (MSV-K) hybrid pair. These homologous hybridization values represent the extent of transcription of viral RNA into complementary DNA.

Table 2

RNA-^{3}H added	Unlabeled DNA added MSV-M	MSV-K	MuLV-R	MuLV-G
Viral Homologous Sarcoma	83	51	66	68
FS-B	21	4	0	0
FS-437	26	0	0	NT
OS-392	22	9	0	0

[a]The values shown are percent hybridization values which have been corrected by subtracting the values observed when calf thymus DNA was annealed with a given radioactive RNA species. These latter values were used as a measure of the non-viral specificity of the annealing reactions. Pancreatic RNase A was used to measure hybrid formation.

The most striking feature of the cross-hybridization data is that positive annealing values were observed only with complementary DNA products synthesized from sarcoma viruses. Cross-hybridization values of 21 to 26 percent were determined with the DNA product of Moloney sarcoma virus (MSV-M) and values of up to 9 percent were noted with the DNA product of Kirsten sarcoma virus (MSV-K). The three high-molecular-weight RNA species released by human sarcoma-cell cultures did not cross-hybridize with either the DNA product of Rauscher leukemia virus (MulV-R) or the DNA product of Gross leukemia virus (MuLV-G) (21).

As far as we are aware, this is the first time that such results have been obtained. These molecular observations are obviously of potential significance, and other parameters of this apparent nucleotide sequence relatedness are under investigation.

In conclusion it can be stated that studies on osteosarcoma in animals of various species have provided a basis for a rational approach to studies on the possible viral origin of human osteosarcoma. Evidence is gradually accumulating that is suggestive of the implication of a virus or viruses in the origin of human bone tumors.

SUMMARY

Biological studies on FBJ osteosarcoma virus in tissue cultures have led to the isolation of murine sarcoma virus. Characteristic type

C-MuLV particles were observed in bone tumors induced by the SD-MSV-M-virus in vitro and in vivo. The SD-MSV-M virus also induced bone tumors in rats of all strains tested, and it has a similar tumor-inducing property in hamsters. Immunoelectronmicroscopic studies showed that envelope antigens of MSV-SD virus in rat bone tumors can be distinguished from those found in hamster bone tumor cells. In tissue cultures of MSV-SD rat bone tumors, two separate cell lines have been established: one of them releases both MSV and MuLV and the other produces MuL virus only. The MuLV in this cell line acts as helper. The different interactions appear to support the concept of control mechanisms for the partial expression of genes which are responsible for neoplastic properties, virus replication, and synthesis of gs-antigens. Biochemical studies on structural rearrangement and subunit composition of RNA released from MSV-SD virus, have shown that there are two forms of the native genome RNA differing in their sedimentation coeffiecients and in subunit composition. In human osteosarcoma tissue culture, type-C viruslike particles are found. In cocultures derived from human osteosarcoma with cells taken from the bone marrow or peripheral blood of patients with different types of leukemia, certain morphological changes are observed which resemble those induced in animal cells by RNA tumor viruses. In osteosarcomas where no cytoplasmic antigen could be proved by an immunofluorescence test, the antigen could be produced by cocultivation with antigen-positive leukemic bone marrow cells. Whole human embryo cells treated with fluid from leukemia bone marrow cultures showed the presence of the cytoplasmic antigen when tested with positive sera, but they showed no morphologic changes.

In high molecular weight RNA species, sedimentation coefficients ranging from 62S to 68S are demonstrated by molecular hybridization techniques. In cross-hybridization experiments, annealing values were observed only with complementary DNA products synthesized from sarcoma viruses. Three particularly high molecular weight RNA species released from human sarcoma cell cultures showed no cross-hybridization with either the DNA product of Rauscher leukemia virus or that of Gross leukemia virus.

This study was supported in part by USPHS Contract No. NO1-CP-33304 within the Virus Cancer Program of the Virus Cancer Program of the National Cancer Institute, USPHS, and by Grants CA-05831 and RR-05511 from the Division of Research Resources, NCI, NIH.

REFERENCES

1. ALBALA, M.M., ESPARZA, A.R.: Transplantable osteogenic sarcoma in inbred AKR mice. Cancer Res. 29, 1519-1522 (1969)
2. BARRETT, M.K., DALTON, A.J., EDWARDS, J.E.: A transplantable osteogenic sarcoma originating in a C_3H mouse. J. nat. Cancer Inst. 4, 389-402 (1944)
3. BASSIN, R.H., SIMONS, P.J., CHESTERMAN, F.C., HARVEY, J.J.: Murine sarcoma virus (HARVEY): characteristics of focus formation in mouse embryo cell cultures and virus production by hamster tumor cells. Int. J. Cancer 3, 265-272 (1968)
4. BISKIS, B.O., FINKEL, M.P.: Electron microscopy of the FBJ osteosarcoma virus. 27th Annual Proceedings of Electron Microscope Society of America (Ed. C.J. Arceneaux), p. 398, 1969

5. BOWEN, J.M., ALLEN, P.T., EAST, J.L., MARUYAMA, K., NEWTON, W.A., GEORGIADES, J., PRIORI, E.S., DMOCHOWSKI, L.: Molecular probes in studies on the relationship of viruses to human neoplasia. Amer. J. clin. Path. 60, 88-99 (1973)
6. BOWEN, J.M., EAST, J.L., ALLEN, P.T., MARUYAMA, K., PRIORI, E.S., GEORGIADES, J., CHAN, J.C., MILLER, M. F., SEMAN, G., DMOCHOWSKI, L.: Comparative morphology, immunology, and biochemistry of viruses associated with neoplasia of animal and man. In: Viruses, Evolution and Cancer: Comparative Virology. (Eds E. KURSTAK, K. MARAMOROSH), Vol. 2. New York; Academic Press 1973
7. CHAN, J.C., EAST, J.L., DMOCHOWSKI, L.: Sarcoma-negative leukemia-positive transformed cell culture established from murine sarcoma virus-induced rat bone tumor. Cancer Res. 35, 2475-2481 (1975)
8. DMOCHOWSKI, L.: Recent studies on leukemia and solid tumors in mice and man. Leukemia in animals and man. Proceedings IIIrd International Symposium on Comparative Leukemia Research, Paris, 1967 (Ed. H. J. BEDIXEN), p. 285. Basle, New York: Karger 1968
9. DMOCHOWSKI, L.: Comparison of leukemogenic and sarcomogenic viruses at the ultrastructural level. Proceedings IVth International Symposium on Comparative Leukemia Research (Ed. R. M. DUTCHER), p. 62. Basle, New York: Karger 1970 (Bibliotheca Haematologica no. 36)
10. DMOCHOWSKI, L.: Studies on the relationship of viruses to leukemia and solid tumors in man. Proceedings of the Tenth International Cancer Congress. Oncology, 1970 (Eds. R. L. CLARK, R. W. CUMLEY, J. C. McCAY), p. 134. Chicago: Year Book Medical Publishers 1971
11. DMOCHOWSKI, L.: Studies on the relationship of RNA viruses to the origin of leukemia and solid tumors of animals and man. In: Unifying Concepts of Leukemia. Proceedings Vth International Symposium on Comparative Leukemia Research (Eds. R. M. DUTCHER, L. CHIECO-BIANCHI), p. 1194. Basle, New York: Karger 1973 (Bibliotheca Haematologica no. 39)
12. DMOCHOWSKI, L., ALLEN, P.T., BOWEN, J.M., EAST, J.L., GEORGIADES, J., MARUYAMA, K., NEWTON, W,A.: Studies on transforming activities from human solid tumor cells following cocultivation with human leukemia bone marrow cells. In: Cellular Modification and Genetic Transformation by Exogenous Nucleic Acids. Monograph of the Sixth Miles International Symposium on Molecular Biology (Eds. R. BEERS, R. C. TILGHMAN), p. 157. Baltimore, Md.: Johns Hopkins University Press 1973
13. DMOCHOWSKI, L., BOWEN, J.M.: The search for a virus in human cancer. Proceedings Seventh National Cancer Conference. American Cancer Society, Inc. 697-710 (1973)
14. DMOCHOWSKI, L., EAST, J.L., BOWEN, J.M., LEWIS, M.L., SHIGEMATSU, T.: Studies on tumorigenicity of rat bone tumor virus (SD-MSV-M) in mice, rats, and hamsters. Tex. Rep. Biol. Med. 30, 301-312 (1973)
15. DMOCHOWSKI, L., GEORGIADES, J., EAST, J.L., ALLEN, P.T., BOWEN, J. M.: Virus retrieval studies in human neoplasia. Proceedings of the VIth International Symposium on Comparative Leukemia Research. Nagoya-Ise Shima. In Comparative Research 1973. Leukemogenesis, p. 431-449 (ed. R.M. Dutcher) University Tokyo Press 1975
16. DMOCHOWSKI, L., GREY, C.E.: Studies on microscopic structure of leukemias of known or suspected viral origin. A review. Blood 13, 1017-1042 (1958)
17. DUNN, T.B., ANDERVONT, H.B.: Histology of some neoplasms and non-neoplastic lesions found in wild mice maintained under laboratory conditions. J. Nat. Cancer Inst. 31, 873-885 (1963)
18. DURAN-REYNALS, F.: The reciprocal infection of ducks and chickens with tumor-inducing viruses. Cancer Res. 2, 343-369 (1942)
19. DURAN-REYNALS, F.: The infection of turkeys anf guinea fowls by the Rous sarcoma virus and the accompanying variations of the virus. Cancer Res. 3, 569-577 (1943)

20. EAST, J.L., ALLEN, P.T., KNESEK, J.E., CHAN, J.C., BOWEN, J.M., DMOCHOWSKI, L.: Structural rearrengement and subunit composition of RNA released from Soehner-Dmochowski murine sarcoma virus. J. Virol. 11, 709-720 (1973)
21. EAST, J.L., KNESEK, J.E., CHAN, J.C., MARUYAMA, K., PRIORI, E.S., DMOCHOWSKI, L.: Structural rearrangement and subunit composition of RNA released from Soehner-Dmochowski murine sarcoma virus. j. Virol. 11, 709-720 (1973)
22. End Results in Cancer. Report No. 4. U.S. Department of Health, Education and Welfare. Public Health Service, National Institutes of Health (Eds. L.M. Axtell, S.J. Cutler, M.H. Myers) DHEW Publication No. (NIH) 73-272, 1972
23. EVANS, D.L., BARNETT, J.W., DMOCHOWSKI, L.: Immunological responsiveness in rats infected with the Soehner-Dmochowski murine sarcoma virus (MSV-SD) Texas Rep. Biol. Med. 32, 449-460 (1974)
24. FINKEL, M.P., BISKIS, B.O.: Experimetal induction of osteosarcomas. Progr. exper. Tumor Res. 10, 72-111 (1968)
25. FINKEL, M.P., BISKIS, B.O., FARRELL, C.: Pathogenic effects of extracts of human osteosarcomas. Arch. Path. 84, 425-428 (1967)
26. FINKEL, M.P., BISKIS, B.O., FARRELL, C.: Osteosarcomas appearing in Syrian hamsters after treatment with extracts of human osteosarcomas. Proc. Nat. Acad. Sci. (Wash.) 60, 1223-1230 (1968)
27. FINKEL, M.P., BISKIS, B.O., JENKINS, P.B.: Virus induction of osteosarcoma in mice. Science 151, 698-701 (1966)
28. FISCHINGER, P.J., SCHAFER, W., SEIBERT, E.: Detection of some murine leukemia virus antigens in virus particles derived from 3T3 cells transformed only by murine sarcoma virus. Virology 47, 229-235 (1972)
29. FRANK, L.M., ROWLATT, C., CHESTERMAN, F.C.: Naturally occurring bone tumor in C57BL/ICrf mice. J. nat. Cancer Inst. 50, 431-438 (1973)
30. FUJINAGA, S., POEL, W.E., DMOCHOWSKI, L.: Light and electron microscope studies of osteosarcomas induced in rats and hamsters by Harvey and Moloney sarcoma viruses. Cancer Res. 30, 1698-1708 (1970)
31. GIRALDO, G., BETH, E., HIRSHAUT, Y., AOKI, T., OLD, L.J., BOYSE, E.A., CHOPRA, H.C.: Human sarcomas in culture. Foci of altered cells and a common antigen; induction of foci and antigen in human fibroblast cultures by filtrates. J. exper. Med. 133, 454-478 (1971)
32. HARTLEY, J.W., ROWE, W.P.: Production of altered cell foci in tissue culture by defective Moloney sarcoma virus particles. Proc. nat. Acad. Sci. (Wash.) 55, 780-786 (1966)
33. HARVEY, J.J.: An unidentified virus which causes the rapid production of tumors in mice. Nature (Lond.) 204, 1104-1105 (1964)
34. HARVEY, J.J.: Replication of murine sarcoma virus Harvey (MSV-H) in tissue cultures of virus-induced sarcomas. J. gen. Virol. 3, 327-336 (1968)
35. HELLSTROM, I., HELLSTROM, K.E.: Studies in cellular immunity and its serum-mediated inhibition in Moloney virus induced mouse sarcomas. Int. J. Cancer 4, 587-600 (1969)
36. HIRAKI, S., CHAN, J.C., HALES, R.L., DMOCHOWSKI, L.: An immunoelectron microscopy study of Soehner-Dmochowski murine sarcoma virus (MSV-SD) following passage in rats and hamsters. Cancer Res. 34, 2906-2910 (1974)
37. HUEBNER, R.J., HARTLEY, J.W., ROWE, W.P., JANE, N.T., CAPPRS, W.J.: Rescue of defective genome of Moloney sarcoma virus from noninfectious hamster tumor and the production of pseudotype sarcoma viruses with various leukemia viruses. Proc. Nat. Acad. Sci. (Wash.) 56, 1164-1168 (1966)
38. IKEMOTO, K., YAMAMOTO, T.: Induction of rat osteosarcoma by inoculation of murine sarcoma virus into bone marrow. Gann. 63, 141 (1972)

39. KANO-TANAKA, K., YOSHIDA, T.O., TANAKA, T., HANAICHI, T.: Establishment of a virus-persistent cell line and deviation of malignant cell clones from rat osteosarcoma induced by a murine sarcoma virus (Moloney). Gann 63, 459-469 (1972)
40. KANO-TANAKA, K., YOSHIDA, T.O., TANAKA, T., KOJIMA, K., HANAICHI, T.: Different neoplastic response of mice and rats to infection by murine sarcoma virus (Moloney). Gann 63, 445-457 (1972)
41. KARPAR, A., TUCKERMAN, E.: Transformation of human fibroblasts with DNA of cultured human rhabdomyosarcoma cells. Lancet 1974 2, 1138-1141
42. KELOFF, G., HUEBNER, R.J., LEE, Y.K., TONI, R., GILDEN, R.V.: Hamster-tropic sarcomagenic and nonsarcomagenic viruses derived from hamster tumors induced by the Gross pseudotype of Moloney sarcoma virus. Proc. Nat. Acad. Sci. (Wash.) 65, 310-317 (1970)
43. KLEMENT, V., HARTLEY, J.W., ROWE, W.P., HUEBNER, R.J.: Recovery of a hamster-specific focus-forming and sarcomagenic virus from "noninfectious" hamster tumor induced by the Kirsten sarcoma virus. J. nat. Cancer Inst. 43, 925-934 (1969)
44. LEVY, J.A., HARTLEY, J.W., ROWE, W.P., HUEBNER, R.J.: Studies of FBJ osteosarcoma virus in tissue culture. I. Biologic characteristics of the "C"-type viruses. J. nat. Cancer Inst. 51, 525-539 (1973)
45. MOLONEY, J.B.: A virus-induced rhabdomyosarcoma of mice, Nat. Cancer Inst. Monograph. 22, 139-142 (1966)
46. NAKAKUKI, K., SHIMOKAWA, K., YAMAICHI, H., OJIMA, A.: A transplantable osteogenic sarcoma in AKR/Ms mice. Proc. Jap. Cancer Ass. 31st Annual Meeting, Nagoya, p. 267, 1972
47. National Cancer Institute Fact Book 1974. DHEW Publication No. (NIH) 74-512, 1974
48. NOMURA, S., FISCHINGER, P.J., MATTERN, C.F.T., PEEBLES, P.T., BASSIN, R.H., FRIEDMAN, G.P.: Revertants of mouse cells transformed by murine sarcoma virus. I. Characterization of flat and transformed sublines without a rescuable murine sarcoma virus. Virology 50, 50-64 (1972)
49. PECK, K., VIOLA, M.V., SMITH, K.L., WIVEL, N.A., MOLONEY, J.B.: Biologic studies on hamster tumors induced by the murine sarcoma virus (Moloney). Cancer Res. 29, 1089-1102 (1969)
50. PRIORI, E.S., WILBUR, J.R., ALLEN, P.T., EAST, J.L., DMOCHOWSKI, L.: Transformation of cells in human bone tumor cultures. Proceedings VIth International Symposium on Comparative Leukemia Research, Nagoya/Ise-Shima, Japan. Comparative Leukemia Research 1973. Leukemogenesis, p. 185 (Eds. R.M. Dutcher, Y. Ito). Univ. of Tokyo Press 1975
51. PYBUS, F.C., MILLER, E.W.: Spontaneous bone tumors of mice. Amer. J. Cancer 33, 98-111 (1938)
52. SARMA, P.S., LOG, T., GILDEN, R.V.: Studies on hamster-specific oncogenic viruses derived from hamster tumors induced by Kirsten murine sarcoma virus. Proc. Soc. exp. Biol. 133, 718-722 (1970)
53. SOEHNER, R.L., DMOCHOWSKI, L.: Induction of bone tumors in rats and hamsters with murine sarcoma virus and their cell-free transmission. Nature 224, 191-192 (1969)
54. SOEHNER, R.L., FUJINAGA, S., DMOCHOWSKI, L.: Neoplastic bone lesions induced in rats and hamsters by Moloney and Harvey murine sarcoma viruses. In: Proceedings IVth International Symposium on Comparative Leukemia Research, (Ed. R.M. Dutcher), p. 539. Basle, New York: Karger 1970 (Bibliotheca Haematologica No. 36)
55. TODARO, G., HUEBNER, R.J.: N.A.S. Symposium: New evidence as the basis for increased efforts in Cancer Research. The viral oncogenic hypothesis' new evidence. Proc. nat. Acad. Sci. (Wash.) 59, 1009-1015 (1972)
56. Unifying Concepts of Leukemia (Eds. R.M. Dutcher, L. Chieco-Bianchi). Basle, New York: Karger 1973 (Bibliotheca Haematologica No. 39)

57. YUMOTO, T., ANDO, K., YOSHIDA, H., OKAMOTO, S., MATSUI, K.: Naturally occurring bone tumor in a NZB mouse. 1974 (in press)
58. YUMOTO, T., POEL, W.E., KODAMA, T., DMOCHOWSKI, L.: Studies on FBJ virus-induced bone tumors in mice. Tex. Rep. Biol. Med. 28, 145-165 (1970)

Immunologic Aspects of Human Sarcomas

D. J. PRITCHARD, J. C. IVINS, and R. E. RITTS, Jr.

INTRODUCTION

Considerable evidence has been accumulated from clinical and laboratory observations to support the concept that host factors influence the development and progression of human sarcomas. There is suggestive evidence that the immunologic response of the patient to his sarcoma is one such factor. Thus, EVERSON and COLE (8), and other authors have cited specific case reports of the spontaneous regression of tumors, including various sarcomas. Conversely, WOODRUFF has cited the sudden appearance of sarcomas after long latent periods, sometimes coinciding with immunosuppressive therapy (36). Other authors (11, 21) noted the failure of circulating tumor cells in autotransplants to metastasize. Others have noted an increased incidence of malignant disease in patients with congenital immunologic deficiency diseases (9) and in those receiving immunosuppressive treatment for renal homografts (14, 23). WILSON et al. noted the regression of disseminated neoplasms after cessation of immunosuppressive drugs in organ transplant patients who inadvertently received tumor allografts from cancer patients (33). The results of a study of patients who survived longer than 10 years after treatment for osteogenic sarcoma suggested that the survivors had better immune responses than did the nonsurvivors (22).

Both humoral and cellular expressions of immunoincompetence in patients with sarcomas have been reported. MORTON and MALMGREN reported the presence of tumor-associated antibodies in the sera of patients with osteogenic sarcoma (20); they also found antisarcoma antibodies in a high percentage of family members and associates of sarcoma patients. Cross-reactivity between several human mesenchymal sarcomas was also demonstrated with the aid of a liposarcoma antigen (18); 92 percent of all sarcoma patients had positive complement-fixation titers to this common sarcoma antigen, whereas 21 percent of normal blood-bank donors reacted positively. With sera from patients who had various other malignancies, no more than 26 percent of sarcoma patients had demonstrable titers. MORTON et al. also demonstrated that this common sarcoma antigen promotes an in-vivo antibody response that is predominantly IgM (17, 19). Furthermore, antigens located on the cell surface render the tumor cells susceptible to in-vitro cytolysis when reacted with specific antibody and complement. The serum factor responsible for cytolysis has been shown to be antibody (35); the cytotoxic reaction is complement-dependent, the reaction is specific, and the cytotoxin is extractable in the γ-globulin fraction of the serum. By the use of indirect immunofluorescence techniques (24, 25, 26) tumor-associated antibodies have also been demonstrated in patients with osteogenic sarcomas. REILLY et al. reported that the sera of 52 of 53 patients with osteogenic sarcoma reacted positively to cryostat-cut sections of osteosarcoma tissue (27).

EILBER and MORTON showed a correlation between the degree of general depression of immunologic responsiveness and the rapidity of growth of sarcomas (6), and they related this to prognosis after surgical therapy. There is a paucity of literature regarding *in-vitro* and *in-vivo* evidence of cellular immunodeficiency in patients with various sarcomas. The few reports of the use of cellular cytotoxicity and colony inhibition tests are not consistent, and the results are inconclusive.

Within the last 10 years, many investigators have shown that the small immunocompetent lymphocyte under regulation by the thymus (the T-cell) is responsible for mediation of cellular immunity. Such specifically sensitized immunocompetent cells undergo blastogenic transformation when placed *in vitro* in contact with a specific antigen to which the cell has been sensitized. In addition, there are nonspecific materials or mitogens, many of them lectins, that are also capable of transforming T-cells or bursa-equivalent cells (B-cells) or both types of cells, presumably because of complementary receptor sites on their membranes. While these mitogens may not show evidence of specific immunologic reactivity, they do permit at least a qualitative estimation of T-cell or B-cell reactivity. Thus, the ability of lymphocytes to undergo transformation when exposed to either phytohemagglutinin or concanavalin A may reflect the potential for activation of predominantly thymus-derived T-cells; lymphocytes that are independent of the thymus (B-cells) undergo blastogenesis when exposed to pokeweed, although it is clear that some T-cells are also transformed. The possibility of using these various plant mitogens to induce lymphocyte transformation allows the study of different populations of lymphocytes and thus to quantitate individually the reactivity of T-cells and B-cells as they vary with the clinical status of the patient. Several studies utilizing lymphocyte transformation as an *in-vitro* correlate of delayed-type hypersensitivity in patients with sarcomas have been reported (1, 15, 10, 32). Some of these studies suggest diminished to absent transformation when lymphocytes are exposed to nonspecific mitogens such as phytohemagglutinin, concanavalin A, and pokeweed. However, the reported results are not comparable and are sometimes conflicting. With other cancers, any defect in cellular immune competency appears to be general, while this defect is approximately proportional to the severity and extent of the malignant process, thus reflecting the correlation of relative anergy with disease progression.

The present study was undertaken to make a quantitative assessment of the immunologic status of patients with sarcomas and to correlate this information with the prognosis.

METHODS AND PROCEDURE

Patients. Forty-seven patients with mesenchymal sarcomas, seen consecutively at the Mayo Clinic, were examined clinically and in the laboratory for evidence of humoral and cellular immunity. Each patient was seen either immediately before treatment or after a 3-month interval between any prior treatment and testing. Two patients had metastasis at the time of the initial laboratory visit. Two others were clinically free of disease but had previously undergone resection of metastatic lesions. One patient presented with a soft-tissue recurrence. All patients were subsequently seen at 3-month intervals, or sooner if the clinical situation dictated. All patients were followed for at least one year or until death. There were 24 males and 23 females, whose ages ranged from 11 to 65 years, with an average of 24.4 years.

The initial visit involved a general medical examination, complete roentgenographic studies, including stereo posteroanterior and lateral chest projections and whole-lung tomograms, and a standard battery of laboratory studies.

Humoral Cytotoxicity Test. Test Sera. Serum samples were stored at -196°C until used.

Target Cells. Cells were obtained from an established osteosarcoma line maintained at 37°C in 5% CO_2 with RPMI 1640 supplemented with 20% fetal calf serum. The target cells were treated with 0.25% trypsin solution, counted, and diluted to 6×10^3 viable cells per ml tissue-culture medium (RPMI 1640 with 20% fetal calf serum) and then seeded into the wells of a Falcon microtiter plastic plate by means of a Hamilton microliter syringe with a semiautomatic dispenser to give approximately 100 cells per well. The distribution on a given plate was relatively uniform, as revealed by counting trials. A nonsealing lid was applied, and the plate was incubated overnight at 37°C to allow adherence of the cells to the wells. The medium was then aspirated, and the cells were washed several times with tissue-culture medium. The medium was replaced with 5 µl per well of the test serum. The outer two rows of wells were used as untreated controls. The middle two rows were used for the addition of known negative and positive control sera obtained from healthy donors. Test serum was then added in duplicate to rows 2 and 7, rows 3 and 8, and rows 4 and 9. After incubation for 60 minutes at 37°C, the test serum was replaced with 5 µl of pooled guinea-pig serum as a source of complement. After a further 2-hour incubation, the complement was removed and the cells were labeled with fluorescein diacetate (which is hydrolyzed by the living cell to produce fluorescence). The plates were washed once in Hanks' balanced salt solution and kept in the dark until reading on a fluorescence microscope. The mean viable cell counts of 12 replicates of test serum were compared with 12 replicates of the negative controls in the same plate to derive a humoral cytotoxic index (34). The humoral cytotoxic index (HCI) is defined by the following formula:

$$HCI = \frac{\text{no. of viable control cells - no. of viable test cells}}{\text{no. of viable control cells}}$$

Thus, an index of 0 represents no cytotoxicity and one of 1.0 represents 100 percent cytotoxicity. A negative index is possible but is considered as a chance deviation from 0 and is recorded as 0.

Delayed-Type Hypersensitivity Skin Tests. Various common antigens were tested for recall. The reagents included purified protein derivative, 0.1 ml (intermediate strength) (Mantoux Connaught Liquid); mumps, 0.1 ml containing 2 CFU ST antigen (Lilly); streptokinase-streptodornase (Varidase) (Lederle Lab), 50 units freshly prepared; *Candida* organisms (*Monilia albicans*), 0.1 ml of 1:100 extract with 50% glycerin (Hollister-Stier Lab); and diluent (PBS). All antigens were applied as intradermal injections in the forearm.

Reactions to the skin tests were determined at 24, 48, and 72 hours. Induration, the hallmark of delayed hypersensitivity skin testing, was measured (mm) in two diameters (major and minor diameters) with calipers, and the average was calculated; the size of the response to the diluent was subtracted from this average.

Skin tests were considered unequivocally positive if reactions showed 5 mm or more of induration. Responses of 1 to 4 mm were considered negative if the diluent yielded a comparable reaction, but any presenting induration was deemed positive if it was greater than that of the diluent site.

Lymphocyte Transformation. Lymphocyte Separation. Thirty ml of heparinized venous blood was allowed to sediment. Lymphocytes were then separated according to the method of Boyum as modified by RITTS (28), a ficoll-Hypaque gradient being used. The viability of the separated lymphocytes was 94 to 97 percent, as determined by trypan blue exclusion.

Mitogens and Lymphocyte Cultures. Duplicate-quadruplicate cultures containing 0.05 ml phytohemagglutinin-M (Bacto-PHA-M) or 0.025 ml pokeweed (Gibco Pokeweed Mitogen) or concanavalin A (25 μg) per 2.5 ml culture (1.25×10^6 cells) and duplicate control cultures (nonstimulated) were incubated for 96 hours at 37°C.

Labeling Procedure. $|^{125}I|$2'-Desoxyuridine was diluted to 5 μCi/ml and 0.1 ml of the diluted isotope was added to each culture 4 hours prior to harvesting (i.e. at 92 hours).

Counting Procedure. Cold uridine was added at the end of a 4-hour "pulse". Cultures were precipitated with 10 percent trichloroacetic acid, and culture tubes containing cell precipitates were placed in a γ-scintillation counter, and counts of ^{125}I per 60 seconds were determined. Counting controls included ^{125}I standard, blank medium, and spontaneous transformation. Decay was corrected back to day 1 of the ^{125}I half-life. Data were expressed as net cpm of incorporated label, as calculated from the average cpm of the stimulated lymphocytes minus the average cpm of the unstimulated lymphocytes or as the ratio of the average cpm of stimulated to average cpm of unstimulated lymphocytes.

RESULTS

The various parameters obtained at the initial visit were studied. Patients were then separated into two groups, depending on whether or not the sarcoma progressed, as evidenced by either metastasis or death; the study involved both the 6-month and the 1-year follow-up. At 6 months, 31 patients remained free of disease (17 females and 14 males, average age 24.9 years) and 16 had progression (7 females and 9 males, average age 23.5 years). At 12 months, 27 patients remained free of disease (15 females and 12 males, average age 21.9 years) and 20 had progression (9 females and 11 males, average age 27.9 years).

Humoral Cytotoxicity Results. The humoral cytotoxicity indices of patients with sarcoma who remained free of disease were compared with those in whom metastasis developed or who died (Table 1). The median

Table 1. Humoral cytotoxicity indices in patients with sarcoma. Significant difference (rank-sum test): *$p<0.01$; †$p<0.01$

Type of patient	No. of patients	Indices Mean	Range	Median
Sarcoma, free of disease at 6 mo (S_1)	31	0.51	0.10-0.93	0.52*
Sarcoma, metastasis or death at 6 mo (S_2)	16	0.06	0.00-0.49	0.03*
Sarcoma, free of disease at 12 mo (S_3)	27	0.48	0.10-0.74	0.51†
Sarcoma, metastasis or death at 12 mo (S_4)	20	0.19	0.00-0.93	0.04†

indices were significantly different: patients with low indices tended to have the worst prognosis. This appears to be a short-term factor, however, since the four patients who developed metastasis or who died between 6 and 12 months all had high indices. There was a moderate overlap of values; the most striking example was the patient with an index of 0.49 who underwent a forequarter amputation because of osteogenic sarcoma and who died 3 months later of widespread metastasis.

Skin Test Results. The number of responses of the delayed-type hypersensitivity skin tests is shown in Table 2. Data from columns 3 and 4 of Table 2 were combined, and the independence of type of patient and number of responses was tested by the use of chi-square. There was a highly significant difference ($p<0.001$).

Table 2. Skin test results in patients with sarcoma. Significant difference (t test): *$p<0.05$; †$p<0.01$

Type of patient	No. of patients	Mean ages (yr)	No. of reponses 0	1	2	3	4	Mean no. of responses
Controls	40	33.2	0	14	10	14	2	2.10
S_1	31	24.9	2	12	8	9	0	1.77*
S_2	16	23.5	6	4	5	1	0	1.06*
S_3	27	21.9	1	9	8	9	0	1.93†
S_4	20	27.9	7	7	5	1	0	1.00†

We investigated further to determine more specifically where the departure from independence was. We found that the patients with progressive sarcoma (S_2 and S_4) were the ones who were different, particularly in that there were fewer nonresponders and fewer responders to three or four antigens in these groups. The patients with nonprogressive sarcomas were not significantly different from the normal.

The mean number of responses was not significantly different for the patients who remained free of disease for 6 or 12 months (S_1 or S_3) than for controls. However, the mean number of responses for the patients who developed metastasis or who died at 6 or 12 months (S_2 or S_4) was significantly different ($p<0.001$) from that of patients with nonprogressive sarcoma (S_1 and S_3); this is confirmed by Table 3.

Patients with sarcoma, especially those with progressive disease, tended to have less pronounced responses to skin testing than did the controls; however, this difference was not significant for mumps (Table 4).

Table 3. Skin test results in patients with sarcoma

Type of patient	No. of patients	No. responding[a] M	PPD	C	SK-SD	% responding[a] M	PPD	C	SK-SD
Controls	40	23	4	19	38	57.5	10.0	47.5	95.0
S_1	31	15	3	15	22	48.4	9.7	48.4	71.0
S_2	16	4	1	5	7	25.0	6.3	31.3	43.8
S_3	27	14	3	14	21	51.9	11.1	51.9	77.8
S_4	20	5	1	6	8	25.0	5.0	30.0	40.0

[a]M, mumps; PPD, purified protein derivative; C, *Candida* organisms; SK-SD, streptokinase-streptodornase.

Table 5. Lymphocyte transformation results (medians and ranges as cpm) in human sarcoma

Type of patient	No. of patients	Con A S-NS	Con A S/NS	No. of patients	PHA S-NS	PHA S/NS	No. of patients	PWM S-NS	PWM S/NS
Controls[a]	26	6,668 (560–13,398)	6.2 (1.8–11.9)	39	6,066 (2,221–23,662)	6.3 (1.7–34.6)	36	5,187 (463–21,137)	5.0 (1.5–16.1)
All S[a]	23	2,162 (0–46,542)	2.5 (1.0–81.0)	41	1,205 (0–36,521)	1.8 (1.0–43.8)	38	2,523 (66–72,932)	2.8 (1.0–31.1)
S_1[b]	15	3,518 (0–46,542)	3.1 (1.0–81.0)	26	1,646 (0–36,521)	2.0 (1.0–43.8)	25	2,269 (111–72,932)	2.8 (1.0–31.1)
S_2[b]	8	547 (0–6,985)	1.2 (1.0–6.6)	15	1,062 (0–7,822)	1.8 (1.0–8.3)	13	2,808 (66–12,846)	2.8 (1.0–13.1)
S_3[c]	14	3,633 (0–46,542)	3.1 (1.0–81.0)	22	1,536 (0–36,521)	1.9 (1.0–43.8)	22	2,902 (111–72,932)	3.2 (1.0–31.1)
S_4[c]	9	711 (0–6,985)	1.3 (1.0–6.6)	19	1,205 (0–7,822)	1.8 (1.0–8.3)	16	1,500 (66–12,846)	1.8 (1.0–13.1)

[a]Controls significantly higher, than other groups, for all 3 mitogens ($p<0.01$).

[b]S_1 significantly greater than S_2 for Con A only ($p<0.05$).

[c]S_3 significantly greater than S_4 for Con A only ($p<0.05$).

Table 4. Skin test results in patients[a] with sarcoma

Type of patient	Mean size of responses[b] M	PPD	C	SK-SD	Range of responses M	PPD	C	SK-SD
Controls[c]	23.6	56.0	27.4	58.1	5-52	40-67	5-52	5-127
S_1[d]	18.1	10.7	15.3	31.1	5-31	8-14	5-33	5-65
S_2[d]	15.8	10.0	13.8	26.9	5-38	10	5-30	9-83
S_3[d]	17.9	10.7	15.3	31.6	5-31	8-14	5-33	5-65
S_4[d]	16.6	10.0	14.0	26.0	5-38	10	5-30	9-83

[a]Patients who responded positively (see Table 3).
[b]Average (mm) major and minor diameters of induration.
[c]Controls significantly different (t test) from all sarcoma groups for PPD, C, and SK-SD.
[d]No significant difference between S_1 and S_2 or S_3 and S_4.

Lymphocyte Transformation Results. The results for concanavalin A, phytohemagglutinin, and pokeweed are shown in Table 5. Examination of the cpm as a measure of lymphocyte transformation revealed considerable variability and skewness. The results were therefore analyzed by use of the rank-sum test instead of the t-test. Because medians are more indicative of the averages in such cases, they are presented instead of means. All three mitogens had differences in cpm for stimulated and nonstimulated lymphocytes that were significantly higher for controls than for the total group with sarcoma ($p<0.01$). This difference was also true when the ratio of stimulated to nonstimulated lymphocytes was considered ($p<0.01$).

Patients with sarcoma classified into S_1, S_2, S_3, and S_4 (as defined) were also compared. Patients in group S_2 or S_4 (with disease at 6 or 12 months) had responses to concanavalin A that were significantly lower than those for patients in S_1 or S_3 (free of disease at 6 or 12 months), respectively. Responses to phytohemagglutinin were similar but not significantly different. There was no significant or consistent difference in the responses to pokeweed.

DISCUSSION

Our study confirms that both the humoral and the cellular parameters of immune responsiveness are affected in sarcoma. The most significant finding is that the degree of diminution of responsiveness tends to be related to the short-term clinical prognosis.

The humoral results are consonant with those obtained previously (35, 7, 25) in studies based on the use of various techniques, including complement fixation, immunofluorescence , and cytotoxicity testing to demonstrate systemic tumor-associated antibodies in patients with sarcoma. MORTON and his group have also suggested that these various tests tend to indicate the extent and progression of the disease (16, 19).

The diminution or absence of delayed-type hypersensitivity or cellular immunity has frequently been noted in different histologic tumor types. In our study, the diminution in delayed-type hypersensitivity, as shown by the failure to respond to recall antigen testing, was especially evident in patients who subsequently developed metastasis or died. All the normal controls responded to at least one microbial antigen, whereas eight patients with sarcoma failed to respond to at least one skin test; seven of the eight had progression of the disease during the first year.

Numerous reports indicate that lymphocyte blastogenic transformation induced by phytohemagglutinin or concanavalin A and, to a lesser extent, by pokeweed as in-vitro correlates of delayed-type hypersensitivity is impaired in patients with cancer. Such impairment is presumably due, at least at an operational level, to a deficit or a malfunction (or both) of the thymus-regulated T-lymphocytes (29). Using morphologic criteria for lymphocyte reactivity, HERSH and OPPENHEIM noted a correlation between phytohemagglutinin-induced lymphocyte reactivity and reactivity to recall skin test antigens (13). CATALONA et al. stated that the evidence appears conclusive that in-vitro lymphocyte reactivity to phytohemagglutinin quantitates in-vivo cell-mediated immune competence and demonstrated the greater incidence of low lymphocyte reactivity in patients with sarcomas as compared to normal persons and to patients with some other malignancies; patients with disseminated sarcoma had the most striking lack of reactivity (1). McMASTER et al. found no impairment in phytohemagglutinin response of lymphocytes from nine patients with various stages of osteosarcoma (15). GOLUB et al. compared lymphocyte transformation with phytohemagglutinin, concanavalin A, and pokeweed in nine patients who had sarcomas in various stages with that in normal persons, and found that there was no significant diminution of phytohemagglutinin response or pokeweed response, but the average response to concanavalin A was significantly reduced (10). TWOMEY et al. compared phytohemagglutinin reactivity in patients with sarcoma before operation with reactivity of cured patients (32). They demonstrated low responsiveness in preoperative sarcoma-bearing patients, whereas cured sarcoma patients showed high reactivity as compared to normals-suggesting either that there is a "heightened in-vitro lymphocyte reactivity" similar to the "overshoot" of lymphocyte responsiveness to phytohemagglutinin (2) or that cured patients might have had normal immune competence before operation, whereas patients with impaired immunity might be the ones who die of recurrent tumor. Our present prospective approach indicates that this is true; i.e. the median value in our study tended to be lower in patients whose clinical prognosis was poor.

The variances and overlap of values shown in the results of any of these tests suggest caution in the interpretation of a single test result. In addition, the exceptions to the median result indicate that other factors may be operative. Many investigators have suggested that the interaction between humoral and cellular immune responses may be of crucial importance. Thus, impressive evidence has been offered in support of the theory that tumor enhancement may result from a humoral blocking factor (12, 3, 4, 5). SINKOVICS et al. have suggested that both humoral and cellular components may be separated by cytotoxic or enhancing ability and that various combinations may exist in a given patient (30, 31). Such factors may help to explain why some patients with high cytotoxic indices subsequently develop disease progression. The application of techniques in a prospective manner, with multiple parameters of immune responsiveness, as suggested by these authors, may allow an even higher correlation of laboratory findings with clinical results.

At our institution, 235 patients with sarcomas have now been tested for multiple parameters of immunologic responsiveness. These patients will be followed prospectively in a manner similar to that described in the present study. Not enough time has elapsed for any definite conclusions to be possible; however, the initial test results for this larger group are similar to those noted in the present group of 47 patients. The tests currently utilized in the assessment of immune competence include an assessment of the numbers of B-cells and T-cells, responsiveness to DNCB skin testing, and procedures included in this report. The current lymphocyte transformation procedure utilizes a microtechnique that allows for the assessment of the optimal mitogen dose and the optimal time of incubation of lymphocytes with the mitogens. We are hopeful that such techniques may help to identify patients with minimal residual disease before it becomes clinically manifest. Such an approach might aid in the selection of patients for the recently accepted clinical trials in which adjunctive chemotherapy or immunotherapy (or both) follows the surgical removal of grossly apparent cancer.

SUMMARY

Forty-seven patients with mesenchymal sarcoma seen at the Mayo Clinic were tested for humoral and cellular immunologic responsiveness by means of a humoral cytotoxicity test, skin tests for delayed-type hypersensitivity, and lymphocyte transformation with concanavalin A, phytohemagglutinin, and pokeweed. Prospective follow-up of the clinical and laboratory results revealed that patients with low humoral cytotoxic indices, anergic skin test responses, or low lymphocyte transformation responsiveness tended to have the worst short-term clinical outlook.

This investigation was supported in part by Research Grant CA-11911 from the National Institutes of Health, Public Health Service.

REFERENCES

1. CATALONA, W.J., SAMPLE, W.F., CHRETIEN, P.B.: Lymphocyte reactivity in cancer patients. Correlation with tumor histology and clinical stage. Cancer 31, 65-71 (1973)
2. CHEEMA, A.R., HERSH, E.M.: Local tumor immunotherapy with in vitro activated autochthonous lymphocytes. Cancer 29, 982-986 (1972)
3. COHEN, A.M.: Host immunity to growing sarcomas. Tumor-specific serum inhibition of tumor-specific cellular immunity. Cancer 31, 81-89 (1973)
4. COHEN, A.M., KETCHAM, A.S., MORTON, D.L.: Cellular immunity to a common human sarcoma antigen and its specific inhibition by sera from patients with growing sarcomas. Surgery 72, 560-567 (1972)
5. COHEN, A.M., KETCHAM, A.S., MORTON, D.L.: Tumor-specific cellular cytotoxicity to human sarcomas. Evidence for a cell-mediated host immune response to a common sarcoma cell-surface antigen. J. Natl. Cancer Inst. 50, 585-589 (1973)
6. EILBER, F.R., MORTON, D.L.: Impaired immunologic reactivity and recurrence following cancer surgery. Cancer 25, 362-367 (1970a)
7. EILBER, F.R., MORTON, D.L.: Sarcoma-specific antigens. Detection by complement fixation with serum from sarcoma patients. J. Natl. Cancer Inst. 44, 651-656 (1970b)
8. EVERSON, T.C., COLE, W.H.: Spontaneous Regression of Cancer. A Study and Abstract of Reports in the World Medical Literature and of Personal Communications Concerning Spontaneous Regression of Malignant Disease. Philadelphia: Saunders 1966
9. GATTI, R.A., GOOD, R.A.: Occurence of malignancy in immunodeficiency diseases. A literature review. Cancer 28, 89-98 (1971)
10. GOLUB, S.H., O'CONNELL, T.X., MORTON, D.L.: Correlation of in vivo and in vitro assays of immunocompetence in cancer patients. Cancer Res. 34, 1833-1837 (1974)

11. GRACE, J.T., Jr.: Clinical aspects of immunity in untreated cancer. Ann. N.Y. Acad. Sci. 114, 736-746 (1964)
12. HELLSTRÖM, I., SJÖGREN, H.O., WARNER, G., HELLSTRÖM, K.E.: Blocking of cell-mediated tumor immunity by sera from patients with ıg growing neoplasms. Int. J. Cancer 7, 226-237 (1971)
13. HERSH, E.M., OPPENHEIM, J.J.: Impaired in vitro lymphocyte transformation in Hodgkin's disease. N. Engl. J. Med. 273, 1006-1012 (1965)
14. MCKHANN, C.F.: Primary malignancy in patients undergoing immunosuppression for renal transplantation. A request for information. Transplantation 8, 209-212 (1969)
15. MCMASTER, J.H., WEINERT, C.R., Jr., DICKENS, D.R.V.: Immunocompetence of lymphocytes from osteosarcoma patients (letter to the editor). Lancet 1, 781-782 (1973)
16. MORTON, D.L.: Cancer immunology and the surgeon (editorial). Surgery 67, 396-398 (1970)
17. MORTON, D.L., EILBER, F.R., JOSEPH, W.L., WOOD, W.C., TRAHAN, E., KETCHAM, A.S.: Immunological factors in human sarcomas and melanomas. A rational basis for immunotherapy. Ann. Surg. 172, 740-747 (1970)
18. MORTON, D.L., HALL, W.T., MALMGREN, R.A.: Human liposarcomas. Tissue cultures containing foci of transformed cells with viral particles. Science 165, 813-816 (1969)
19. MORTON, D.L., HOLMES, E.C., EILBER, F.R., WOOD, W.C.: Immunological aspects of neoplasia. A rational basis for immunotherapy. Ann. Intern. Med. 74, 587-604 (1971)
20. MORTON, D.L., MALMGREN, R.A.: Human osteosarcomas. Immunologic evidence suggesting an associated infectious agent. Science 162, 1279-1281 (1968)
21. NADLER, S.H., MOORE, G.E.: Clinical immunologic study of malignant disease. Response to tumor transplants and transfer of leukocytes. Ann. Surg. 164, 482-489 (1966)
22. O'HARA, J.M., HUTTER, R.V.P., FOOTE, F.W., Jr., MILLER, T., WOODARD, H.Q.: An analysis of thirty patients surviving longer than ten years after treatment for osteogenic sarcoma. J. Bone Jt. Surg. (Am.) 50, 335-354 (1968)
23. PENN, I., STARZL, T.E.: Malignant tumors arising de novo in immunosuppressed organ transplant recipients. Transplantation 14, 407-417 (1972)
24. PRIORI, E.S., WILBUR, J.R., DMOCHOWSKI, L.: Immunofluorescence tests on sera of patients with osteogenic sarcoma. J. Natl. Cancer Inst. 46, 1299-1308 (1971)
25. PRITCHARD, D.J., REILLY, C.A., Jr., FINKEL, M.P.: Evidence for a human osteosarcoma virus (letter to the editor). Nature (New. Biol.) 234, 126-127 (1971)
26. PRITCHARD, D.J., REILLY, C.A., Jr., FINKEL, M.P., IVINS, J.C.: Cytotoxicity of human osteosarcoma sera to hamster sarcoma cells. Cancer 34, 1935-1939 (1974)
27. REILLY, C.A., Jr., PRITCHARD, D.J., BISKIS, B.O., FINKEL, M.P.: Immunologic evidence suggesting a viral etiology of human osteosarcoma. Cancer 30, 603-609 (1972)
28. RITTS, R.E., Jr.: Tests for immune function of lymphocytes, pp. 381-400. In Laboratory Procedures in Clinical Microbiology. Boston: Little, Brown & Co. 1974
29. RITTS, R.E., Jr., NEEL, H.B., III: An overview of cancer immunology. Mayo Clin. Proc. 49, 118-131 (1974)
30. SINKOVICS, J.G., CABINESS, J.R., SHULLENBERGER, C.C.: Disappearance after chemotherapy of blocking serum factors as measured in vitro with lymphocytes cytotoxic to tumor cells. Cancer 30, 1428-1437 (1972)

31. SINKOVICS, J.G., WILLIAMS, D.E., KAY, H.D., CAMPOS, L.T., HOWE, C.D.: Intensification of immune reactions of patients to cultured sarcoma cells (abstract). In: Symposium on Neoplasm Immunity: Theory and Application, Chicago, September, 11, 1974
32. TWOMEY, P.L., CATALONA, W.J., CHRETIEN, P.B.: Cellular immunity in cured cancer patients. Cancer 33, 435-440 (1974)
33. WILSON, R.E., HAGER, E.B., HAMPERS, C.L., CORSON, J.M., MERRILL, J.P., MURRAY, J.E.: Immunologic rejection of human cancer transplanted with a renal allograft. N. Engl. J. Med. 278, 479-483 (1968)
34. WOOD, W.C., MORTON, D.L.: Microcytotoxicity test. Detection in sarcoma patients of antibody cytotoxic to human sarcoma cells. Science 170, 1318-1320 (1970)
35. WOOD, W.C., MORTON, D.L.: Host immune response to a common cell-surface antigen in human sarcomas. Detection by cytotoxicity tests. N. Engl. J. Med. 284, 569-572 (1971)
36. WOODRUFF, M.: The challenge of osteosarcoma. Ann. roy. Coll. Surg. Engl. 44, 299-307 (1969)

BIBLIOGRAPHY

(References not cited in text)

CHRETIEN, P.B., CROWDER, W.L., GERTNER, H.R., SAMPLE, W.F., CATALONA, W.J.: Correlation of preoperative lymphocyte reactivity with the clinical course of cancer patients. Surg. Gynecol. Obstet. 136, 380-384 (1973)

EILBER, F.R., MORTON, D.L.: Demonstration in sarcoma patients of anti-tumour antibodies which fix only human complement (letter to the editor). Nature 225, 1137-1138 (1970a)

EILBER, F.R., MORTON, D.L.: Immunologic studies of human sarcomas. Additional evidence suggesting an associated sarcoma virus. Cancer 26, 588-596 (1970b)

GARRIOCH, D.B., GOOD, R.A., GATTI, R.A.: Lymphocyte response to P.H.A. in patients with non-lymphoid tumours (letter to the editor). Lancet 1, 618 (1970)

HUMPHREY, L.J., LINCOLN, P.M., GRIFFEN, W.O., Jr.: Immunologic response in patients with disseminated cancer. Ann. Surg. 168, 374-380 (1968)

KRANT, M.J., MANSKOPF, G., BRANDRUP, C.S., MADOFF, M.A.: Immunologic alterations in bronchogenic cancer. Sequential study. Cancer 21, 623-631 (1968)

LYTTON, B., HUGHES, L.E., FULTHORPE, A.J.: Circulating antibody response in malignant disease. Lancet 1, 69-70 (1964)

MOORE, M.: Tumour-specific antigens. Their possible significance in the etiology and treatment of malignant disease. J. Bone Jt Surg. (Br.) 53, 13-22 (1971)

MORTON, D.L.: Immunologic studies with human neoplasms. J. Reticulo-endothel. Soc. 10, 137-160 (1971)

MORTON, D.L., MALMGREN, R.A., HALL, W.T., SCHIDLOVSKY, G.: Immunologic and virus studies with human sarcomas. Surgery 66, 152-160 (1969)

PIESSENS, W.F.: Evidence for human cancer immunity. A review. Cancer 26, 1212-1220 (1970)

PINSKY, C.M., OETTGEN, H.F., EL DOMEIRI, A., OLD, L.J., BEATTIE, E.J., BURCHENAL, J.H.: Delayed hypersensitivity reactions in patients with cancer. Proc. Amer. Cancer Res. 12, 100 (1971)

PREHN, R.T., MAIN, J.M.: Immunity to methylcholanthrene-induced sarcomas. J. Natl. Cancer Inst. 18, 769-778 (1957)

SUTHERLAND, R.M., INCH, W.R., MCCREDIE, J.A.: Phytohemagglutinin (PHA)-induced transformation of lymphocytes from patients with cancer. Cancer 27, 574-578 (1971)
VÁNKY, F., STJERNSWÄLD, J., NILSONNE, U.: Cellular immunity to human sarcoma. J. Natl. Cancer Inst. 46, 1145-1151 (1971)

The Immune-Status in Patients with Bone and Soft-Tissue Sarcomas

R. KOTZ, W. RELLA, and M. SALZER

As the sarcoma develops in most cases at a stage of life when there is sufficient immunity, namely during the first three decades, immunological testing of sarcoma-bearing patients is extremely interesting. A further reason for examining sarcoma patients is the rapid development of metastases in this illness. This suggests that observation of the development over a short period will suffice for an assessment of the prognosis (8, 16). If careful clinical examination 6 months after actual treatment does not reveal metastases, the chances of survival are considerably better than if metastases are discovered.

So far immunotherapy in cases of bone tumor has not been really successful, although positive results have been described sporadically in the literature (4, 10, 12, 13) in cases where clinical developments were taken as positive criteria. These developments as such, however, cannot lead to a clarification of the very complex immunologic process. Therefore it seems necessary to gain an insight into the immunity situation before immunotherapy is applied and to analyze changes in the course of the disease. According to the results so far (3, 6, 14, 17), successful checking of the anti-tumor-defense seems to be effective by applying cell-mediated cytotoxicity, bringing examinations of cellular immunity into the focus or our interest.

MATERIAL

It has been possible to carry out immunological examinations in 50 sarcoma patients in the last two years. The diagnosis was established histologically in all these cases. The histologic diagnoses were made by Dr. Mechthild SALZER-KUNTSCHIK. The tumors under discussion comprised 40 bone and 10 soft-tissue sarcomata (Table 1). The average age of the patients was 24.5 (± 15.4) years. Clarification of the diagnosis, therapy and regular control were carried out at our clinic. Radical surgery was performed in 17 of 19 patients suffering from osteosarcoma and two received radiation therapy. Out of 17 round-cell sarcoma patients all but three who had radical resection received radiation therapy. Radical surgery was performed in all other cases of sarcoma. To avoid tumor-cell showers, cytostatic polychemotherapy with four substances (cyclophosphamide, vinblastine, 5-fluorouracil, and mitomycin C) was applied as a routine intraoperative measure even in cases where a biopsy alone was being performed. In cases of osteo- and Ewing's sarcoma, prophylactic measures consist of six further infusions at weekly intervals, which are then continued at monthly intervals over a period of one year. Nine patients (4 with Ewing's sarcomata, 3 with osteosarcomata, 2 with chondrosarcomata) received monthly BCG inoculations (0.1 mg lyophilized organisms, Institut Pasteur) instead of monthly prophylaxis after initial cytostatic chemotherapy.

Table 1. Diagnoses of 50 sarcoma patients

Primary malignant bone tumors			40
Osteosarcoma			19
Round-cell sarcoma (glycogen-positive)	11	"Ewing's sarcoma"	15
Round-cell sarcoma (glycogen-negative)	4		
Monocyte sarcoma			1
Reticulosarcoma			1
Chondrosarcoma			4
Primary malignant soft-tissue tumors			10
Polymorphic-cell sarcoma			3
Fibrosarcoma			2
Malignant synovialoma			2
Myxosarcoma, rhabdomyosarcoma, hemangiopericytoma			3

The immunological screening was regularly carried out before the operation and was checked again four to eight weeks after the operation. In cases of osteosarcoma and Ewing's sarcoma, the immune status was also checked at intervals of three months over a period of one year. An interval of at least one week was always observed after the last cytostatic intermittent high dose.

Table 2. Methods for examination of cell-mediated tumor immunity in man

In-vivo methods:

1. Nonspecific skin tests
   a) DNCB (epicutaneous): primary response
   b) recall antigens (intradermal): secondary response (streptococci, Candida, tuberculin, mumps)
2. Specific skin tests: with tumor antigen (autologous or homologous)
   a) cells (irradiated or treated with cytotoxic agents)
   b) extracts (KCl, NaCl, phenol extracts)

In-vitro methods:

1. Nonspecific reactions
   Stimulation of lymphocytes by phytohemagglutinin, pokeweed, PPD, concanavalin A
2. Specific reactions
   a) cytotoxicity test: colony inhibition (modified), release of chromium 51
   b) inhibition of migration
   c) mixed lymphocyte-tumor culture

Delayed hypersensitivity was checked in skin tests <u>in vivo</u> with the following substances:

1. <u>DNCB</u> (2,4 dinitrochlorobenzol) to test the immunological primary response. Before the operation the patients were sensitized epicutaneously with 2000 mg in 0,1 ml acetone. The challenge was carried out 14-60 days later with 100, 50, 25, or 12.5 μg per 0,1 ml. The reaction was observed between 48 and 72 hours later; erythema and induration were assessed as positive reactions;

2. Recall antigens to test the immunological response. Antigens were applied intracutaneously in 0,1 ml:
   a) mixed streptococci (F1) Bencard testing solution
   b) Candida albicans 0.5% Bencard testing solution
   c) Tuberculine GT 10 IU Behring
   d) mumps skin test antigen (2 CFU) Lilly

   These reactions were also assessed after 48-72 hours by measurement of the diameter of the urtica (erythema without induration or hematoma were not considered to be positive). Measurements carried out 48 and 72 hours later revealed differences only in one-third of the cases (18 out of 51 tests). The differences were 1-2 mm with deviations above or below. Checks after 48 as well as 72 hours thus seemed justified and comparable. If the diameter of the urtica was less than 4 mm, cases were classified as negative or liminally anergic. Reactions with urtica of over 4 mm in diameter were classified as positive.

In-vitro Methods: To check the immunological reactivity of the lymphocytes, 20-40 ml blood was taken at the time of the skin test. Lymphocytes were separated from the other blood cells via a Fikoll-Ronpacon gradient (Cilag-Chemie) after Perper. The capacity for stimulation by phytohemagglutinin (PHA) was measured with the aid of an enclosed radioactive thymidin. The stimulation index (SI) thus derived was compared to that of healthy control subjects. In addition, the lymphocytotoxicity (LT) in homologous sarcoma-cell lines (SA) marked by tritium was determined and compared with that in fibroblast cultures (FI):

$$\%\ \text{PHA stimulation} = \frac{\text{SI patient} - \text{SI control}}{\text{SI control}}\ ;$$

$$\%\ \text{cytotoxicity} = \frac{\text{LT Pat/Sa} - \text{LT Ko/Sa}}{\text{LT Ko/Sa}} - \frac{\text{LT Pat/Fi} - \text{LT Ko/Fi}}{\text{LT Ko/Fi}}\ ;$$

Tumor-cell - lymphocyte ratio = 1:50 - 1:500 (concentration of lymphocytes was of negligible influence on cytotoxicity).

RESULTS

DNCB. A total of 43 patients were tested with DNCB, in 16 of whom the initial reaction (14 days after the operation) was positive; in the remaining 27 patients the initial reaction was negative. It was possible to test 22 patients during the course of their disease (Table 3). Out of 12 patients who are without a tumor at present, 7 were "positive" and 5 "negative," and out of 10 patients with metastases, recurrences or exitus, 6 were "positive" and 4 "negative". Three patients showed more signs of reaction to DNCB in the course of their disease, but, this was of no prognostic value: one patient is free of tumors 14 months after operation, one has metastases, and one patient has metastases and local recurrence.

Recall Antigens. In an earlier analysis of the case histories of 33 sarcoma patients (9), an urtica with a diameter of at least 10 mm in the case of streptococci, candida, and mumps, and of 5 mm in the case of tuberculine was classified as "positive". It was not possible to establish a correlation between development of tumor, therapy, and skin tests at that time. Since urtucae 4-5 mm diameter were most frequent (Table 4), the criterion for classification as "positive" intracutaneous tests had already been fixed at a 4-mm diameter of characteristic urticae, which approaches very closely the data given by HOLLINSHEAD for liminally positive recall antigen tests (7). An urtica of less

Table 3. Follow-up after DNCB skin tests (minimum observation period 6 months)

First test (postoperative)	Test during course	Clinical observation
Pos. 9	Pos. 9	5 disease-free
		4 with metastases
	Neg. 0	
Neg. 13	Pos. 4	2 disease-free
		2 with metastases
	Neg. 9	5 disease-free
		4 with metastases

Table 4. Recall-antigen tests in 50 sarcoma patients (128 intracutaneous tests)

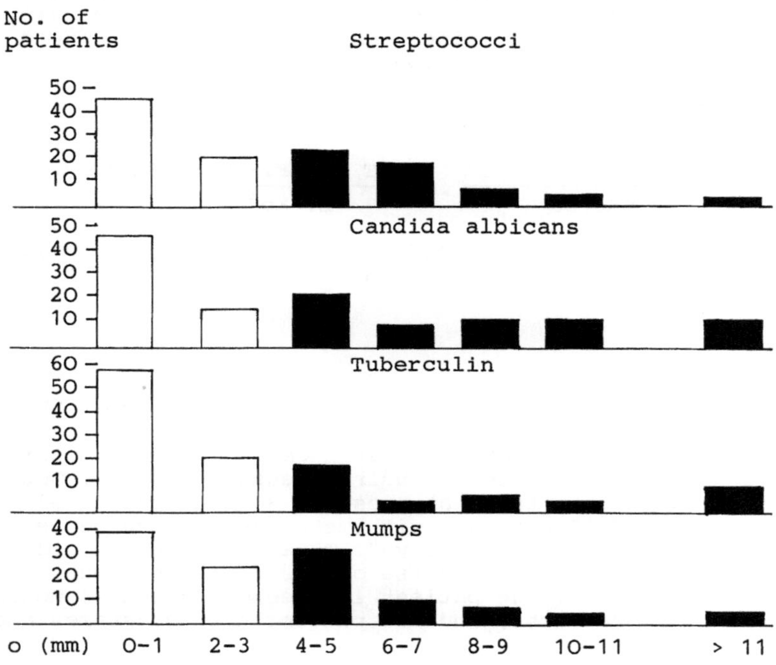

than 4 mm in diameter is not easy to differentiate from nonspecific skin reactions, so this reaction was considered negative.

The battery of intradermal tests was verified with 50 patients, 35 of whom were "positive" before treatment and 15 "negative." It was possible to test 31 of them in the course of their disease (Table 5). All fourteen currently tumor-free patients who had been observed for at least 6 months but for an average of 12.6 (+ 3.6) months showed a positive

Table 5. Follow-up after recall-antigen skin test (minimum observation period: 6 months)

Preoperative test	During course	Clinical observation
Pos. 25	Pos. 22	10 disease-free
		12 with metastases
	Neg. 3	
Neg. 6	Pos. 5	4 disease-free
		1 with metastases
	Neg. 1	1 with metastases

reaction in one of the tests. The remaining patients had metastases, recidivation or exitus, and 13 of them had positive and 4 had negative reactions. Of those cases who were originally negative according to skin tests and had become positive by the time the tests were repeated, five out of six are at present free of tumors and one has metastases. The originally positive patient who became negative in the course of his disease also has metastases.

<u>PHA STIMULATIONS OF THE LYMPHOCYTES</u>

Although the PHA stimulation of lymphocytes of patients is evaluated in relation to those of control persons, a numerical comparison proves difficult because of the broad spread of physiological reactions of lymphocytes to PHA. Only differences of more than 50 percent of PHA stimulations were considered as an alteration in the evaluation of the results. Despite massive deviations of tests results, in all groups a similar distribution of good and bad therapeutic results was observed (Table 6).

Table 6. Follow-up after PHA stimulation (minimum observation period: 6 months)

	Clinical observation
9 patients with similar lymphocyte stimulation in course of disease	4 disease-free
	5 with metastases
7 patients with distinctly increased lymphocyte stimulation	3 disease-free
	4 with metastases
8 patients with distinctly reduced lymphocyte stimulation	3 disease-free
	5 metastases

Correlations: Correlation checks between the DNCB and PHA stimulation in 40 examinations at a time, and also between recall antigen tests and PHA stimulation in 58 examinations at a time, revealed no consistency. A comparison between DNCB and PHA showed a congruent reaction in 20 cases (either DNCB and PHA test positive or both negative), while in 20 cases the results of the two tests were different. Recall antigen reaction and PHA stimulation were congruent in 39 cases and contrary in 19.

CYTOTOXICITY TEST [1]

It was possible to test 19 patients at 1.3 monthly intervals during their disease. Clinical observation also extended over at least six months after actual treatment. In 14 cases the development of the disease correlated with test results (Table 7). Of 8 patients with positive cytotoxicity in the course of their disease, 7 proved to be tumor-free. Of 11 patients with negative cytotoxicity test, 7 had metastases. In 5 patients with negative cytotoxicity test did not correlate with the course of the disease: 4 of them show negative results in the cytotoxicity test and have been tumor-free for 18, 17, 14, and 12 months. One patient proved positive according to the cytotoxicity test and has a solitary lung metastasis. Fig. 1 shows that the course of the disease correlates to a high degree with the immunological situation.

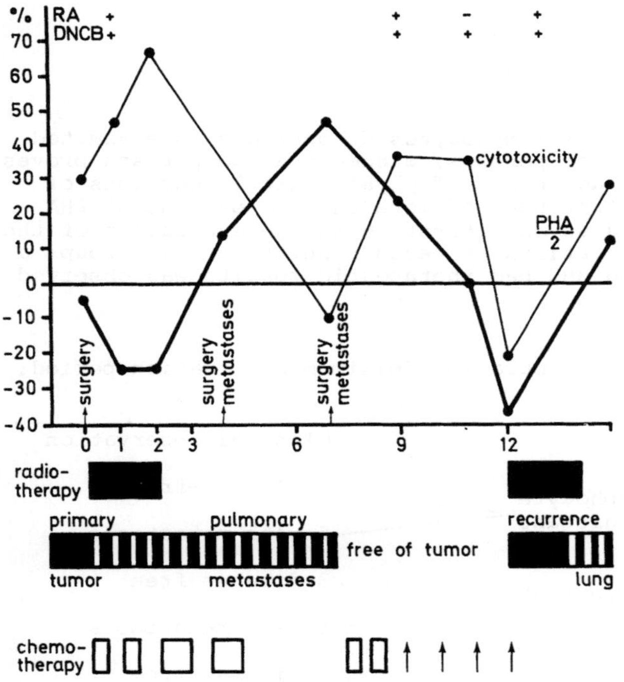

[1] Cytotoxicity of more than 25% is classified as positive, and cytotoxicity of less than 25% as negative.

Table 7. Follow-up after cytoxicity test (minimum observation period: 6 months)

Initial test (preoperative)	During course	Clinical observation
Pos. 7	Pos. 4	4 disease-free
	Neg. 3	1 disease-free
		2 with metastases
Neg. 12	Pos. 4	3 disease-free
		1 with metastasis
	Neg. 8	3 disease-free
		5 with metastases

Pos. and disease-free 7 Pos. with metastasis 1
Neg. and disease-free 4 Neg. with metastases 7

DISCUSSION

For in-vivo examinations only tests which are nonspecific in respect to the tumor were used. Most sarcoma patients showed an anergic reaction to DNCB. In a population free from disease, however, a positive reaction is expected in 90 percents of the subjects (2). Comparison with the course of the illness showed no correlation. The expected positive reaction in tumor-free patients and the switch-over to an anergic test reaction as soon as metastases develop were not observed. In both groups (positive and negative DNCB test) the distribution of favorable cases is even. The recall antigen tests also showed no clinically applicable correlation with the development of the tumor. It is true that all anergic patients had metastases, mainly in the final stage of the disease, but half the patients who had positive results in the recall antigen test belonged to the prognostically unfavorable group of patients with metastases. Our own observations in the case of sarcoma patients are incompatible with data quoted with regard to the course of the illness in tumor patients described in literature on the subject of correlations between clinical and unspecific immunological reaction abilities (1, 5). The evaluation of the development in the case of the PHA stimulation as nonspecific in-vitro test also showed no correlation (either positive or negative) with the development of tumors. Nor have correlations checks between the DNCB test and the PHA stimulation and between the recall antigen test and PHA stimulation shown any correspondence. Thus none of the three tests seems to be characterteristic with regard to development of tumors and immune situation. There is an amazingly high correlation between the course of disease and the cytoxicity of patients' lymphocytes on homologous sarcoma-cell lines. In all cases with positive test results in the course of disease, the development of the illness could be influenced positively by combined therapeutic measures (operation, radiation, cytostatic chemotherapy). The cytotoxicity test as a tumor-specific immune test allows assessments that are of importance for further action. This test can be regarded as a report of an individual case. The battery of unspecific immune tests offers fewer contributions towards a prognosis than a simple check of the sedimentation rate.

Further pointers to the complex immunological processes might be expected from tumor-specific skin tests. Non-tumor-specific intradermal tests might then be used as a control for tumor-associated antigen tests, since no intradermal reaction is to be anticipated for tumor antigens in the case of completely negative recall antigen tests (11).

SUMMARY

The immunologic status of 50 sarcoma patients was established. It was possible to apply the DNCB test and the recall antigen test in most cases during the course of the illness. The PHA stimulation of the lymphocytes and their cytotoxicity on homologous sarcoma cell lines were also correlated with the course of the illness. Nonspecific tests related neither to each other nor to the development of the illness while the tumor-specific cytotoxicity test correlated closely with the course of the disease.

REFERENCES

1. AL-SARRAF, M., WONG, P., SARDESAI, S., VAITKEVICIUS, V.K.: Clinical immunologic responsiveness in malignant disease. Cancer 26, 262-268 (1970)
2. BRUN, F.E.: Die kutan-allergische Spätreaktion auf 2, 4-Dinitrochlorobenzol bei Krebspatienten unter zytostatischer Chemotherapie. Schweiz. med. Wschr. 101, 1235-1243 (1971)
3. COHEN, A.M., KETCHAM, A.S., MORTON, D.L.: Tumor-specific cellular cytotoxicity to human sarcomas: evidence for a cell-mediated host immune response to a common sarcoma cell-surface antigen. J. nat. Cancer Inst. 50, 585-589 (1973)
4. COLEY, W.B.: The treatment of inoperable sarcoma by bacterial toxins. Proc. roy. Soc. Surg. Sed. 3, 1 (1909)
5. EILBER, F.R., MORTON, D.L.: Impaired immunologic reactivity and recurrence following cancer surgery. Cancer, 25, 362-367 (1970)
6. HELLSTRÖM, I., HELLSTRÖM, K.E., SJÖGREN, H.O.: Demonstration of cell-mediated immunity to human neoplasms of various histological types. Int. J. Cancer 7, 1-16 (1971)
7. HOLLINSHEAD, A.C., STEWART, H.M., HERBERMANN, R.B.: Delayed-hypersensitivity reactions to soluble membrane antigens of human malignant lung cells. J. nat. Cancer Inst. 52, 327-337 (1974)
8. KOTZ, R., SALZER-KUNTSCHIK, M., ZWEYMÜLLER, K., SALZER, M.: Therapy and prognosis of the Ewing-sarcoma. Öst. Z. Onkol. 1, 15-22 (1974)
9. KOTZ, R., RELLA, W.: Überprüfung der zellulären Abwehrlage bei Patienten mit Knochentumoren. Verh. dtsch. Ges. Path. 58. 471-474 (1974)
10. MARCOVE, R.C., MIKÉ, Valerie, HUVOS, A.G., SOUTHAM, C.M., LEVIN, A.G.: Vaccine trials for osteogenic sarcoma. A preliminary report. Ca. Cancer J, Clin. 23, 74-80 (1973)
11. MAVLIGIT, G.M., AMBUS, U., GUTTERMAN, J.U., HERSH, E.M., MCBRIDE, C.M.: Antigen solubilized from human solid tumours: lymphocyte stimulation and cutaneous delayed hypersensitivity. Nature New Biol. 243, 188-190 (1973)
12. MENDOZA, C.B., MOORE, G.E., WATNE, A.L., HIRAMOTO, R., JURAND, J.: Immunologic response following homologous transplantation of cultured human tumor cells in patients with malignancy. Surgery 64, 897-900 (1968)

13. NADLER, S.H., MOORE, G.E.: Immunotherapy of malignant disease. Arch. Surg. 99, 376-381 (1969)
14. PERLMANN, P., O'TOOLE, D., UNSGAARD, B.: Cell-mediated immune mechanism of tumor cell destruction. Fed. Proc. 32, 153-155 (1973)
15. PERPER, R.J., ZEE, T.W., MICHELSON, M.M.: Purification of lymphocytes and platelets by gradient centrifugation. J. lab. clin. Med. 72, 842-848 (1968)
16. SALZER, M., SALZER-KUNTSCHIK, M., ZHUBER, K., PRICE, C.H.G., WILLERT, H.G., IMMENKAMP, M., GROH, P., MATEJOVSKY, Z., KEYL, W.: Therapie und Prognose des kindlichen Osteosarkoms. Z. Orthop. (in press)
17. VÅNKY. F., STJERNSWÄRD, J., NILSONNE, U.: Cellular immunity to human sarcoma. J. nat. Cancer Inst. 46. 1145-1151 (1971)

Laboratory Models of Minimal Residual Cancer; Development and Preliminary Immunotherapy Studies

CH. M. SOUTHAM

INTRODUCTION

In introducing his paper on "Semimalignant bone lesions", Dr. Uehlinger (7) delightfully begged forgiveness for his indecisive terminology by pointing to a similar indecisiveness amongst theologicans, who solved their dilemma by creating an intermediate state between damnation and blessedness. I would like to extend the analogy.

The quality of malignancy or benignity may indeed be intrinsic to a tumor and immutable, like the quality of those souls assigned for eternity (whether by God, priest, or Dante) to the inferno or paradiso. But the progress of souls in purgatorio is not predestined solely by their inherent qualities; it is influenced by certain extrinsic factors (including perhaps the prayers of their kin). So too, as oncologists, we must consider the possibility that the clinical course of many neoplasms might depend in part on factors which are extrinsic to the tumor cell, such as the patient's immunologic mechanisms.

Bone tumors are characterized by a high rate of recurrence after what is planned as curative treatment of a localized lesion. Chondrosarcomas and fibrosarcomas commonly recur locally. Osteosarcomas recur as distant metastases in the great majority of patients, even though the primary tumor is completely removed by amputation. These local recurrences or distant metastases develop from deposits of tumor cells too small to be detected by any method currently available; the clinical situation which is aptly described as minimal residual cancer.
The need for adjuvant forms of treatment to supplement surgery is apparent to every clinician who treats malignant bone tumors. One possibility is immunotherapy.

Unfortunately, this paper deals with connective tissue fibrosarcomas rather than osteosarcomas, because the experiments described were planned before this symposium, but I think the principles of pathogenesis and immunotherapy with which I am concerned apply equally to all malignant tumors, regardless of histologic origin.

ARGUMENT

During the past few years a great enthusiasm for cancer immunotherapy has replaced the nihilism of the previous four decades. The present enthusiasm is based on impressive and extensive evidence that tumor cells often differ antigenically from normal cells of the same (or a genetically identical) individual, and that the host develops an antitumor immune reaction which confers a certain degree of resistance against growth of that tumor. Most of the evidence comes from in-vitro and transplantation studies of experimental animal tumors, but less extensive data from studies of patients and human cancer cells give assurance that these are universal phenomena, not merely laboratory artifacts. Thus there is a real basis for the renaissance of interest in tumor immunology. However, the degree of enthusiasm and the blind faith that immunologic reactivity can be equated to clinical immunotherapy are not justified by the kind or amount of data yet available. There have not yet been adequate demonstrations of actual therapeutic effects against cancer as it is seen in clinical practice. This deficiency is due largely to the inherent difficulties and restrictions of experimental clinical trials and the lack of experimental animal models which accurately mimic the clinical situation of treating the patient who has cancer. It is to the problem of developing and testing such a system that the ongoing studies reported in this pager have been addressed.

Tumor transplantation studies in several species of inbred experimental animals have clearly shown that excision of a syngeneic tumor is often followed by resistance to subsequent implantation of that same tumor. The degree of that resistance is low in comparison to the resistance which can be developed against microbial infections or tissue homografts (as might be predicted since syngeneic tumor cells are antigenically identical with the host cells except for those new antigens which appeared concomitantly with neoplastic transformation). Nevertheless, the resistance is real, reproducible and quantifiable; and it is antigenically specific. A comparable degree of tumor-specific transplantation immunity can be induced in healthy syngeneic animals by intact nonviable tumor cells or, in some experimental systems, by tumor-cell homogenates or extracts. Clearly, this raises the possibility of a tumor vaccine if the massive problems of obtaining the desired tumor-specific antigens in effective form and amounts can be solved.

We must recognize that there is a tremendous difference between induction of an immune response in a healthy animal and induction of an immune response in a cancer patient which is sufficient in quality and quantity to reverse the progressive growth of an established tumor. It is in the latter situation, an only the latter, that we need immunotherapy. A patient who has cancer will be completely cured if every cancer cell is removed or destroyed by his primary treatment, and such a patient has no need of immunotherapy. (Many of us suspect that in some patients who are cured by surgery or other primary treatment, immunologic defense mechanisms may in fact contribute to the cure by destroying some few cancer cells remaining after the primary treatment. Data illustrating that such cases do indeed occur have been recorded, but such patients do not need immunotherapy because their defenses were adequate without additional stimuli.) If cancer recurs, it is obvious that the cancer cells were not completely removed by the primary treatment but that some had escaped detection or resisted destruction and had continued to propagate either locally at the primary site or in some distant sites to which they had spread before the primary tumor was treated. These are the patients whose only chance for cure is further treatment, and amongst the methods to be considered are the immunologic methods, i.e. immunotherapy.

Two points now deserve emphasis: (1) It can be regarded as axiomatic that immunotherapy has a greater probability of success if the amount of cancer to be eliminated is small, i.e. that the earlier one institutes treatment the better is the chance of therapeutic success. This is the reason for emphasizing immunotherapy and chemotherapy during the period of minimal residual cancer ; (2) The patient whose cancer recurs after primary treatment is a "two-time loser". His immune mechanisms failed to respond adequately when the cancer originated, and a second time when most of the cancer had been removed or destroyed by the primary treatment. In a patient who has twice failed to respond adequately when his "tumor burden" was minimal, there is reason to doubt that he will be able to respond adequately to attempts to further stimulate his own immune response. For this reason, the immunologist must consider not only vaccines and immunopotentiators, but passive and adoptive and "instructional" methods of immunotherapy.

Very few laboratory studies of tumor immunotherapy have utilized models which reproduce the clinical situation. Propylactic immunization of a healthy animal and subsequent challenge by inoculation of a transplantable tumor is obviously inappropriate as a model for therapy. Animals which have recently been injected with a rapidly growing and rapidly lethal syngeneic tumor are comparable only to the most aggressive kinds of human cancer. The animal has too little time to develop an immune response before it is overwhelmed by disease. In terms of my opening analogy, such animals are irrevocably commited to the inferno, and if Dante had been a pathologist, he probably would have assigned these tumors to circle eight malebogia seven.

What is needed is an experimental animal system in which a biologically and antigenically uniform tumor can be initiated in groups of individuals with growth of a primary (transplantable) tumor which can be treated in a manner analogous to potentially curative clinical cancer therapy (surgical excision, local radiation, or systemic chemotherapy), but leaving a uniform residuum of viable tumor cells sufficient in number to produce recurrence of the tumor in a majority of the animals. Such an experimental animal model would truly mimic the situation encountered by the clinician in a population of patients who undergo putatively curative primary treatment but have a predictable high rate of recurrence. In such a model it will be possible to initiate experimental therapeutic studies not only when recurrence is actually demonstrable, but even during the period of minimal residual cancer before recurrence is detectable.

This paper is a report of some studies leading to the development of such experimental models, and preliminary attempts to apply a novel experimental approach to provide adoptive and passive immunotherapy during the period of minimal residual cancer.

EXPERIMENT

Development of the Experimental Models

The experimental work leading to the development of laboratory models for minimal residual cancer will be presented stage by stage to allow consideration of the several prerequisites for suitable models, and their fulfillment.

To mimic precisely the problem of human cancer, it would of course be necessary to use animals with autochthonous tumors. This should be feasible, but it would be technically tedious and difficult to achieve uniformity and reproducibility, so efforts to date have been limited to transplantable syngeneic tumors.

The first prerequisite is reproducibility of the experimental tumors. We have induced fibrosarcomas in inbred lines of rats (Fisher) and mice (C57BL/6) by subcutaneous or intramuscular injection of methylcholanthrene. Autochthonus tumors were isografted for one or two passages and then established in tissue culture in order to have inocula with greater viability and uniformity and reproducibility of tumor growth than could be achieved by preparing inocula directly from tumor tissue. Cultures were quite easily established as monolayers on glass. We have permanent lines of 10 mouse fibrosarcomas and two rat fibrosarcomas, representing a success rate of about 50 percent.

It is of course necessary to prove that a culture from a tumor really is a culture of tumor cells. It is quite possible to establish a cell line from nonmalignant components of a tumor mass. Proof of malignancy is easily obtained (for these experimental animal tumors) by syngeneic transplantation. Table 1 shows the results of quantitative transplantation studies with some of the culture lines of mouse and rat tumors, performed simultaneously by various routes. All of them induced subcutaneous tumors in almost all recipients at a dose of 100,000 cells; and 10,000 cells caused a few tumors. Only one cell line (S-11) grew subcutaneously from inocula of 1,000 cells. Intraperitoneal transplantation required the same number of cells or occasionally fewer (S-8 and S-9). The results of intravenous transplantation are noteworthy because there was clearly a greater resistance to transplantation of three of the cell lines (S-9, S-10 and S-11). Transplantation studies with the two rat-tumor lines gave similar results.

The second prerequisite is that the experimental tumor be immunogenic, i.e. it must carry tumor-specific transplantation antigens. Tables 2 and 3 show representative results of immunogenicity studies of a few of our sarcoma lines. Both the rat lines and two of the three mouse lines were antigenic, as evidenced by host resistance to challenge after total excision of a primary subcutaneous transplant of the same tumor line. Mouse tumor S-9 gave no indication of immunogenicity in thee studies. Tumors S-11 and MCF4 were "strongly" antigenic, as shown by complete resistance of the immunized animals to the challenge doses. Tumors S-8 and MCF5 were moderately antigenic; as shown by a significantly lower number of takes in the immunized animals but not complete resistance. (As expected of these chemically induced tumors, the tumor-specific transplantation antigens are unique to each individual tumor, i.e. their tumor antigens do not cross-react.)

Table 1. Transplantability of MC-induced fibrosarcomas to syngeneic recipients (C57BL/6 mice or fischer rats) by various routes, number of cells indicated as $\log_{10}$. Ten-fold dilutions from 10^6 to 10^3 cells were tested; 5 or more animals per group. 4/5 takes is tabulated as TD_{90}.

	SC		IP		IV		IM	
Tumor	MTD	TD_{90}	MTD	TD_{90}	MTD	TD_{90}	MTD	TD_{90}
Mouse S-4	4	5	5	5	?	5	?	5
Mouse S-8	4	5	<=3	4	?	5	<=5	>5
Mouse S-9	4	5	3	4	5	>5		
Mouse S-10	4	5	4	5	6	>6		
Mouse S-11	3	5	3	5	6	>6		
Mouse S-12	4	5	4	4	?	5	?	4
Rat MCF4	5	6			5	<6		
Rat MCF5	?	<=6			6	<6		

Table 2. Individual tumor-specific immunogenicity of MC-induced fibrosarcomas in C57BL/6 mice (mice with tumors at 5 weeks/total number of mice).

Immunized[a] with	S.C. challenge with tumor line S-8	S-9	S-11
	inoculum 1,000,000 cells		
S-8	31/40	20/20	
S-9	19/20	40/40	
S-11	20/20	20/20	0/40[b]
Nothing	10/10	10/10	10/10
	inoculum 100,000 cells		
S-8	4/10	10/10	10/10
S-9	10/10	10/10	
S-11	10/10	10/10	0/20
Nothing	20/20	20/20	10/10

[a]Immunized by excision of S.C. tumor 14 days before challenge
[b]Also resisted challenge by 10^7 cells (0/10).

Table 3. Individual tumor-specific immunogenicity of MC-induced fibrosarcomas in Fischer rats

Immunized against	S.C. challenge 10^6 cells MCF4	MCF5
MCF4	0/7	5/5
MCF5	4/4	3/9
Nothing	30/30	10/10

The third prerequisite is that the immunogenicity be not so strong that tumor resistance develops concurrently with growth of the primary tumor to such a degree that it prevents dissemination or local recurrence. (As clinical oncologists, we would welcome such strong resistance, but in an experimental model for the study of immunotherapy it would defeat our purpose.) This question was investigated in studies which included the techniques which we now use to produce experimental models of minimal residual tumor. A primary subcutaneous tumor was produced by isotransplantation of a tumor line, and some time later a quantitated challenge dose of the same tumor-cell line was injected either subcutaneously or intravenously. In one of the experimental groups, the primary tumor was not removed. Comparison of the frequency of tumor takes with that in a simultaneously inoculated nonimmune control group provided a test for tumor resistance concurrent with growth of the primary tumor. In another group, the primary tumor was excised immediately before the challenge, as a test of the ability of a relatively small number of cells to cause recurrence. Still other groups had their primary tumor excised two weeks before the challenge, as a positive control for the immunogenicity of the tumor. Only the two rat tumors have been studied so far. Results with MCF4 are shown in Table 4. In the normal control rats, 10^6 cells caused subcutaneous (SC) tumors in all rats, and intravenous injection of this dose caused lung tumors in four of eight rats. Resistance to transplantation was clearly evident in the immunized groups. Surprisingly, the experimental group which was challenged immediately (4 hours) after excision of the primary transplant, and the group which was challenged without removal of the primary transplant also showed resistance. Apparently this tumor was so antigenic that it rapidly induced a degree of resistance such that it was impossible to produce either local recurrence or distant metastases by this experimental approach.

Table 4. Tumor growth and immunity: MCF-4 sarcoma of fisher rats

Status of recipients	Growth[a] of Challenge Inoculum 10^6 Cells SC	10^6 Cells IV	10^5 Cells SC	10^5 Cells IV
Unimmunized	10/10	4/8	1/9	5/8
Immunized with 10^7 γ-irradiated cells	0/4	1/5	0/8	0/5
1° implant excised 14 days before challenge	0/2	0/6	0/10	0/4
1° implant excised 4 hours before challenge	0/3	0/6	0/10	0/9
1° implant still in place	0/7	2/7	X	3/6

[a]Group in bottom line observed for only 3 weeks after challenge (when growth in unimmunized controls was 8/10), because of deaths from the primary implants. All others observed for 12 weeks.

The preliminary studies of the immunogenicity of the rat tumors (Table 3) had suggested that the MCF5 line was less immunogenic than MCF4, so we repeated the attempts to establish a model of minimal residual cancer using MCF5. Results of this experiment a presented in Table 5. The results of subcutaneous and intravenous challenge in the rats which had been immunized (by excision of subcutaneous tumors two weeks before challenge, or by injection of γ-irradiated cells) confirmed that this tumor is immunogenic, but less so than MCF4. In the other two experimental groups, the results were interestingly different. there was no evidence of concomitant immunity in the group of tumor-bearing rats. In the group which was challenged immediately after excision of the primary tumor mass the challenge did produce tumors, evidently overwhelming whatever tumor immunity had developed. The inoculum dose of 10^6 cells represents about 1 mg of tissue, an amount which is undetectable on clinical examination, but enough (of this particular tumor line) to cause recurrence of tumor growth. Nevertheless, immunologic resistance was detectable, as shown by the lower frequency of takes in these groups as compared to the unimmunized control group. It is evident, therefore, that the reinitiation of tumor growth in the experimental groups did not occur because of an absence of immunity. It occurred because immunity which had developed during grouwth of the primary tumor was insufficient, i.e. the small amount of residual tumor was sufficient to overwhelm the week immunity. This interpretation is also

Table 5. Tumor growth and immunity: MCF-5 sarcoma of fischer rats

Status of recipients	Growth[a] of Challenge Inoculum 10^6 Cells S.C.	10^6 Cells I.V.
Unimmunized	10/10 (100%)	2/7 (29%)
Immunized with 10^7 γ-irradiated cells	3/8 (38%)	0/7
1° implant excised 14 days before	3/9 (33%)	0/11
1° implant excised 4 hours before	10/24 (42%)	1/7 (14%)
1° implant still in place	5/8 (63%)	0/12

[a]Group in bottom line observed for only 3 weeks after challenge (when growth in unimmunized controls was 8/10), because of deaths from the primary implants. All others observed for 12 weeks.

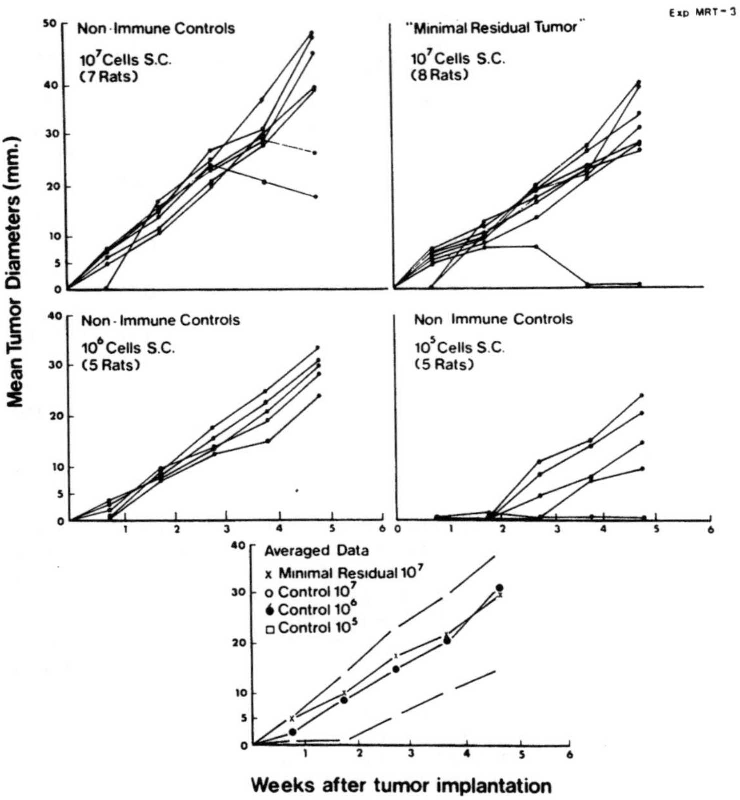

Fig. 1. Comparison of regrowth of subcutaneous tumor from a "minimal residuum" of tumor cells, and growth of primary tumor implant from an equal or lesser inoculum of tumor cells. Data from experiment MRT-3 of BOWER et al. (2), MCF5 tumor in Fischer rats

supported by the data shown in Fig. 1 and 2, in which the grwoth curves of tumors in individual rats are shown. In the experiments shown in Fig. 1, the rate of growth of MCF 5 tumors in animals which had had a primary implant excised one hour before challenge (the minimal residual tumor group) was appreciably less than that in the nonimmune controls which were given the same dose of cells, more closely resembling that in nonimmune animals given an inoculum of one tenth the dose of cells. In the experiment shown in Fig. 2, six of nine rats which were inoculated with 10^7 cells immediately after excision of their primary implant rejected the challenge inoculum after a short period of growth, whereas in the nonimmune control groups an inoculum of either 10^7 or 10^6 cells caused progressive tumor growth in all recipients. In the three animals in the minimal residual tumor model which did sustain progressive growth of the challenge tumor, the rate of growth was comparable to that produced by an inoculum of one tenth the dose of cells in the nonimmune group.

Exploratory Immunotherapy Studies

Rational progression to trials of various methods of immunotherapy required, in addition, proof that the tumor could in fact be restrained

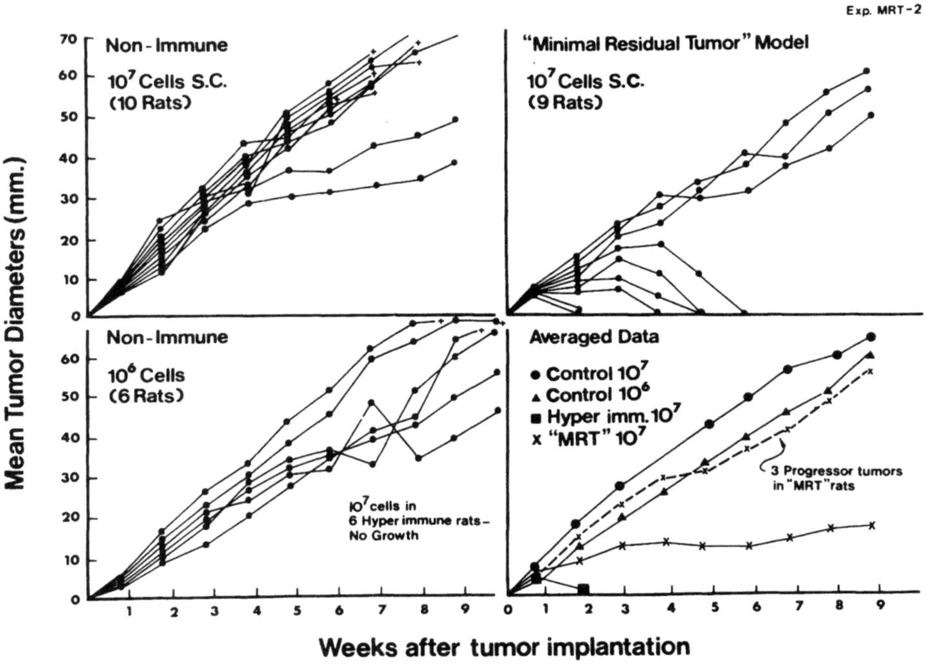

Fig. 2. As Fig. 1. Data from experiment MRT-2 of BOWER et al. (2)

by immunologic mechanisms initiated after the tumor was established. Attempts to investigate this prerequisite by the use of tumor-specific vaccines or nonspecific immunopotentiators would introduce an additional variable of which we had no knowledge - the ability of the host's immune mechanisms to effectively increase its own response to the tumor antigens. It is possible to avoid this unknown variable by studying adoptive or passive immunotherapy, i.e. treatment by transfer of sensitized immunocytes and antiserum from a specifically immunized donor. (It will be noted that we could use adoptive or passive immunotherapy in this experimental system because it is completely syngeneic, thus guaranteeing that the immune reactions are tumor-specific.) Obviously, for our purpose, we wanted a maximum degree and duration of treatment, so we utilized the technique of parabiosis, uniting our "patients" to "immunized donors." Under ether anesthesia the left abdominal wall of the patient was excised from the lateral border of the rectus muscle to the posterior axillary line and from the costal margin to the pelvic brim, widely exposing the peritoneal cavity. The same procedure was performed on the right side of the donor. The two animals were then sutured together, muscle to muscle and skin to skin, providing an extensive cross-circulation of plasma and blood cells through the vasculature of skin and muscles and via the common peritoneal cavity.

That cells (as well as serum) were in fact exchanged between the donor and the patient was demonstrated by injecting ^{51}Cr-labeled syngeneic erythrocytes intravenously into the donor members of two parabiotic pairs, and comparing the levels of radioactivity in the donors and patients. By two hours after injection, the labeled cells were present in blood of the uninjected member of the pair at approximately one third the concentration which was found in the injected animal. At 24 hours the concentration of labeled erythrocytes in blood of the patient was almost as high as in the injected member of the pair. The labeled cells were also demonstrated in liver, spleen and tumor of the patients (3).

The next step was to see whether immunotherapy, as provided by parabiosis to a hyperimmunized donor, would inhibit the growth of a primary tumor transplant. This may seem like a regressive step because it is not the clinical model to which our efforts are directed, but treatment of animals during growth of a primary transplant is technically simpler and answers the immediate question concerning the transfer of antitumor immunity. Data from these studies are shown in Table 6 and 7.

Data from three experiments with the mouse tumor line S-11 were quite uniform, so they are combined in Table 6. Transmission of tumor resistance from immunized donor to normal recipients is dramatically shown by failure of tumors to grow when transplantated two days after the parabiotic union was established (i.e. after prophylactic parabiosis). As therapy, parabiosis is equally effective if initiated one day after tumor implantation, and it had a significant but lesser effect when initiated two or four days after tumor implantation. Even if delayed seven days after tumor implantation, parabiosis to a hyperimmunized donor inhibited the rate of tumor growth but could not stop it.

Table 6. Effect of parabiosis to hyperimmunized syngeneic "donors" on growth of primary transplants of sarcoma S-11. Combined data from mouse experiments 1-3 of CURRIE *et al*. (3)

	Tumor takes/ Total no. of mice	Mean tumor diameters (mm) at 6 weeks
Normal controls	14/15	17
Parabiosed to nonimmunized mouse	6/6	17
Prophylactic parabiosis (2 days before tumor implant)	1/8	2
Therapeutic parabiosis		
1 day after tumor implantation	0/6	0
2 days after tumor implantation	2/3	9
4 days after tumor implantation	4/6	11
7 days after tumor implantation	8/8	13

Table 7. Effect of parabiosis to hyperimmunized syngeneic "donors" on growth of primary transplants of rat sarcoma line MCF5. Combined data from rat experiments 1, 3, 4 of CURRIE *et al.* (3)

	Tumor takes/ total no. of rats	Mean tumor diameter (mm at 6 weeks)	Mortality at 10 weeks
Normal controls	16/16	35	8/16
Parabiosed to nonimmunized rat	9/9	32	3/9
Prophylactic parabiosis (2 days before tumor inplant)	2/4	0	0/4
Therapeutic parabiosis			
1 day after tumor implantation	9/10	12	2/10
4 days after tumor implantation	10/10	27	2/10
7 days after tumor implantation	15/16	29	0/16

The same type of experiment was also performed in rats, the MCF5 tumor line being used, with similar results. Selected data from CURRIE et al. (3) are presented in Table 7. As in the mouse experiments, transmission of tumor resistance was clearly accomplished when parabiosis was performed prior to implantation of the tumor. Of four animals treated in this way, only two developed palpable tumor nodules and these regressed completely by six weeks. As therapy, parabiosis exerted a significant effect on tumor growth if performed one day after tumor transplantation, as shown by complete regression of tumor in several rats, which was reflected by the low mean tumor size at six weeks. Parabiosis performed four or seven days after tumor implantation had only a minimal effect on the rate of tumor growth, but death from the tumors was delayed, as reflected in the lower mortality at 10 weeks. The lesser efficacy of immunotherapy by parabiosis for the rat tumor probably is explained by the fact that whereas S-11 was a highly immunogenic tumor, this MCF5 rat tumor was only moderately immunogenic (see Tables 2 and 3).

In some very preliminary studies of immunotherapy in the "minimal residual tumor" system in rats (2), parabiosis was used in the manner just described as a means of transferring serum and immunocytes from the immunized donors to the "patient", but in these experiments the patient had residual subcutaneous tumor cells following excision of the primary tumor. The first of three experiments with this experimental protocol is illustrated in Fig. 3. Parabiosis to a hyperimmunized donor immediately after excision of the primary tumor and introduction of the residuum of tumor cells caused regression in six of the seven

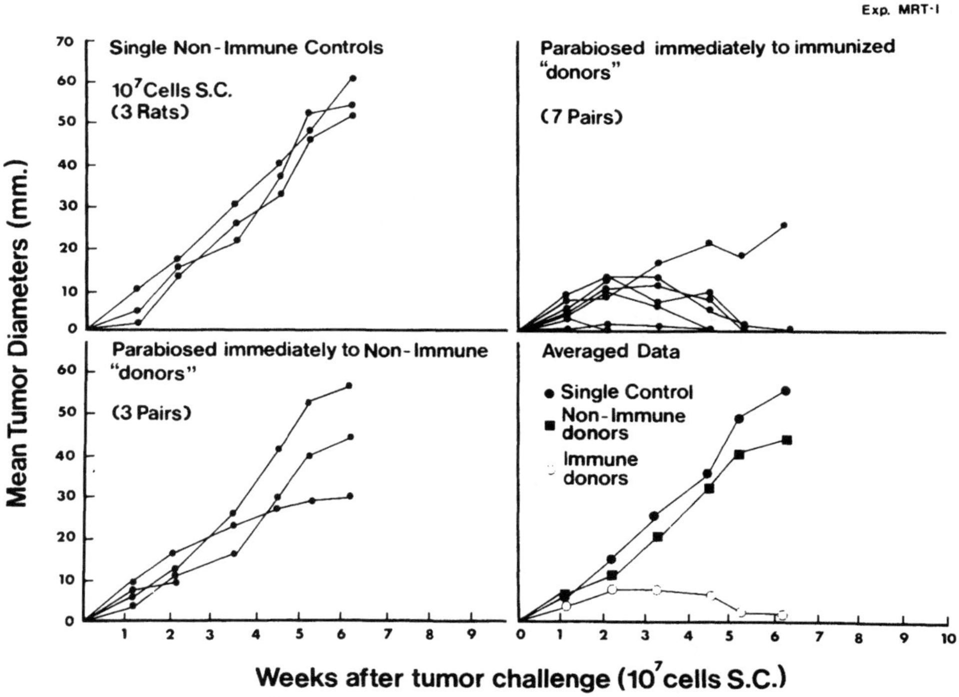

Fig. 3. Immunotherapy for minimal residual cancer following excision of the primary tumor (MCF5 sarcoma in Fischer rats). Adoptive/passive immunotherapy achieved by parabiosis to a hyperimmunized syngeneic "donor." Data from experiment MRT-1 of BOWER et al. (2)

patients whereas parabiosis to nonimmune donors had no significant effect on tumor growth as compared to tumor growth in single nonimmune control rats. In two additional experiments designed to monitor several additional variables, similar results were obtained in larger experimental groups. We have not yet undertaken immunotherapeutic studies with the model system in which the residual tumor is hematogenously disseminated, nor have we studied active methods of immunotherapy.

DISCUSSION

Recognition of the need for experimental tumor systems which resemble clinical cancer is not new, but little progress has been made in developing satisfactory models. For many years, MARTIN (5) has been advocating studies in which tumor-bearing animals would be treated initially by incomplete excision followed by chemotherapy and/or immunotherapy, but his own results were unimpressive because of the low efficacy of his chemotherapeutic agents and immunostimulants and because he used nonsyngeneic tumors. ALEXANDER and his co-workers (1) performed adoptive immunotherapy studies in autochthonous sarcomas (chemically induced) of rats after subtotal tumor excision. While no fault can be found with the biological factors in this system, the inherent biological variability is great, and reproducibility of the residual tumor burden is poor. Recognizing the need for better models, the World Health Organization recently convened an expert commitee to consider tumors of domestic animals as models for research (8). Numerous potentially useful animal tumors are described. Some of those which are induced by viruses have already been used in fruitful immunoprophylactic experiments, but as yet none has been utilized for immunotherapy studies.

The MCF5 model of minimal residual cancer in rats which was developed in the studies reported here does seem to fulfill the prerequisites for a laboratory model of clinical cancer suitable for immunotherapy studies. It gives a high degree of reproducibility in replicate groups of a single experiment, and is fairly reproducible in repeated experiments. Although it requires considerable labor with a variety of techniques, most of the procedures are neither difficult nor fastidious. Local recurrences from the quantitated "residual" tumor cells can be produced in nearly 100 percent of animals with a dose of cells which is only slightly above the threshold dose required for regrowth. The model of hematogenous "metastases" following surgical cure of the primary tumor is much more time-consuming; to date it has given less consistent results, and evaluation must be delayed until the animals are autopsied. Nevertheless, it promises to be a technically feasible and biologically appropriate model for human tumors such as osteosarcomas, which characteristically recur as pulmonary metastases after the primary lesion has been successfully removed by surgery.

It is now our intention to utilize the MCF5 model of minimal residual cancer for further therapeutic studies by a variety of immunologic methods and in combination with chemotherapy, and to continue development of model systems, using moderately immunologic mouse fibrosarcoma lines. Of particular interest to this group is the possibility of developing similar models for the virus-induced osteosarcoma of rats (6) or mice or hamsters (4).

SUMMARY

It is the author's contention that if we wish to investigate immunotherapy for cancer in laboratory models, the model must reproduce or at least mimic the biological conditions which are encountered in clinical oncologic practice. The usual experimental animal tumor systems do not satisfy this requirement. They are usually studied as primary transplants of rapidly progressive tumors which kill in a few weeks, and experimental treatments are usually started within a day or two after implantation, before the tumor is detectable by ordinary methods of examination. In clinical oncology the existence of cancer is seldom suspected until it reaches a clinically detectable mass, and it is then treated by various established methods which, if not curative, at least reduce tumor mass temporarily before the tumor recurs locally or at distant sites. A cancer patient, therefore, has a rather prolonged exposure to his tumor and an opportunity to develop immune and other biological responses to it. Present animal models are therefore inadequate for immunotherapy research.

This paper examines the prerequisites for more accetable experimental tumor models for immunotherapeutic research, describes a step-by-step investigation leading to the development of what to seems to be more appropriate models, and describes preliminary immunotherapy studies in one of the models, in which parabiosis is used as a means of transferring antitumor resistance to the "patients" from specifically immunized donors.

REFERENCES

1. ALEXANDER, P., et al.: The proliferation and spread of neoplastic cells. Williams and Wilkins Press 1968
2. BOWER, E., SOUTHAM, C.M., BABCOCK, V.I.: Immunotherapy of rat sarcomas by parabiosis in aminimal residual tumor system. (Submitted for publication 1976)
3. CURRIE, V.E., SOUTHAM, C.M., BABCOCK, V.I.: Immunotherapy by parabiosis for syngeneic mouse and rat sarcomas. (Submitted for publication 1976))
4. FINKEL, M., REILLY, C.A., BISKIS, B.O.: Pathogenesis of radiation and virus induced bone tumors. This Volume
5. MARTIN, D.S., HAYWORTH, P., FUGMANN, R.A., ENGLISH, R., McNEIL, H.W.: Combination therapy with cyclophosphamide and zymosan on a spontaneous mammary cancer in mice. Cancer Research 24, 652-654 (1964)
6. SOEHNER, R.L., DMOCHOWSKI, L.: Induction of bone tumors in rats and hamsters with murine sarcoma virus and their cell-free transmission. Nature 224, 191-192 (1969)
7. UEHLINGER, E.: Problems of semi-malignancy and of malignant transformation in primary benign bone tumors. This Volume
8. WORLD HEALTH ORGANIZATION: Naturally occurring tumors in domestic animals as models for research: Parts 1 and 2. Bulletin of WHO, Vol-49, p. 81-91 and 205-213 (1973)

The author acknowledges with gratitude the participation of the following for their participation in various phases of the studies summarized in this paper: VIRGINIA I, BABCOCK, EDWARD BOWER, VIOLANTE CURRIE, ADRIENNE TANZI.

The Treatment of Malignant Bone Tumors by Conservative Surgery

R. C. MARCOVE

The purpose of conservative surgery is to avoid an amputation. In the case of a malignant bone tumor, conservative surgery consists in the excision of the tumor along with its peripheral tissue by cutting through the normal surrounding structures, thereby keeping away from the tumor itself. If the tumor is seen during this surgical procedure, it is practice to close the wound and notify the patient that the operation is a failure. After a failure of this kind ablation of the tumor can usually be performed later by amputation at a more proximal point; with a change of instruments it could even be done at same operative intervention.

It must be emphasized that proper conservative surgery does not mean removal of a tumor by merely shelling it out at the level of its pseudocapsule; surgery of that type is doomed to failure.

Another method of conservative surgery to salvage a limb is the use of cryosurgery to necrose the tumor and surrounding tissue by the application of liquid nitrogen. This is done merely by pouring liquid nitrogen through a funnel directly onto, then into, the neoplasm, which is surgically cavitated. The type of surgery should be monitored by thermocouples and it can also be checked by a further biopsy a few weeks later to determine whether all the tumor is indeed necrosed. The cryosurgical technique is usually used either on so-called benign tumors which recur locally (often infrequently metastasizing tumor), or on low-grade lesions such as some chondrosarcomas, where the usual manifestation of a surgical failure is a local recurrence in the primary area before a metastasis would become evident. Combinations of these two methods of surgery - local radical excision and cryosurgery - can be performed where cryosurgery can remove a soft-tissue mass and allow a more local but nevertheless radical procedure to be performed later, by this means enabling one to salvage a limb from ablation. Occasionally an artery graft is needed (6, 14).

In my experience, the frequently quoted rule of "amputate any malignant tumor presenting below the elbow or knee" is not necessarily valid. Cases should be studied individually. The other rule, that "any malignant osseous tumor should have its entire length of primary bone excised", has many exceptions, and even in an osteogenic sarcoma (where skip areas have been definitely observed) reasonable cure rates have been reported with lesser surgery (Mayo Clinic); perhaps patients who do have skip areas in the primary bone always have a particularly bad prognostic presentation. As better techniques for ancillary medical care develop, even the more aggressive malignant tumors may be conquered by local resections. For example a lysed-cell autogenous vaccine has helped to improve the cure rate for osteogenic sarcoma from 17 percent to 42 percent (9, 12). Chemotherapy may improve the cure rate for this disease even further, and also shrink the primary tumor area

(15, 16). Perhaps, in the future, combinations of vaccine and chemotherapy will give the highest cure rates of all. Even if vaccine therapy only shortens the necessary duration of chemotherapy, this will be helpful. Further salvage can even be obtained by multiple local pulmonary wedge resections in sarcomas, even if the disease is bilateral and appears repetitively (7, 13).

The preoperative work-up should be careful when a conservative radical procedure is planned. Routine physical findings and roentgenograms can be supplemented by soft-tissue studies (xerography and arteriography) and bone-tumor distribution details should be carefully studied with bone scans (radioactive fluorine and/or strontium). Tomography and even open biopsy in the distal, presumably normal area, can also be performed to determine whether local surgery can be undertaken.

Summary. The indications for local radical en-bloc resection are discussed. The preoperative work-up and the aspects to be considered before surgery are detailed, and specific diseases, operations, and experences are illustrated.

REFERENCES

1. BIESECKER, J.L., MARCOVE, R.C., HUVOS, A.G., MIKE, V.: Areurysmal bone cysts: a clinicopathologic stud of 66 cases. Cancer 26, 615-625 (1970)
2. HUVOS, A.V., MARCOVE, R.C.: Chondroblastoma of bone - a critical review. Clin. Orthop. related Res. 95, 300-312 (1973)
3. HUVOS, A.G., MARCOVE, R.C., ERLANDSON, R.A., MIKÉ, V.: Chondroblastoma of bone-a clinicopathologic and electron microscopic study. Cancer 29, 760-771 (1972)
4. MARCOVE, R.C.: The management of bone tumors. Memorial Sloan-Kettering Cancer Center Clinical Bulletin 1, 7-10 (1971)
5. MARCOVE, R.C., HUVOS, A.V.: Cartilaginous tumors of the ribs. Cancer 27, 794-801 (1971)
6. MARCOVE, R.C., KHAFAGY, M.M.: Total femur and knee replacement using a metallic prosthesis. Memorial Sloan-Kettering Cancer Center Clinical Bulletin 4, 69-71 (1974)
7. MARCOVE, R.C., LEWIS, M.M.: Prolonged survival in osteogenic sarcoma with multiple pulmonary metastases. J. Bone Jt. Surg. 55A, 1516-1520 (1973)
8. MARCOVE, R.C., LYDEN, J.P., HUVOS, A.G., BULLOUGH, P.B.: Giant cell tumors treated by cryosurgery: an analysis of 25 cases. In: Seventh National Cancer Conferences Proceedings, p. 951. New York: American Cancer Society, Inc. (1973)
9. MARCOVE, R.C., MIKE, V., HUVOS, A.G., SOUTHAM, C.M., LEVIN, A.G.: Autogenous lysed cell vaccine in the treatment of osteogenic sarcoma - a preliminary report on fifteen cases. Colston Papers, Vol. 24, p. 313. London: Butterworths Scientific Publications (1973) pp. 313-323.
10. MARCOVE, R.C., MILLER, T.R.: Treatment of primary and metastatic localized bone tumors by cryosurgery. Surg. Clin. N. Amer. 49, 421-430 (1969)
11. MARCOVE, R.C., SADRIEH, J.L., HUVOS, A.G., GRABSTALD, H.: Cryosurgery in the treatment of solitary or multiple bone metastasis from renal cell carcinoma. J. Urol. 108, 540-547 (1972)
12. MARCOVE, R.C., SOUTHAM, C.M., LEVIN, A.G., HUVOS, A.G.: Autogenous vaccine in the treatment of osteogenic sarcoma. Cont. Surg. 2, 54-55 (1973)

13. MARTINI, N., HUVOS, A.G., MIKÉ, V., MARCOVE, R.C., BEATTIE, E,J.: Multiple pulmonary resections in the treatment of osteogenic sarcoma. Ann. Thorac. Surg. 12, 271-280 (1971)
14. MIRRA, J.M., BULLOUGH, P.G., MARCOVE, R.C., JACOBS, G., HUVOS, A. G.: Malignant fibrous histiocytoma and osteosarcoma in association with bone infarcts: report of four cases, two in caisson workers. J. Bone Jt. Surg. 56A, 932-940 (1974)
15. ROSEN, G., SUWANSIRIKUL, S., KWON, C., TAN, C., WU, S.J., BEATTIE, E.J., MURPHY, M.L.: High-dose methotrexate with citrovorum factor rescue and adriamycin in childhood osteogenic sarcoma. Cancer 33, 1151-1163 (1974)
16. ROSEN, G., WOLLNER, N., TAN, C., WU, S.J., HAJDU, S.I., CHAM, W., D'ANGIO, G.L., MURPHY, M.L.: Disease-free survival in children with Ewing's sarcoma treated with adjuvant four-drug sequential chemotherapy. Cancer 33, 384-393 (1974)
17. SHOJI, H., KOSHINO, T., MARCOVE, R.C., THOMPSON, T.C.: The role of the lateral ligaments and the periosteum at that lateral malleolus for lateral stability of the ankle - an experimental study. J. Jap. Orthop. Ass. 46, 51-56 (1972)
18. SHOJI, H., KOSHINO, T., MARCOVE, R.C., THOMPSON, T.C.: Subperiosteal resection of the distal portion of the fibula for aneurysmal bone cyst: report of two cases. J. Bone Jt. Surg. 52A, 1472-1476 (1970)
19. SOUTHAM, C.M., MARCOVE, R.C., LEVIN, A.G., BUCHSBAUM, H.J., MIKÉ, V.: Clinical trial of autogenous tumor vaccine for treatment of osteogenic sarcoma. Seventh National Cancer Conference Proceedings, p. 91. New York: American Cancer Sociaty, Inc. (1973)

Management of Osteogenic Sarcoma at the Mayo Clinic

J. C. IVINS and D. J. PRITCHARD

In the literature on osteogenic sarcoma, the classic paper by FRIEDMAN and CARTER (3) stands as a masterpiece of data collection and scrutiny, and its extensive bibliography lists all the important references. Among other things, these authors made recommendations about the structure of future studies devoted to osteogenic sarcoma. Thus, in reviewing the management of osteogenic sarcoma at the Mayo Clinic, we make no attempt to review the literature further. Instead, we shall relate some of our experiences, unpublished previously, with specific points emphasized by FRIEDMAN and CARTER and then give a report of a controlled study that we believe fulfills the criteria suggested by FRIEDMAN and CARTER (3), who stated that "Immunologic factors appear to play a significant role in this disease and the potential role of immunotherapy needs to be seriously considered."

MAYO CLINIC EXPERIENCE

Most of the interest in osteogenic sarcoma at the Mayo Clinic has been directed toward clinical management and reports of retrospective studies. However, etiologic factors have also been studied. For example, a study of beryllium-induced osteogenic sarcoma in rabbits showed that splenectomy was required before the tumors would form in all animals. It was later found that the tumors failed to form when the beryllium supplied for the experiments was free of all trace metals (6). This led to further work examining the significance of this finding. Although such sarcomatous tissues contain different amounts of eight trace metals than do normal tissues, no conclusions are yet possible; however, such work may eventually yield support for the importance of Furst's metal-binding hypothesis (4) of cancer etiology.

Collaborative work with regard to the viral etiology of osteogenic sarcoma has been carried on at the Argonne National Laboratory (10).

About 900 patients with osteogenic sarcoma have been seen and treated at the Mayo Clinic. In recent years, the management of all patients with osteogenic sarcoma has been under the direction of an osteogenic sarcoma study group comprising the following members: a pathologist, a radiologist, an orthopedic surgeon, a thoracic surgeon, a medical oncologist, an immunologist, a virologist, and a statistician. An orthopedic oncology laboratory was established in 1972; this laboratory, among other things, has carried out pretreatment and post-treatment immunologic surveillance on all osteogenic sarcoma patients.

A careful study of 430 patients with osteogenic sarcoma was reported by COVENTRY and DAHLIN in 1957 (1). In 1967, a detailed study of 600 cases was published by DAHLIN and COVENTRY (2). In this latter report, osteogenic sarcoma was defined as any sarcoma containing malignant cells that produce osteoid substance, even if in only small foci. Three histologic types were recognized, depending on the dominant cellular differentiation, About 50 percent were osteoblastic in type, about 25 percent were fibroblastic, and about 25 percent were chondroblastic. Some of the findings of this study of 600 patients are summarized in Fig. 1. Anatomically, more than one-half of the tumors developed either just above or just below the knee; the upper humerus was the third most common site. Most of the tumors were of high-grade malignancy. The prognosis varied, depending on histologic type, but it was distinctly better when the tumor was located distal to the elbow or knee (Table 1). Treatment was consistent with the commonly accepted method, i.e., early diagnosis, amputation between two tourniquets, and no postoperative adjunctive treatment of any kind. If the lesion was distally located, a cross-bone amputation was usually performed; for proximal lesions, disarticulation or girdle amputation was used. The 5-year survival for the entire group was 20.3 percent.

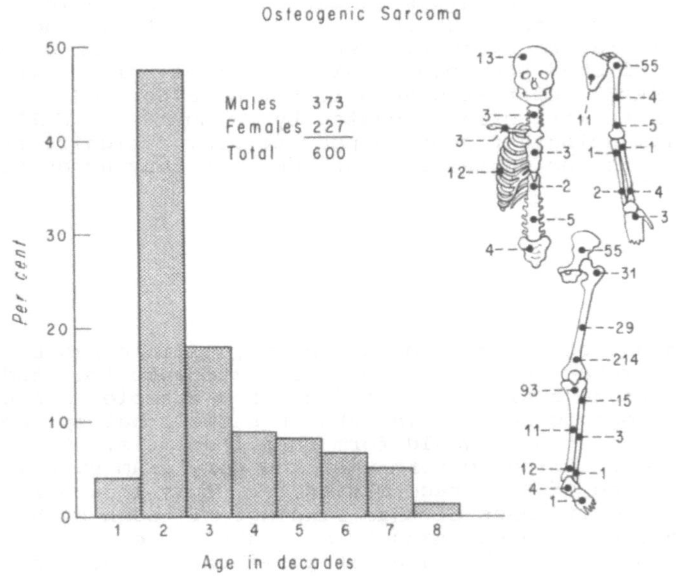

Fig. 1. Skeletal, age, and sex distribution of 600 cases of osteogenic sarcoma. (From DAHLIN D.C., COVENTRY, M.B. (2), by permission)

A study of this report and similar reports from other institutions raises a question concerning differences in survival that can be illustrated by two brief case reports.

Case 1. - A 14-year-old girl complained of pain about her left hip for only 3 weeks. Biopsy of a lesion in the left femoral neck revealed a grade-3 osteogenic sarcoma; veins in the specimen were filled with tumor. Because the high-grade lesion was in a proximal location and because of a small chance of cure, the primary lesion in the neck of the femur was irradiated (tumor dose: 7,320 rad); both (negative) lung fields were also irradiated (1,500 rad). About 6 months after completion of radiation therapy, the femoral head and neck were resected and a Mat-

Table 1. Survival in osteogenic sarcoma. From DAHLIN, D.C., COVENTRY, M.B. (2), by permission

	Total	Traced	Lived 5 years or more No.	Percent of traced patients
Overall group				
Total	410	408	83	20.3
Male	258	256	55	21.5
Female	152	152	28	18.4
Osteoblastic	217	216	37	17.1
Chondroblastic	94	94	21	22.3
Fibroblastic	99	98	25	25.5
Tumors distal to upper end of humerus and upper end of femur	282	280	71	25.4
Tumors below elbows and knees	107	106	38	35.8

chett-Brown type of intramedullary prosthesis was inserted. Recovery was excellent. Still alive more than five years after onset, she is an active college girl with little or no functional disability.

Case 2. - An 11-year-old girl complained of pain about the right hip for 3 months. At biopsy, a grade-3 osteogenic sarcoma was found in the right femoral neck. Because of the prognosis of this proximally located tumor, the neoplasm was irradiated (6,000 rad), as were the negative lung fields (1,500 rad). About 4 months later, a mass lesion appeared in the left lung. This was resistant to irradiation and chemotherapy, and she died about one year after the start of her treatment.

The reason why, under these closely similar circumstances, one of these two girls should die and the other survive, obviously has little to do with the clinical examination or the mode of treatment. Other factors, most probably immunologic, must be of paramount importance.

CONTROL OF PULMONARY METASTASES

Osteogenic sarcoma characteristically causes death through the development of secondary deposits in the pulmonary parenchyma. At the moment, we have no reliable way of predicting which patients will develop this complication and we have no uniformly effective form of treatment for it once it has developed.

Whole-Lung Irradiation. It is generally agreed that pulmonary metastatic seeding occurs continuously and that it has been initiated long before the patient sees the doctor for the first time. Assuming that malignant seeding of the lungs occurs in all patients with osteogenic sarcoma, one can postulate that, in some patients, perhaps removal of the primary lesion allows re-establishment of a more favorable immune defense so that malignant cells in the pulmonary parenchyma are phagocytized or otherwise destroyed. Efforts to detect subclinical pulmonary metastatic deposits have been unrewarding. Neither pulmonary function studies nor radioisotope lung scans have proved helpful, and careful radiographic examination of the lungs, including the usual stereoscopic and lateral views and whole-lung tomograms made with 1-cm cuts, may fail to disclose metastatic lesions if their greatest diameter is less than 1 cm.

In 1969, we began a prospective study designed to test the effect of so-called prophylactic whole-lung radiation in preventing the appearance of pulmonary metastatic lesions. Patients with proven osteogenic sarcoma and with negative radiographs of the lung fields were randomized into two groups, treated and control, and the study was stratified with respect to anatomic location of the primary lesion. In approximately 2.5 years, 53 patients were registered in this study. Anatomic sites affected and histologic types were similar in the two groups. The patients in the treated group received a 1,500-rad tumor dose to the whole of both lungs in divided doses. In an attempt to potentiate the effect of the irradiation, oxygen at ambient pressure was administered to each patient for 10 minutes before and during each treatment session, and actinomycin D (usual dose, 0.5 mg) was also injected intravenously at each treatment session (usual dose, 0.5 mg i.v.). Both groups were followed carefully, with frequent conventional radiographs and also with whole-lung tomograms every 3 months. In no case was there ever any discernible harmful effect to the pulmonary parenchyma.

It soon became evident that we were not influencing the course of the disease by this approach and the study was stopped. There was no statistically significant difference in the disease-free interval between the two groups, and somewhat more than half the patients in each group developed radiographic evidence of pulmonary lesions at about the expected time. At the time these patients were reviewed, approximately half of the patients in each group had died, death occurring a little over one year after treatment. All the patients now alive and well have been followed for more than two years (9).

Thoracotomy. In the report of 600 cases seen at the Mayo Clinic (2), it was noted that 14 patients underwent an operation for metastatic pulmonary disease. Two patients underwent a pulmonary operation more than five years after amputation, and both subsequently died from widespread bilateral pulmonary involvement. Whether or not the pulmonary metastatic lesion can, itself, metastasize to produce lesions elsewhere is now debatable. In any event, it seems that the earlier the metastatic lesion is excised, the greater is the chance for cure - hence our advice to our patients to have chest roentgenograms monthly, at least for the first two years after treatment.

Stimulated by the experience at Memorial Hospital for Cancer and Allied Diseases, New York, and other centers (5, 7, 8), we recently began to take a much more aggressive surgical approach to the treatment of pulmonary metastatic lesions. Of the 26 patients who were treated with whole-lung irradiation, nine (17%) had one or more thoracotomies with wedge resections, and three are living. Currently, 18 other patients whose cases have not been reported have undergone single or multiple thoracotomies. Among these patients, 13 (72%) are living but have been treated too recently to allow any conclusions. Moreover, for patients treated by thoracotomy we are just initiating a controlled study of post-thoractomy adjunctive treatment with combination chemotherapy. We hope this more vigorous approach will produce an improved survival rate. We are enthusiastic about surgical removal of pulmonary metastatic lesions; we believe that resection alone will save many lives that otherwise would be lost. Recently, our thoracic surgeons have been removing bilateral lesions by median sternotomy with single surprisingly little morbidity (11).

PREOPERATIVE IRRADIATION OF THE PRIMARY LESION

Not all patients with osteogenic sarcoma can be persuaded to submit to amputation as the immediate primary treatment. With some patients, who have a high-grade lesion in a proximal location, it has seemed unwise to press the issue; and, in some patients, because of the anatomic location of the tumor, the operation is not technically possible. Finally, every surgeon knows of the patient who has sought advice in several different hospitals and will consent to treatment only at the hands of the surgeon who promises not to amputate right away. For these and for other reasons, we have occasionally applied high-dose radiation directly to the primary lesion, with amputation or excisional surgery planned to follow in the absence of roentgenographic evidence of pulmonary metastatic spread. The following account of our experience with this form of therapy, however, is anecdotal and should not be regarded as representing any controlled randomized study.

We have experience with preoperative irradiation in 32 patients, but this account will consider therapy only in the 26 who have now been followed for more than two years and for up to 4.5 years after treatment. No patients with Paget's sarcoma or sarcoma arising in a postirradiated bone are included. There was nothing remarkable about the sex and age distribution or anatomic location of the lesion in these patients. With respect to the tumors, 22 of the sarcomas were of the osteoblastic type and all but one were either grade 3 or grade 4. The radiation therapy in most instances took the form of a split-course technique, the source of radiation being either cobalt or a linear accelerator; the dose varied from 5,000 to 8,000 rad. After the radiation therapy had been completed, all patients were carefully observed, and, as long as good function remained and radiographic examination of the primary lesion showed no new activity, surgery was deferred. There were, however, three exceptions. Two patients who had not completed the course of therapy had to undergo amputation early because of pathologic fracture, and both these patients died. The third patient, who also had a pathologic fracture, refused amputation before the radiation course was completed and he died 6 months later.

Of the 26 patients, seven underwent no surgical procedure because of early appearance of pulmonary metastases, and one underwent no surgical procedure because of an inaccessible lesion located in the sacroiliac joint with much of the lesion on the sacral side. The remaining 18 patients were treated by either amputation or resection from 6 days to 2 years after irradiation; most of them had an operation from 6 to 9 months after completion of radiation therapy. Of these patients, 10 are alive and free of disease, the remainder having died from metastatic spread. The 10 patients who are alive have all been followed for more than 2 years, but two of them have had thoracotomies during this period. Only three of these 10 patients had lesions below the knee and these lesions were of grades 1 through 3 in only three of the 10. This rather crude analysis indicates, therefore, that 10 of the 26 patients (about 38%) whose planned treatment was preoperative irradiation and delayed surgery completed the planned treatment and survived and that two of those who survived underwent pulmonary wedge resection.

This experience with preoperative irradiation and delayed surgery has been instructive, and we can draw the following pertinent conclusions about this therapeutic regimen:

1. the course of radiation therapy is time-consuming and expensive for the patient and is occasionally followed by considerable morbidity;

2. this combined approach does nothing to lessen the psychologic impact of the disease. The patient realizes that amputation or some form of surgical procedure is inevitable and is only being delayed;

3. in every patient but one in this group, viable tumor was found at operation. The one exception was a girl with a grade-4 primary osteogenic sarcoma in the ilium. The lesion was resected after irradiation with 8,000 rad, and she is now alive and well 5 years later, having had one thoractomy for resection of a single pulmonary metastatic nodule;

4. there is some suggestive evidence, which is so far unproven, that irradiation affects the patient's immune response unfavorably;

5. on the basis of past experience, it is reasonable to expect that, as we continue to follow these patients, more of them will appear with pulmonary metastatic lesions. Despite this, one must sometimes take this conservative approach; one can fairly promise the patient and the family that it is no worse and perhaps no better than early primary amputation.

As is evident from earlier reports, when the appearance on an initial chest roentgenogram is suspect or when there are any of a variety of other reasons, this technique may be effective in saving limbs if not in saving lives.

IMMUNOLOGIC STUDIES

About three years ago, the Orthopedic Oncology Research Laboratory was created at the Mayo Clinic. This laboratory is equipped and staffed to provide immunologic surveillance of our patients with cancer. Most of the experience has concerned cutaneous melanoma and osteogenic sarcoma, though we are now monitoring an increasing number of soft-tissue sarcomas as well. Working on the assumption that the techniques of early diagnosis and surgical treatment had reached a penultimate state of effectiveness and that something else was needed if the cure rate in osteogenic sarcoma was to be improved, we began to accumulate data relating to several immunologic considerations. We had a twofold purpose in doing this. First, we wanted to accumulate reliable data on which to base an immunotherapy program; second, we wanted to attempt to discover any trends that might be helpful in predicting prognosis and perhaps guide us eventually in selecting proper therapy.

The various immunologic tests are described in detail elsewhere in this volume (PRITCHARD et al.).

In the light of these various studies, we concluded that some form of immunologic manipulation should be evaluated in a prospective study for its effect in improving prognosis. After considering many possible approaches, we elected to try one form of passive immunotherapy: the use of transfer factor (TF). We did this for two reasons: (1) early trials of TF in immunodeficiency states and bacterial diseases gave promising results; and (2) of all agents that can be considered, TF inconveniences the patient least. We decided to use only specific TF (i.e., TF obtained from patients cured of osteogenic sarcoma), and we began to harvest it by Lawrence's technique about 2 years ago. We expect to compare the results of TF therapy with those of therapy with methotrexate plus adriamycin plus vincristine (MAO).

Protocol for TF and MAO. The Parent Study: In July 1974, after more than 2 years of preparation, we started a prospective study of osteogenic sarcoma. It is so new that all that can be done at this point is to outline the plan briefly. It is based on two forms of treatment, TF (schedule A) and the MAO combination (schedule B). The study is designed to give an early assessment of the results compared with those obtained in the past by using historical controls.

1. Requirements for inclusion in the study. For entry into the study, the patient must have an operable lesion and be free of any metastatic spread, and there must be histologic proof of the diagnosis of osteogenic sarcoma; informed consent also must be obtained.

2. Contraindications. Absolute contraindications include a low leukocyte count; elevation of the creatinine or bilirubin concentration; evidence of heart disease; infection; an unhealed wound; prior treatment with any chemical, any agent that is a source of radiation, or any immunologic agent; poor nutrition; or poor veins.

3. Prerandomization examination. Prior to randomization, a complete general medical examination is carried out and a pretreatment immune file is completed.

4. Stratification. Stratification is based on the tumor histologic type inasmuch as there is, according to our figures, a somewhat better prognosis with the fibroblastic type. Stratification also includes the anatomic site of the primary lesion and the response of the patient to immune testing.

5. Randomization. Each patient is randomly assigned to treatment with either TF or the combination of chemotherapeutic agents.

6. Schedule A (TF). For patients on schedule A, donors are selected who have a strongly positive reaction for one of the skin tests that was negative in the patient. TF (0.1 ml) is given subcutaneously and the skin test is repeated on both arms. If the marker has been successfully transferred, nothing else is done except to test the patient's skin every 3 months and to repeat the dose of TF from the same donor as long as the marker remains positive. If the marker is not successfully transferred, a new donor is chosen; however, a maximum of three new injections from three different donors is permitted. If there is no conversion, the patient is reclassified to receive MAO.

Follow-up investigations include a chest roentgenogram every month and a complete physical examination every 3 months for the first 3 years and then every 4 months for the ensuing 2 years. The complete examination includes evaluation with whole-lung tomograms and immunologic studies.

7. Schedule B (MAO). Randomized patients receive the three drugs as follows: (1) methotrexate is given in a dose of 3,500 mg/m^2 as a 4-

hour infusion, followed within 30 minutes of completion of the infusion by calcium leucovorin (15 mg) given intravenously, and, later, by calcium leucovorin (12 mg) given orally as indicated; (2) vincristine, in a dose of 1.4 mg/m^2 intravenously; and (3) adriamycin, in a dose of 40 mg/m^2 intravenously. The MAO program is started on the 15th postoperative day and is repeated every 4 weeks to a total of 12 treatments.

Follow-up investigations include chest roentgenography monthly for the first year, bimonthly for the second year, quarterly for the third year, and 4-monthly during the fourth and fifth years, as well as a complete physical examination, including whole-lung tomograms and immunologic studies, every 3 months.

8. Study analysis. For both schedules, the following factors are monitored carefully: (i) the interval from surgery until the first appearance of pulmonary metastatic spread; (ii) the interval from surgery until death; (iii) the changes in immune status; (iv) the effect of the initial immune status on response to treatment; and (v) the disease-free interval.

9. Failure. Failure is signified by radiographic evidence of a pulmonary metastatic lesion. The patient is then excluded from the study. Thoracotomy is performed, after which the patient is treated by chemotherapy; the schedule is followed exactly as directed in the protocol. Subsequent thoracotomies are performed as long as the patient's condition is operable. When, because of multiple bilateral pulmonary lesions, surgical resection can no longer be performed, the patient will be treated with whatever investigational chemotherapy program is then available; this of course, changes from time to time.

CONCLUSION

The experience we have gained permits some reasonable conclusions. Surgical treatment of osteogenic sarcoma seems to have reached its penultimate state, i.e. early recognition of the lesion and accurate diagnosis by open biopsy followed by surgical ablation of the primary lesion cannot be expected to improve the cure rate. Something else is needed. There is suggestive evidence that osteogenic sarcoma has a viral cause. Before this is completely worked out, however, it seems certain that the enzymologist(or molecular biologist) and the geneticist will become heavily involved; and it is equally certain that, because we do not now understand the etiology, prevention of the tumor by some sort of vaccination seems to be an utopian dream.

At present, we believe that the primary lesion should be excised as soon as possible. We do not advocate the use of a tourniquet. Surgical removal of the tumor should be followed by some form of adjunctive treatment; and immunotherapy or chemotherapy, or both, seems to hold the the most promise. With respect to secondary lesions, there seems to be no doubt about the life-saving value of an aggressive attitude toward resection of pulmonary metastatic lesions. We firmly believe that thoracotomy should be performed whenever possible and that the surgical removal of all pulmonary metastatic lesions should be followed by some form of adjunctive treatment. We also believe that immune surveillance is a most important part of the examination and follow-up care of patients with osteogenic sarcoma. As more data are gathered about these patients, we may soon be able to identify those patients who will do poorly. In this circumstance, one then might be able to make a better case for temporizing in the treatment of the primary lesion by some form of nonsurgical treatment in order to avoid futile loss of limbs. On the other hand, continued immune surveillance may show that early surgical removal of the primary lesion is indicated in order to relieve the host of its antigenic burden and that this, followed by some form of immunologic manipulation, will result in unexpected cures.

In any event, we can again strongly agree with the conclusion of FRIEDMAN and CARTER (3) that, "It is more than appropriate at this time to attempt a multidisciplinary approach which will hopefully lead to an improvement of the cure rate of this dread tumor."

SUMMARY

In a Mayo Clinic prospective study of metastasis from osteogenic sarcoma, so-called prophylactic whole-lung irradiation (a 1,500-rad tumor dose to the whole of both lungs, in divided doses, with oxygen and actinomycin) proved ineffective. 14 patients underwent an operation for metastatic pulmonary disease. The earlier the excision of a metastatic lesion, the greater the chance of an effective cure. Preoperative irradiation of the bone tumor had no positive effect. The primary lesion should also be excised as soon as possible. Surgical removal of a tumor should be followed by immunotherapy or chemotherapy or both. The rate of reliably "cured" cases could be improved by extensive studies of immunologic reaction before and after surgical intervention.

REFERENCES

1. COVENTRY, M.B., DAHLIN, D.C.: Osteogenic sarcoma: A critical analysis of 430 cases. J. Bone Joint Surg. (Am.) 39, 741-757 (1957)
2. DAHLIN, D.C., COVENTRY, M.B.: Osteogenic sarcoma: A study of six hundred cases. J. Bone Jt Surg. (Am.) 49, 101-110 (1967).
3. FRIEDMAN, M.A., CARTER, S.K.: The therapy of osteogenic sarcoma: Current status and thoughts for the future. J. Surg. Oncol. 4, 482-510 (1972)
4. FURST, A.: Chelation and Cancer: A Speculative Review on Metal Binding in Medicine. In: Proceedings of a Symposium sponsored by the Hahnemann Medical College and Hospital, p. 336. Philadelphia: Lippincott 1960
5. ISHIHARA, T., IKEDA, T., YAMAZAKI, S., SHIBATA, H.: Treatment for pulmonary metastasis arising from osteogenic sarcoma. Keio J. Med. 20, 195-202 (1971)
6. JANES, J.M., MCCALL, J.T., ELVEBACK, L.R.: Trace metals in human osteogenic sarcoma. Mayo Clin. Proc. 47, 476-478 (1972)
7. MARTINI, N., HUVOS, A.G., MIKÉ, V., MARCOVE, R.C., BEATTIE, E.J., Jr.: Multiple pulmonary resections in the treatment of osteogenic sarcoma. Ann. thorac. Surg. 12, 271-278 (1971)
8. MORTON, D.L., JOSEPH, W.L., KETCHAM, A.S., GEELHOED, G.W., ADKINS, P.C.: Surgical resection and adjunctive immunotherapy for selected patients with multiple pulmonary metastases. Ann. Surg. 178, 360-365 (1973)
9. RAB, G.T., IVINS, J.C., CHILDS, Jr., D.S., CUPPS, R.E., PRITCHARD, D.J.: Elective whole lung irradiation in the treatment of osteogenic sarcoma. In press, Cancer

10. REILLY, C.A., Jr., PRITCHARD, D.J., BISKIS, B.O., FINKEL, M.P.: Immunologic evidence suggesting a viral etiology of human osteosarcoma. Cancer, 30, 603-609 (1972)
11. SPANOS, P.K., PAYNE, W.S., IVINS, J.C., PRITCHARD, D.J.: Pulmonary Resections for Metastatic Osteogenic Sarcoma. Paper to be presented at American Academy of Orthopaedic Surgeons, February 2, 1976

Surgical Treatment of Solitary Bone Cysts

H. H. MATTHIASS and M. IMMENKAMP

The term "bone cyst" is commonly used quite inappropriately to designate a variety of conditions of bones that are characterized by a circumscribed, sharply delineated area of radiolucency. Only gas- or fluid-filled intraosseous cavities that are encapsulated can be designated as bone cysts according to the definition. A clear distinction must be made between actual cystic lesions of bone and solid tumors that give a cystic appearance radiographically. When biopsy material from one of these solid tumors is referred to the pathologist as being from a cystic condition, even though there is no true bone cyst from the morphological standpoint, it gives rise to many misunderstandings and much confusion among clinicians and pathologists. According to SALZER-KUNTSCHIK (10), primary bone cysts (i.e. solitary bone cyst and aneurysmal bone cyst), representing a clinically and morphologically distinctive entity of unknown origin, must be separated from the secondary bone cysts and dysontogenetic bone cysts. These comprise a variety of bone cysts of known origin: (1) cystic cavities due to regressive changes in bone tumors; (2) osteoarthritic cyst; (3) subchondral cyst, synovial cyst, intraosseous ganglia; (4) developmental epithelial cyst; (5) traumatic epithelial cyst; (6) echinococcal cyst; (7) hemophilic pseudotumors.

The solitary bone cyst is by far the most common tumor-like lesion of bone in early childhood and adolescence. It is a unicameral, usually fluid-filled, slightly expansile bone cyst that is lined by a thin membrane of connective tissue. There is a definite preponderance of males among the patients in the proportion of about 2 : 1. The sites of predilection are the upper humerus and femur. In larger series the cyst is located in these skeletal sites in rather more than two-thirds of cases. Usually the lesion embraces the full width of the affected metaphysis, the regional cortex being attenuated and expanded.

According to JAFFÉ and LICHTENSTEIN (7), a solitary bone cyst that abuts on the epiphyseal cartilage plate is "active" and prone to show a marked tendency to progressive enlargement and to recur, while cysts that are separated from the plate by an interval of normal bone are "latent," with less tendency to grow and to recur. On our experience the validity and practicability of applying this concept therapeutically is less important since the proportion of recurrences has been shown to be only slightly higher in the active groups. There is no standard treatment for solitary bone cyst. It must be borne in mind that the solitary bone cyst is a completely benign lesion that will never transform to a malignant tumor. The clinical course, however, reveals a high tendency to infraction or pathologic fracture (60 - 70 percent according to GARCEAU and GREGORY (4) and NEER *et al.* (8)). These fractures are thought to heal in a short time, but one or more repeated fractures will often occur during a period of observation, because the cyst normally continues to enlarge. Spontaneous obliteration or disappearance of a cyst after a pathologic fracture is extremely rare and takes place over several years if at all. These findings suggest that there is little to be gained by nonoperative treatment.

Operative treatment of bone cysts enables us to obtain a histologic diagnosis and to reinforce the affected part mechanically by means of a bone graft, which gives the best chance of complete and prompt rehabilitation. The generally accepted surgical treatment for a solitary bone cyst is curettage of the cyst lining followed by packing of the cavity with bone chips. Additional chemical cauterization of the cyst wall after curettage has been advocated by some surgeons. According to most authors this procedure did not affect the cure rate. Since the majority of cysts occur in the young, in whom the sources for autogenous bone grafts are often not adequate, there may be problems in filling up a large defect. There is a great risk of damaging the growth plate of the iliac bone when bone grafts are taken out. Freeze-dried cancellous allograft has been used in the treatment of 177 bone cysts (11). The authors pointed out that the overall healing rate in their series is comparable to that of other authors using only autogenous or homologous grafts.

Successful eradication of a solitary bone cyst is difficult to achieve. Recurrence rates following conventional surgery (i.e. curettage and bone graft) are definitely too high. In our series of 53 solitary bone cysts, including some cases that were first treated elsewhere, the recurrence rate was 34 percent. Recurrence rates as high as 50 percent have been reported in the literature (12: 50 percent; 11: 45 percent; 6: 40 - 50 percent). In our opinion it is permitted to question the validity of a treatment that is followed by such a high failure rate. Incomplete obliteration of the cyst after surgery, the so-called asymptomatic and static "filling defects" may gradually disappear with time; on the other hand these filling defects can be shown in many cases to give rise to true recurrences with reappearance and enlargement of a cyst, causing expansion and thinning of the cortex and fracture even after a period of several years. In one case recurrence was observed after three years. Recently some authors described subtotal (9, 2) and total segmental resection (13, 3, 5) for patients with active cysts leading to repeated pathologic fractures in a weight-bearing long bone or with progressive cyst enlargement. This mode of treatment had already been mentioned in 1967 (1). During the age of growth, especially when local conditions allow preservation of the periosteum, segmental resection can be carried out to advantage, because of the high osteogenetic potency of the periosteum in adolescence. After subperiosteal resection of diaphyseal or metaphyseal segments of any length, reconstruction of the entire bone due to subperiosteal activity can be expected. If an autoplastic or homoplastic fibula graft is interposed after segmental resection of a cyst, the defect will be bridged and stabilized within eight weeks. The fibula is especially suitable for the bridging of large osseous defects: it is sufficiently stable to maintain the distance of the bony ends after being interposed into the defect, while in addition it can be taken out without any very great impairment, since its main function is to serve as a point of insertion of muscles. The fibula defect is bridged in a short time when the graft is removed subperiosteally. The regenerated fibula can even be used a second time as a graft: we have seen this done in a case of monomelic fibrous dysplasia.

At the upper humerus the fibula is carefully inserted into the medullary cavity of the distal diaphyseal part of the affected bone, while proximally the anchoring of the graft is achieved by transfixation of a Kirschner wire connecting the lateral fragment of the humeral head with the transplanted fibula (Fig. 1). Thus, bending and shearing stresses can be eliminated (Fig. 2). Rotational stability is given by two transversely inserted Kirschner wires, which should not be shortened too much, so that they can be removed through a short incision afterwards. In most cases, Kirschner wires are enough to lock the graft securely in place. This form of minimal internal fixation should be performed in such a way that osteogenesis will not be disturbed (Fig. 2). On no account should internal fixation with medullary nails or blade plates anchored into the humeral head be done, as some authors have proposed. The anterior deltoid approach to the upper end of the humerus provides an excellent exposure of the proximal humerus. The periosteum is incised longitudinally. Thus the cyst and a portion of the adjacent normal shaft at each end is exposed subperiosteally. A full transverse saw cut is then made. The proximal cut should be performed carefully so that no damage to the adjacent epiphyseal cartilage plate is incurred. As the involved area of bone is exposed widely, a maximum effort can be made to curette the remnants of the cyst wall adjacent to the cartilage plate gently and under thorough scrutiny. An attempt is then made to reapproximate and to suture the periosteum over the graft. It is very important that the long axes of the graft correspond to the axes of the affected portion of the shaft, in order to guarantee an axial stress on the graft from the very beginning. An abduction thoracobrachial plaster cast is applied and left in place for six weeks to immobilize the extremity and to counteract muscle spasm. After this, union and strength of the humerus is usually sufficiently advanced to permit active and passive motion. The splint is retained for protection during the first one or two weeks of exercise. Bone portions that are exposed to an axial strain with no bending and shearing stresses are suited to segmental resection. The bridging of the defect can be performed by either an autologous or a homologous graft; the homologous graft, however, generally requires a much longer time for union and remodeling.

Since the mechanical stresses brought to bear upon the lower extremities, especially on the proximal femur, are much greater than those on the upper extremities, grave situations may arise, resulting in serious pathologic fractures, deformities and pseudarthroses. These findings suggest that operative treatment is necessary in any case of cyst in the upper femur, but the particular anatomical construction of the femoral neck makes it difficult to perform segmental resection. In practice, these cases necessitate recourse to thorough curettage of the cyst wall lining, followed by packing of the cavity with bone graft, or to subtotal resection even though the possibility of recurrence persists. In some cases, however, segmental resection seems to be inevitable. For example a 6-year-old boy showing a typical solitary unicameral bone cyst of the proximal femur received conservative treatment in the hope of spontaneous obliteration of the cyst (Fig. 3). On admission to our clinic 30 months later he showed a severe varus deformity of the femoral neck. We performed a segmental resection, carefully avoiding the epiphyseal plate of the femoral head. The apophysis of the trochanter major and the trochanter minor unfortunately had to be removed. In general, complete subperiosteal resection of the lesion at this location is practically not feasible. Closure of the periosteum over the graft could not be achieved. In this case subperiosteal new bone formation was not sufficient, as we had expected. Eventually we had to perform another operation, consisting in packing of autogenous bone strut grafts. The follow-up of this case demonstrated that at least the growth of the epiphyseal plate of the femoral head had progressed normally. It should be stressed that full segmental resection of the upper femur should be performed only in exceptional cases, since reconstruction of the exact anatomic structure is very difficult to achieve.

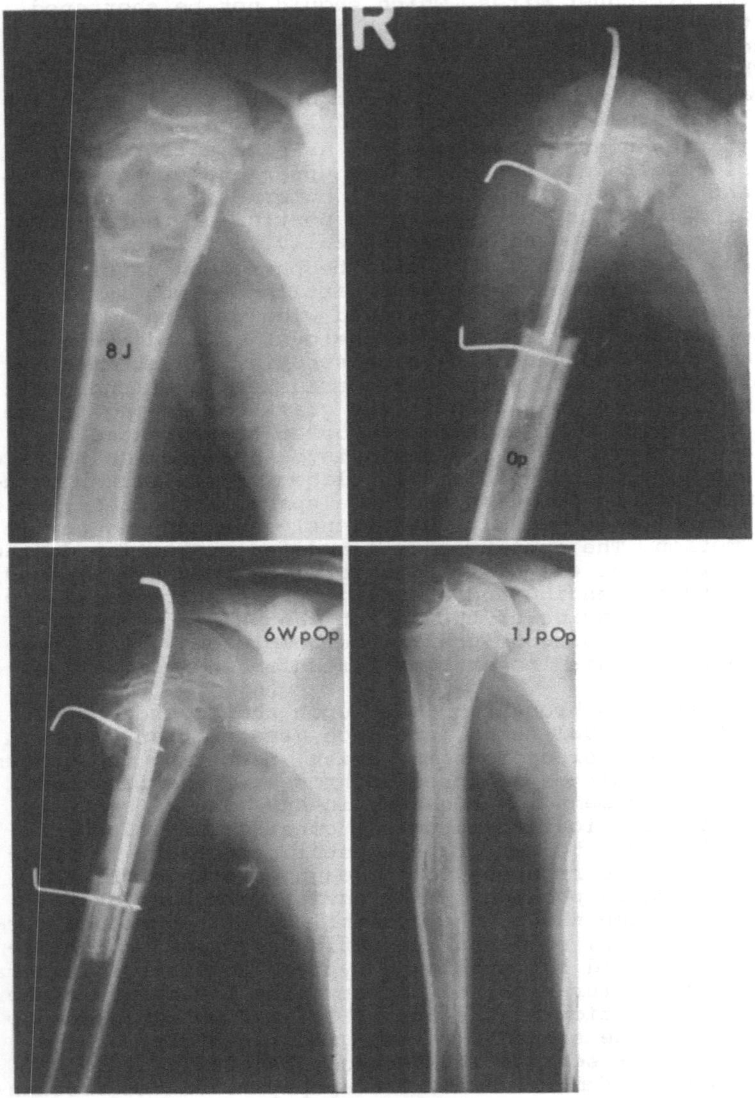

Fig. 1. K.H. (918/73) A typical humeral solitary bone cyst in an eight-year-old girl. Operative treatment was performed without delay, and consisted in subperiosteal segmental resection bridged by an autogenous fibula graft. Full stability was obtained within six weeks. Complete reconstruction of both the fibula (at the donor site) and the humerus was achieved

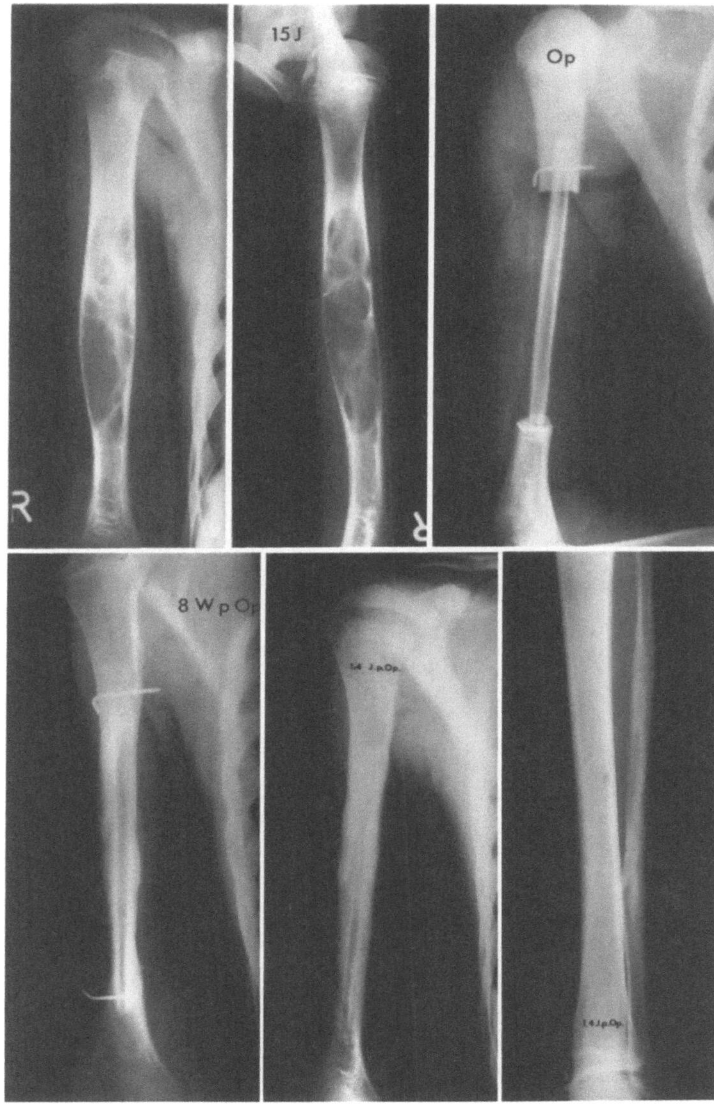

Fig. 2. E.Ch. (7107/72) A complete segmental subperiosteal diaphysectomy bridged by an autogenous fibula graft in a fifteen-year-old boy who displayed a large "latent" solitary cyst of the humerus. Union of the graft and recovery of stability were obtained within eight weeks. Follow-up revealed complete reconstruction of the humerus and the fibula, from where the graft had been taken

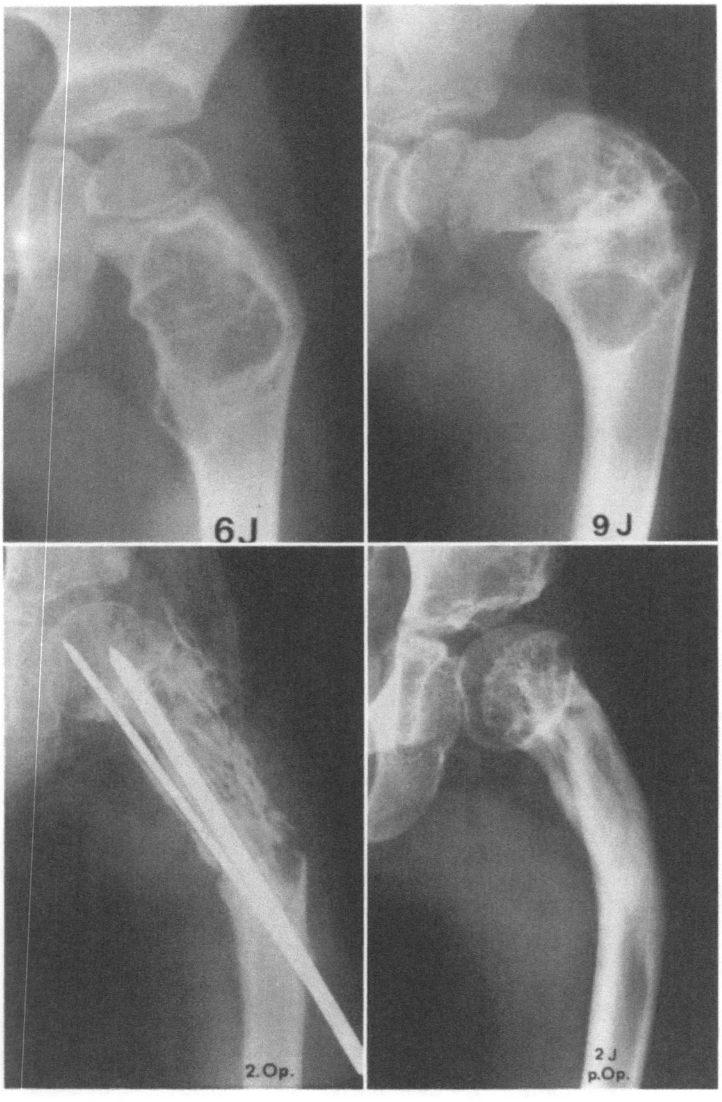

Fig. 3. G. V. (5749/71) A typical histologically proven solitary bone cyst in a six-year-old boy. Operative treatment was delayed in anticipation of spontaneous cyst obliteration. Several pathologic fractures occurred resulting in a severe shepherd's-crook deformity of the upper femur. In this exceptional case, segmental resection even of the femoral neck was deemed necessary. The periosteum could not be fully preserved, and bridging of the defect was thus only achieved by two operations, consisting in fibula grafting and packing of the defect with autogenous bone strut grafts. At least the growth of the epiphyseal plate of the femoral head had progressed normally

We have also found subperiosteal segmental resection beneficial in other benign tumors or tumor-like lesions. It has been performed in osteoid osteoma, aneurysmal bone cyst and fibrous dysplasia, and in some giant-cell tumors or chondromas. In each of 16 cases of solitary bone cyst we were able to achieve a cure without residual filling defects or recurrences. Subperiosteal segmental resection is only a little more extensive than curettage of a cyst, but the possibility of late recurrence is eliminated.

SUMMARY

A special method of subperiosteal segmental resection is described as an operative treatment for solitary bone cysts in long bones. This procedure exploits the high osteogenetic potency of the periosteum in adolescence. An autogenous or homologous fibula bone graft locked between the ends of the cyst serves to maintain the length of the bone fragments and acts as a guiding rod for continued subperiosteal new bone formation. There is full reconstruction of bone stability and function at both the cyst region and the donor region (fibula).

REFERENCES

1. BECKER, F., BECKER, W.: Operative Behandlung der Tumoren der Knochen, der Gelenke und Weichteile des Stützgewebes. In: Therapie maligner Tumoren (Ed. E. Holder), Vol. 2: Die operative Behandlung der Geschwülste. Stuttgart: Enke 1967
2. FAHEY, J.J., O'BRIEN, E.T.: Subtotal resection and grafting in selected cases of solitary unicameral bone cyst. J. Bone Jt Surg. 55A, 59 (1973)
3. GANZ, R., NOESBERGER, B., BOITZY, A.: Die juvenile Knochenzyste und ihre Behandlung. Helv. chir. Acta 40, 155 (1973)
4. GARCEAU, G.J., GREGORY, F.: Solitary bone cyst. J. Bone Jt Surg. 36A, 267 (1954)
5. IMMENKAMP, M.: Operative Behandlung der gutartigen Tumoren im Schulterbereich. Orth. Praxis (in press)
6. JAFFE, H.L.: Tumors and Tumorous Conditions of the Bones and Joints. p. 63. Philadelphia: Lea and Febiger 1958 cit. NEER et al.: Current concepts on the treatment of solitary unicameral bone cyst. Clin. Orthop. 97, 40 (1973)
7. JAFFE, H.L., LICHTENSTEIN, L.: Solitary unicameral bone cyst. Arch. Surg. 44, 1004 (1942)

   NEER, Ch. S., FRANCIS, K.C., JOHNSTON, A.D., KIERNAN, H.A.: Current concepts on the treatment of solitary unicameral bone cyst. Clin. Orthop. 97, 40 (1973)
9. ROBINS, P.R., PETERSON, H.A.: Management of pathological fractures through unicameral bone cysts. J. Amer. med. Ass. 222, 80 (1972)
10. SALZER-KUNTSCHIK, M.: Zysten im Knochen. Wien. klin. Wschr. 122, 425 (1972)
11. SPENCE, K.F., SELL, K.W., BROWN, R.H.: Solitary bone cyst: treatment with freeze-dried cancellous bone allograft. J. Bone Jt Surg. 51A, 87 (1969)
12. WILBER, M.C., HYATT, G.W.: Bone cysts: results of surgical treatment in 200 cases. In: Proceedings of the American Academy of Orthopedic Surgeons. J. Bone Jt Surg. 42A: 879 (1960) cit. NEER et al.: Cur-

rent concepts on the treatment of solitary unicameral bone cyst. Clin. Orthop. 97, 40 (1973)

13. WITT, A.N., WALCHER, K., ZENKER, H.: Die Resektionsbehandlung rezidivierender juveniler Knochencysten. Arch. orthop. Unfall-Chir. 74, 105 (1972)

Resection of Malignant Bone Tumors

M. SALZER and K. KNAHR

When indications for a radical surgical procedure become apparent in connection with a malignant bone tumor, amputation or enucleation of the extremity concerned is usually chosen. The most imperative task of surgeons involved in oncology should therefore be the search for alternatives to amputation. One such alternative seems to have arisen in connection with radical resectioning of the tumor.

Resection operations must be divided into radical and nonradical on the basis of macroscopic and histologic examinations. With a radical resection the tumor must be surrounded on all sides by a layer of normal tissue and must not extend to the incision surface at any point. If the tumor cannot be removed as a whole ("resection" of a vertebral body), or if there are macroscopic or histological tumor tissues on the incision surface, nonradical resection is performed. Because the anticipated results are not so good with nonradical resection, such cases must be classified distinctly apart from radical resections.

At every resection operation, one must aim to preserve an extremity capable of functioning. This is much more advantageous for the patient than the provision of an optimal prosthesis after amputation. Tumor resection has been mentioned in the literature since the beginning of this century (6, 7, 10), but such communications have remained rare up to the present. There are several possible reasons for this:

1. resection is technically more difficult and a more time-consuming operation than amputation;
2. the greater danger of non-radicality makes the results of the operation less certain;
3. most monographs on bone tumors and their treatment are by pathologists, among whom radical treatment automatically means amputation.

INDICATIONS

A resection can be carried out if the results of a morphological examination indicate a radical surgical procedure and suggest that radical resection is possible. Histologic examination must therefore be made before each resection. This can be done either on a biopsy section taken before the operation or on a frozen section taken during the operation. To avoid more than one operation, the frozen-section examination is preferred. In this way it is almost always possible to ascertain the nature of the tumor and thus to decide on the further therapeutic procedure.

Should a radical resection appear technically feasible, this procedure should then be carried out in all instances of primary malignant bone and soft-tissue tumors. This also applies to irradiation-sensitive Ewing's sarcomata, for recurrences can appear even after sufficient irradiation.

Bone metastases then are an indication for this type of operation only when metastases are solitary or when the retention of an extremity capable of functioning is not probable by means of smaller stabilizing operation or irradiation (Fig. 1). In cases of benign bone tumors a resection is only seldom necessary; with giant-cell tumors it is indicated only when there is no basic loss of function of the extremity. Therefore, with the giant-cell tumors frequently found in the knee-joint area, meticulous excochleation and bone-grafting are preferred as primary treatment. A similar procedure is also applied in the case of chondroma of tubular bones. Close postoperative observation is a necessity with both semimaligant groups of tumors. After the appearance of a recurrence a radical procedure is indicated.

Assessment of the technical feasibility of a radical resection requires an accurate preoperative diagnosis. Angiography and scintigraphy have proved to be valuable methods of examination, and both should be carried out in all cases. With angiography (Figs. 2, 6, 7), depiction of the delineation of the tumor in relation to the surrounding soft tissues is usually quite successful (9). Scintigraphy (Fig. 2) makes the delineation of the tumor in the marrow of tubular bones possible and is of special importance for the level of bone section (5). These mandatory examinations make accurate preoperative planning of the procedure considerably easier. Additional information can often be gained by the use of ultrasonic tomography (Fig. 3), which makes it possible to obtain cross-section pictures of an extremity and thereby also to achieve a better recognition of the extent of a soft-tissue tumor and its relationsship to bone (11).

OPERATIVE PROCEDURE

The skin incision must be made in such a manner that the operating area can be displayed distinctly (Fig. 4). Earlier surgical scars and, especially, sites of exploratory incisions should be widely cut around. The tumor and all its parts must be covered with a wide, healthy layer of tissue. The tumor itself must not be visible anywhere during the operation. Opening of the tumor and piecemeal removal of the tumor are to be avoided at all costs.

STABILIZATION MEASURES

After each resection, the question arises as to whether and by what means the function of the extremity can be restored. The radicality of resection is not permitted to be limited in any way by the problems of ensuing stabilization.

In the upper extremities good functional results are often achieved even without restoration of stability. This concerns primarily the function of the hand after shoulder resection.

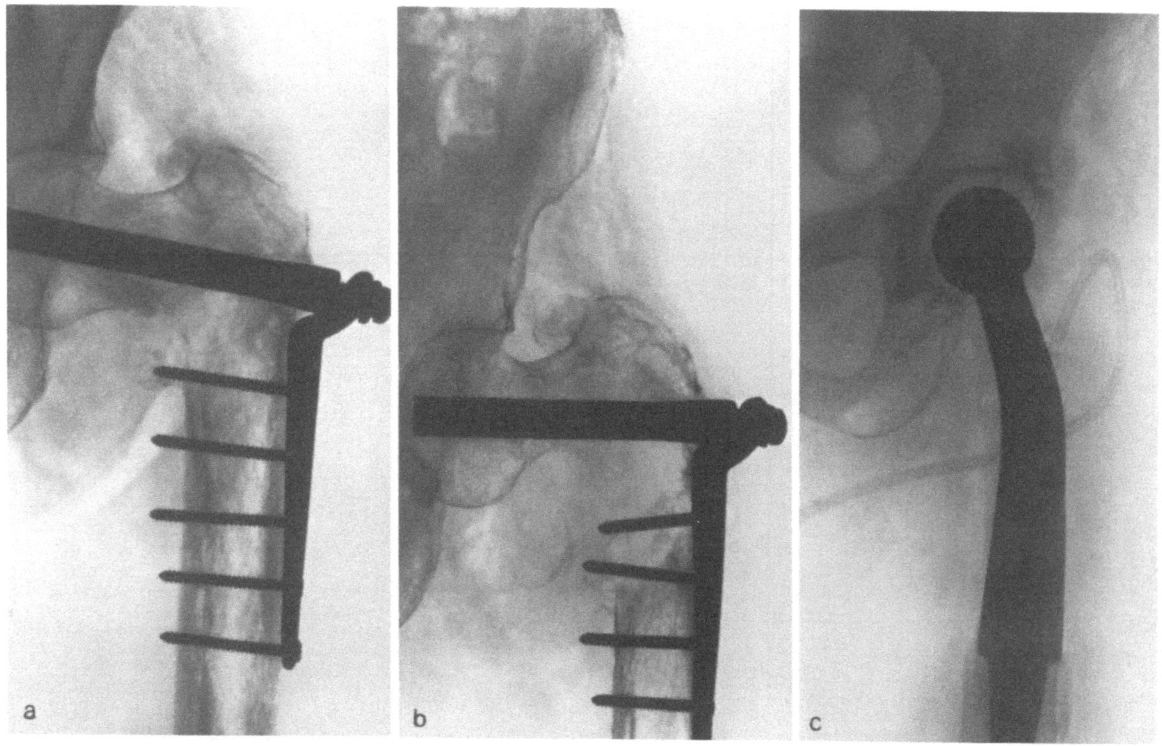

Fig. 1. W.J., f., 68 yrs. Intertrochanteric metastasis from thyroid cancer: (a) first stabilization (b) progression of lesion, breaking of nail, 2 years later (c) special total hip prothesis

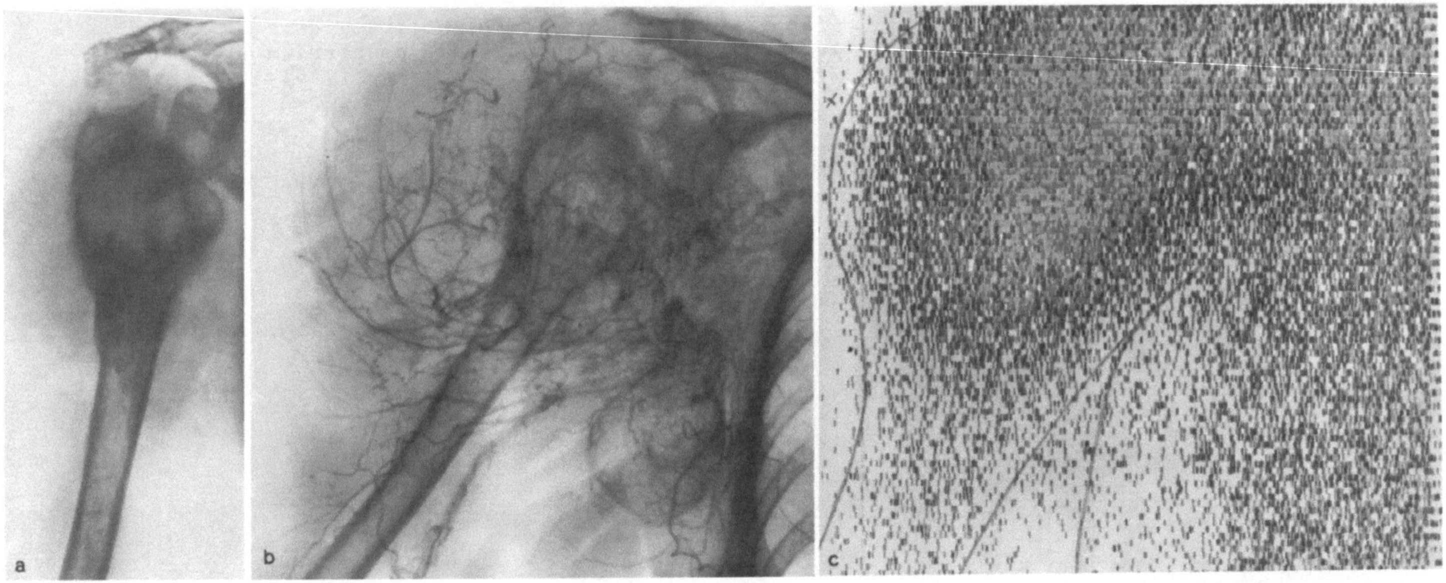

Fig. 2. E.W., f., 69 yrs. Large chondrosarcoma of the proximal humerus (a) X-ray showing bone destruction (b) angiography: clear delineation of soft-tissue mass, axillary lymph-node metastasis (c) scintigraphy with acticity in the proximal third of the shaft

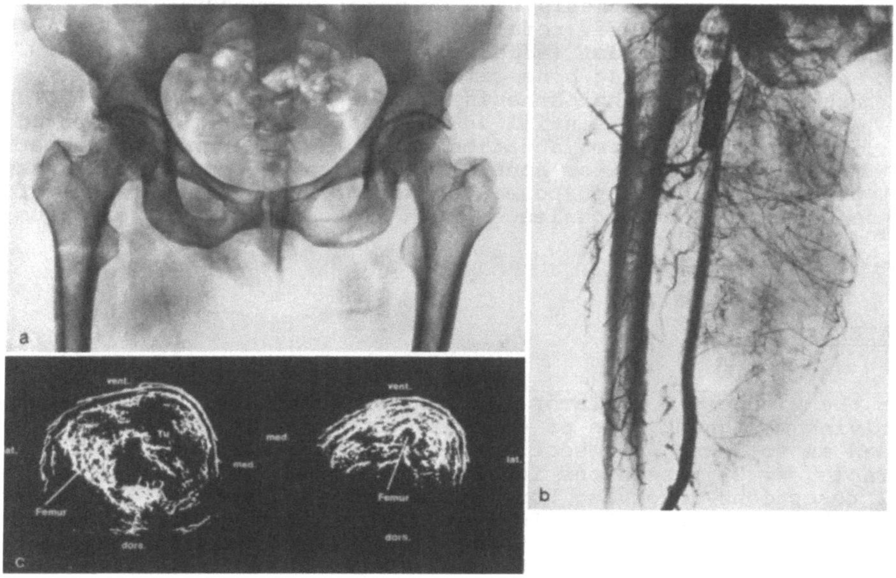

Fig. 3. B.J., f., 58 yrs. Soft-tissue fibrosarcoma of right proximal thigh (a) indistinct soft-tissue mass in the right adductor region (b) angiography: clear delineation of the soft-tissue mass (c) ultrasonic tomography with cross-section of both thighs: on the left, cystic tumor almost completely surrounding the femur

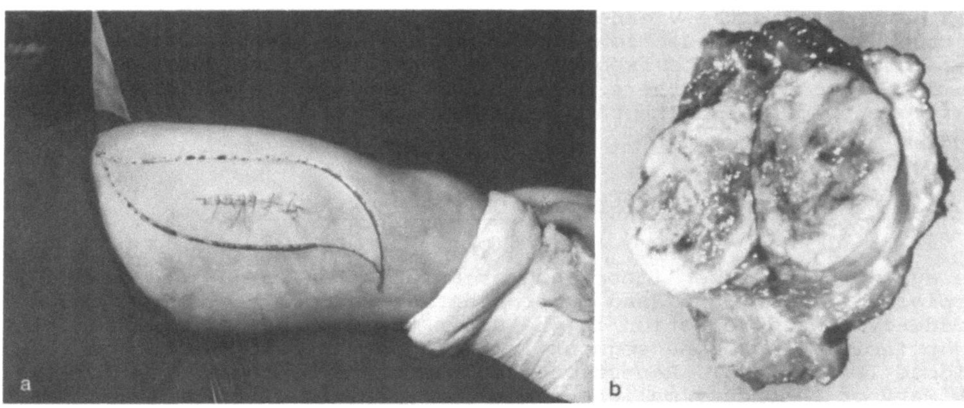

Fig. 4. P.L., f., 14 yrs. Soft-tissue fibrosarcoma of right thigh (a) skin incision widely surrounding the biopsy incision (b) cut specimen covered by normal tissue

The following methods of reconstruction appear possible:

1. autologous bone grafting for the bridging of defects and possible arthrodesis of neighboring joints (2);
2. use of autologous or homologous bone along with supplementary medullary pins or plates (3). This method is considered especially after resections in the knee-joint area. Postoperative treatment proves to be very lengthy in any event;

3. fitting of a prosthesis made of metal or sythetic materials (1, 4). With this procedure, total replacement of the joint nearest the defect is most usual (especially hip and shoulder joints). The use of autopolymerizing bone cement has proved to be necessary (Fig. 1);
4. fitting of an endoprosthesis made of "bio-ceramics (8)". This new material - which is still in the testing stages - offers advantages over traditional implantation materials. The good biocompatibility makes it possible for bone to grow into grooves which are specially provided for this purpose. The use of bone cement is therefore unnecessary. Some experiences with bio-ceramics are very promising (see below).

MATERIAL

At the Viennese Bone Tumor Registry 92 resections were carried out involving malignant bone of soft-tissue tumors in extremities. They break down as follows: 41 resections involving primary malignant bone tumors (Table 1), 29 resections involving malignant soft-tissue tumors, and 22 resections involving bone metastases. Analysis of the resected primary bone tumors by histology yielded 15 osteosarcomata, 9 chondrosarcomata, 6 fibrosarcomata, 5 round-cell sarcomata, and one each of malignant synovialoma, adamantinoma, Paget's sarcoma, myeloma, reticulosarcoma, and rhabdomysarcoma. Chronological analysis revealed that with increasing experience more and more resections took place in relation to amputations: of the 92 resections, 9 were carried out more than 5 years ago, while other 83 operations took place within the last 5 years. A similar picture is seen in connection with resections due to malignant shoulder tumors, for which three operations were carried out more than 5 years ago and 27 within the last 5 years. This increase in resection operations is due mainly to the larger number of tumor patients who have come to the Viennese Bone Tumor Registry. However, a comparison of the numbers of resections and of amputations shows that amputations were considerably more frequent than resections some years ago, while in more recent years there have been 27 shoulder resections as against only one primary interthoracoscapular amputation.

POSSIBILITY OF RADICAL RESECTION ON UPPER EXTREMITIES

Because of its lesser importance as a supporting organ and of the irreplaceability of the hand by prosthetic methods, there is a greater tendency toward resection in the upper than in the lower extremities. In principle, any bone segment in the upper extremities can be resectioned (Figs. 2, 5). Resection must therefore be considered for every primary or secondary malignant bone or soft-tissue tumor. The localization distribution of malignant tumors, the incidence being highest in the shoulder region, means that resections will ensue most often in this area. Because of anatomic factors, removal of even very large tumors is possible in this region (Fig. 8), whereby no consideration must be given to the restoration of stability. If the radicality of an operation proves to be absolute, postoperative irradiation is not necessary even with appearance of Ewing's sarcoma. The delayed effects of massive radiotherapy, in the form of fibrosis and bone necrosis, are often very damaging, since severe impairment of functional and cosmetic results can occur.

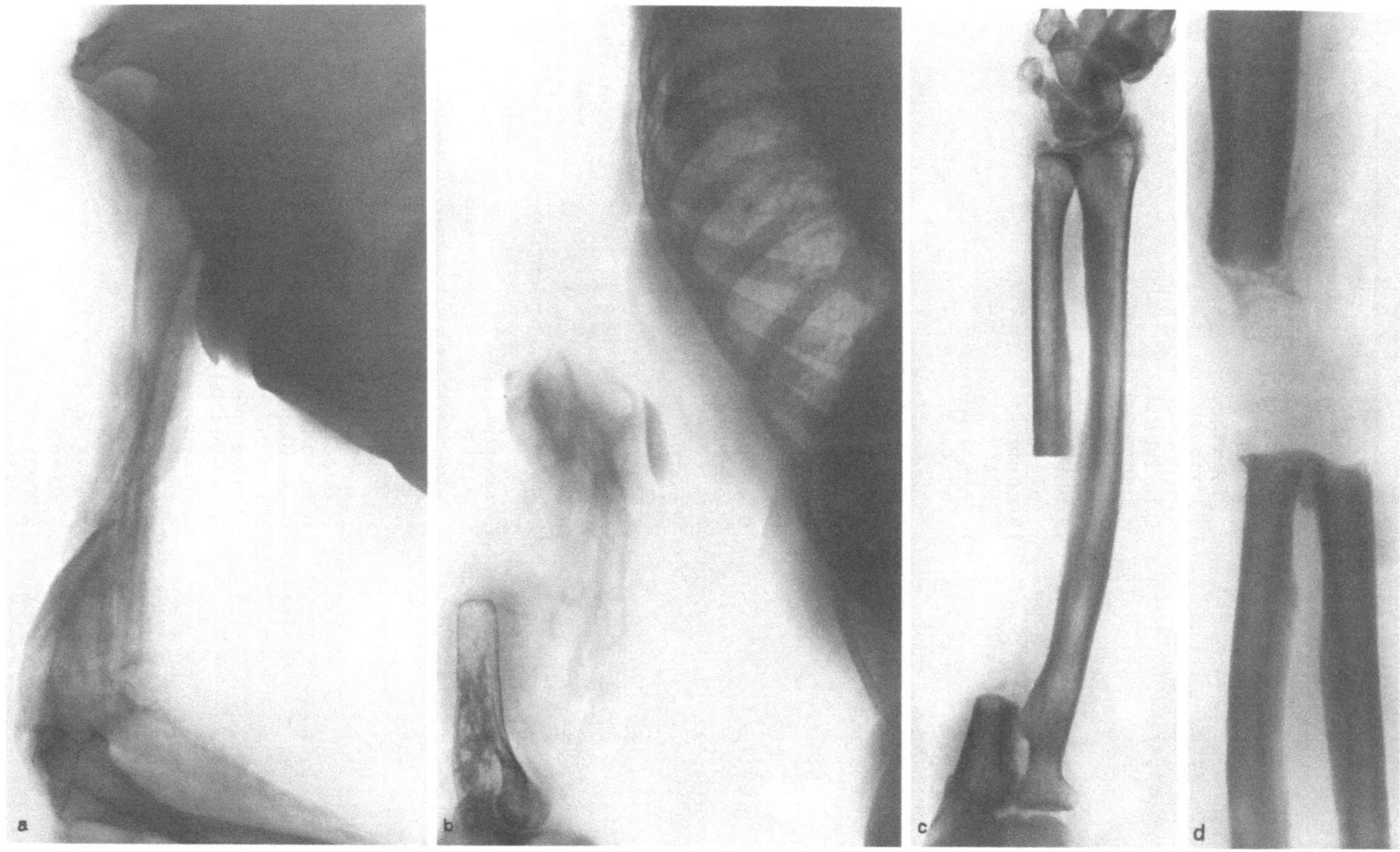

Fig. 5. Resections in upper extremity (a) T.A., f., 86 yrs: large rhabdomyosarcoma with destruction of humerus: total resection of humerus (b) E.W., f., 69 yrs. (see Fig. 2) Tickhor-Linberg resection of the shoulder with 2/3 resections of humerus (c) G.W., f., 74 yrs: fibrosarcoma of the proximal ulna diaphysis with resection of the affected part (d) St.K., m., 60 yrs: malignant synovialoma of the elbow joint 6 months after total joint resection

Table 1. Resection treatment in 41 primary malignant bone tumors

	Patients age (yrs), Sex	follow-up after	recurrence	therapy
Osteosarcoma			Radical	
Humerus	14, f.	16 months, deceased	-	-
Humerus	18, m.	15 months, deceased	-	-
Pelvis	47, f.	15 months, deceased	-	-
Femur	16, f.	96 months, alive	-	-
Fibula	29, f.	32 months, alive	-	-
Humerus	15, f.	18 months, alive	-	-
Femur	8, m.	10 months, alive	-	-
			Nonradical	
Femur	66, m.	3 months, deceased	-	-
Humerus	15, m.	12 months, alive	-	-
Humerus	20, f.		no follow-up	
Clavicula	64, m.	9 months, deceased	-	postoperative irrad.
Astragalus	57, f.		-	amputation after 15 days
Radius	13, m.	96 months, deceased	-	amputation after 19 days
Humerus	47, f.	18 months, deceased	recurrence	amputation after 12 months
Tibia	30, m.	42 months, alive	recurrence	amputation after 20 months
Chondrosarcoma			Radical	
Scapula	62, m.	72 months, deceased	-	-
Scapula	25, m.	9 months deceased	-	-
Scapula	64, m.	8 months, deceased	-	-
Femur	59, f.	25 months, alive	-	-
Scapula	73, m.	24 months, alive	-	-
Femur	42, m.	14 months, alive	-	-
Humerus	69, f.	12 months, alive	-	-
Pelvis	22, m.	12 months, alive	-	-

Table 1. (continued)

	Patients age (yrs), sex	follow-up after	recurrence	therapy
			Nonradical	
Pelivis	60, m.	1 month, alive	-	-
Fibrosarcoma			Radical	
Humerus	56, f.	48 months, deceased	-	-
Femur	23, m.	60 months, alive	-	-
Humerus	39, m.	24 months, alive	-	-
			Nonradical	
Ulna	74, f.	42 months, alive	recurrence	amputation after 36 months
Humerus	24, f.	24 months, deceased	recurrence	amputation after 16 months
Humerus	70, m.	9 months, deceased	recurrence	postoperative irradiation amputation after 6 months
Round-cell sarcoma			Radical	
Humerus	14, f.	30 months, deceased	-	-
Scapula	9, f.	1 month, deceased	-	-
Humerus	12, m.	50 months, alive	-	-
Scapula	13, m.	24 months alive	-	-
			Nonradical	
Rib	15, m.	5 months, deceased	-	postoperative irradiation
Other tumors			Radical	
(Myeloma) Femur	62, m.	26 months, deceased	-	-
(Paget's Sarcoma) Humerus	85, m.	21 months, alive	-	-
(Rhabdomyosarcoma) Humerus	86, f.	9 months, alive	-	-

Table 1. (continued)

	Patients age (yrs), sex	follow-up after	recurrence	therapy
			Nonradical	
(Adamantinoma) Tibia	21, m.	45 months, alive	-	-
(Malignant synovialoma) Calcaneus	16, m.	40 months, deceased		amputation after 5 days
(Reticulosarcoma) Metacarpal bone	74, f.	21 months, alive	-	postoperative irradiation

With patients who are old or not very intelligent, a resection must be carefully considered. An unsuitable extremity presents difficulties in dressing and undressing, and the patient will not be aware of the functional gain of a hand that is fully capable of functioning.

The possibility of atypical resection in the upper extremities arises in cases of extensive tumors of the humerus diaphysis. Excellent results can be achieved - with intelligent patients - even after total or partial removal of the humerus (Fig. 9).

POSSIBILITIES OF RADICAL RESECTION IN LOWER EXTREMITIES

Attempts to preserve the supportive functions of a lower extremity by performing resections without endoprosthetic replacement are possible only rarely (for example, with tumor localization in the area of the pelvis (Fig. 6), fibula (Fig. 7) and the bones of the middle foot). Because of the difficulty of stabilization measures when the tumor is in the distal femur and tibia, the possibility that the patient would be more quickly and better taken care of with an amputation should also be considered.

Typical resections in the lower extremities are those of tumors of the ilium and of the proximal end of the femur (Fig. 1). In the case of localization of the latter type, replacement must be carried out by means of a special endoprothesis. Replacement of only the proximal end of the femur is fairly certain to result in painful arthritis.

Atypical operations in the lower extremities must be carefully considered before being carried out. In one case of an extensive Ewing's sarcoma of the fibula, the tumor was radically resectioned and the peroneal nerve was removed. Postoperative irradiation was waived (Fig. 7), so rehabilitation was much easier. This patient has been under prophylactic chemotherapy and symptom-free for 32 months so far.

With malignant tumors of the distal end of the femur, we generally prefer the primary thigh amputation. In one exceptional case we carried out radical resection. In order to retain an actively moveable "knee joint" for the child, a reconstruction operation was carried out, involving shortening and a 180-degree inversion of the lower leg with subsequent internal fixation between tibia and femur. Then after appropriate muscle transplantation, the ankle joint functioned as a

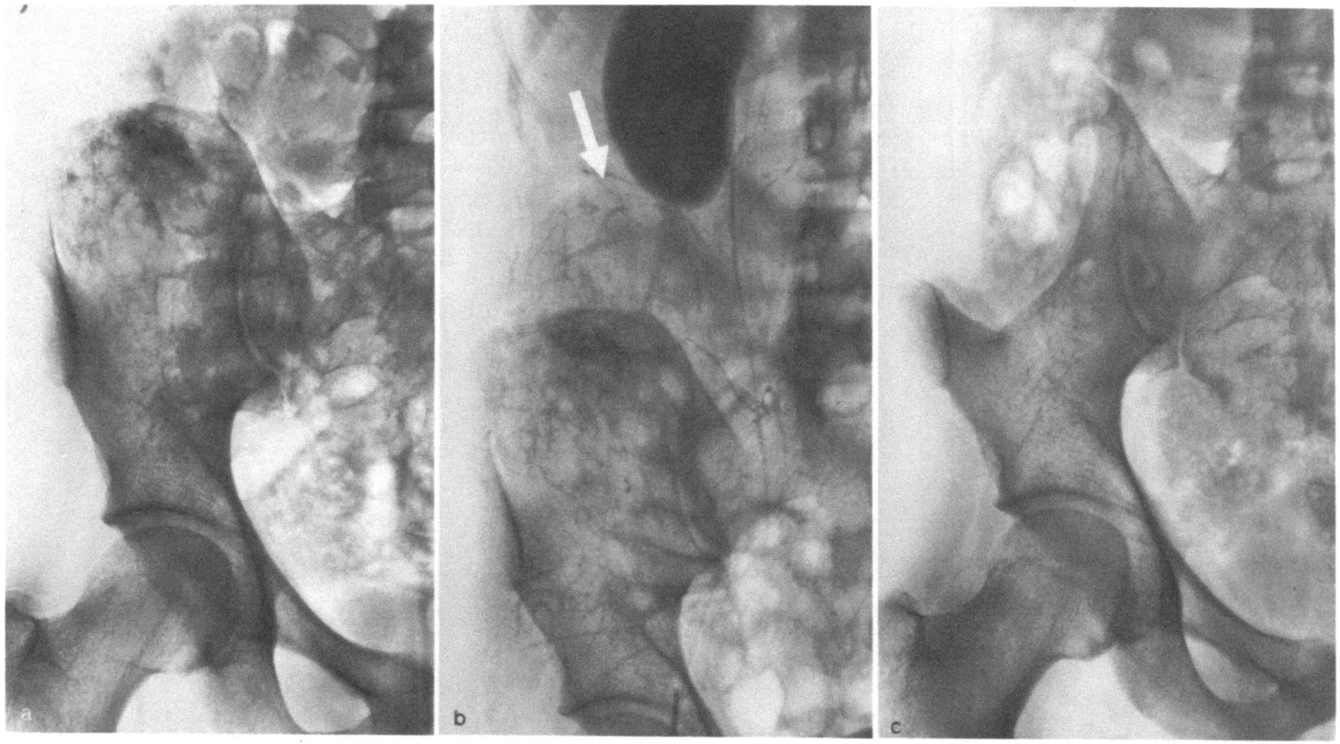

Fig. 6. M.R., m., 22 yrs. Chondrosarcoma innominate bone: (a) X-ray showing bone destruction (b) angiography: soft-tissue mass up to the kidney (→) (c) one year after radical resection

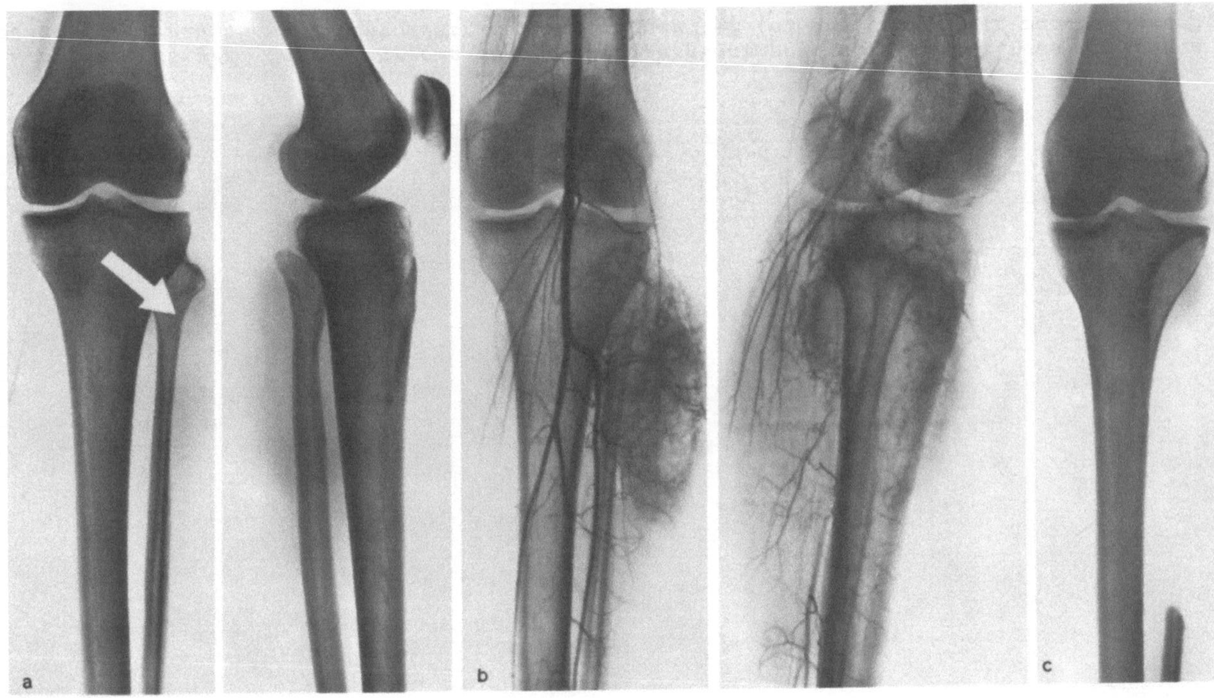

Fig. 7. K.E., 29 yrs. Ewing' sarcoma of proximal fibula, (a) X-ray showing only faint destruction of the cortex (→), (b) angiography: clear-cut delineation of the soft-tissue mass, (c) two years after radical resection

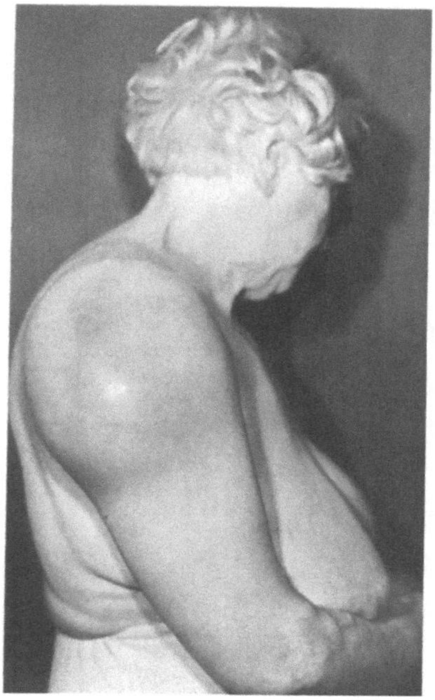

Fig. 8. E.W., f., 69 yrs. Lateral view of the large tumor (see Fig. 2)

knee joint (Fig. 10). The results of this operation are very encouraging; with a modified lower-leg prosthesis the patient can walk excellently and with active knee firmness.

As an alternative solution to traditional endoprosthetic replacement of the resectioned bone segment, bio-ceramic (AL_2O_3) prostheses have been used in some cases. This method has proved successful in the upper arm as well as in the distal radius and in the proximal femur (Fig. 11).

RESULTS OF RESECTION WITH PRIMARY BONE TUMORS (Table 1)

Each specimen was examined quite minutely for radicality. Resection was denoted as unmistakably radical in 25 cases. Of these, one earlier case was irradiated afterwards nevertheless. No postoperative treatment was carried out in any other case, and no local recurrences were observed.

With 16 resections due to primary malignant bone tumors, the tumor was opened intraoperatively or reached the incision on an encircled segment during the morphologic examination. In these cases the operation was classified as nonradical. Connecting amputations ensued in three cases and massive radiotherapy in four. In five patients local recurrences appeared over a period of 6 to 36 months, making a secondary amputation necessary. Of the seven nonprimary or secondary amputees four were still living without detectable recurrences at the time of the postoperative examination. The other three patients succumbed with multiple metastases with no evidence of local recurrences.

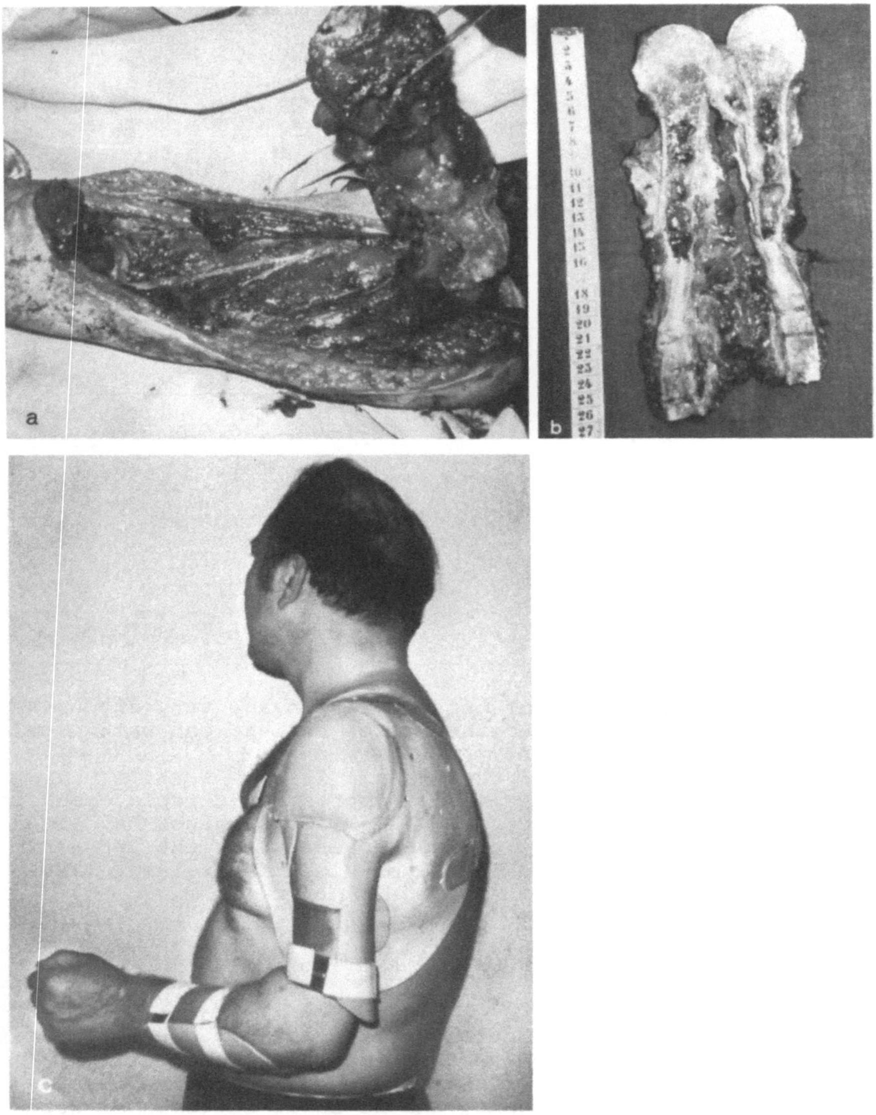

Fig. 9. E.J., m., 39 yrs. Fibrosarcoma of the shaft of the humerus, (a) mobilization of the tumor, (b) cut specism with extent of the tumor in the proximal part of the shaft, (c) good function of the hand with brace

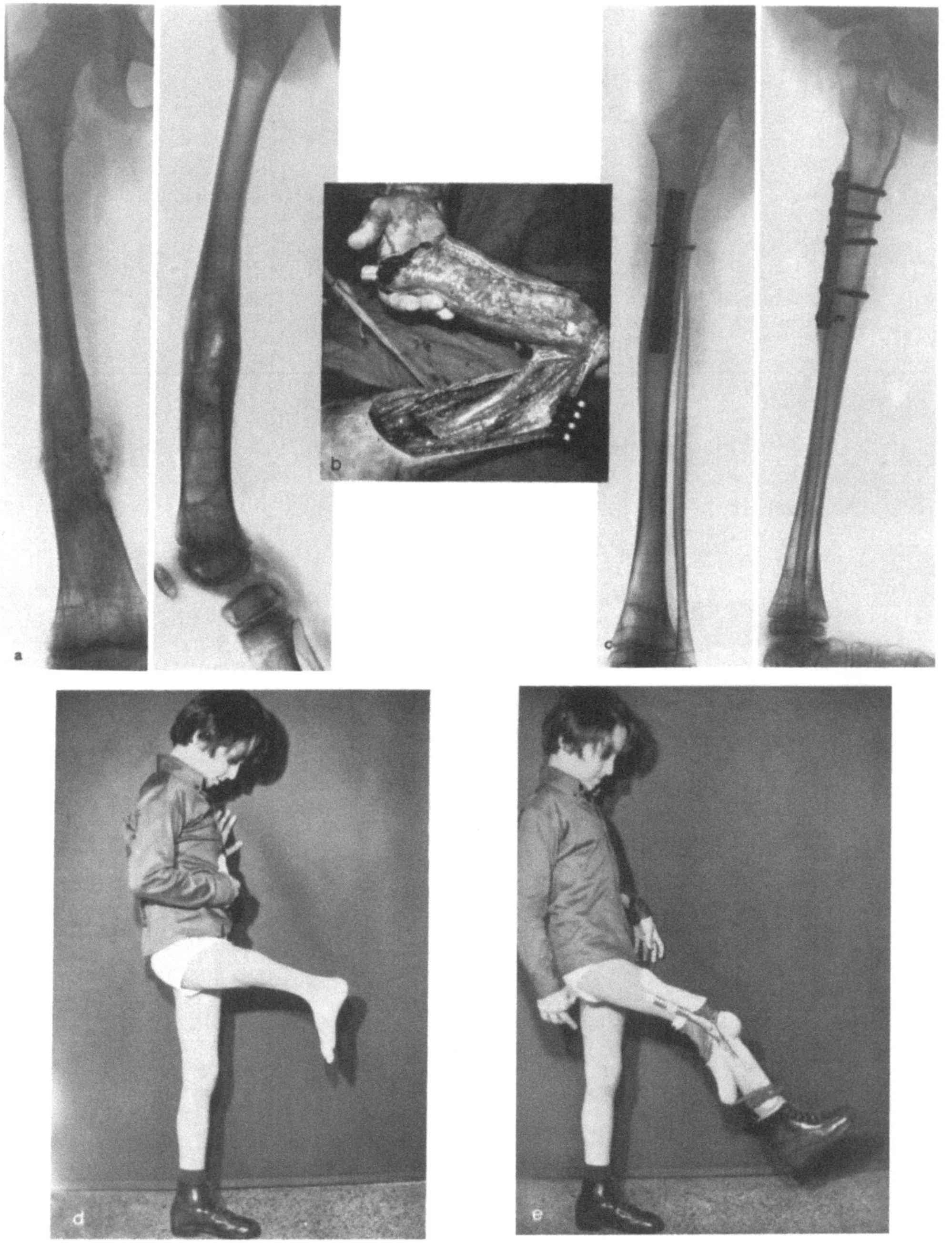

Fig. 10. G.M., m., 8 yrs. Osteosarcoma of the distal shaft of the femur, (a) preoperative X-ray, (b) mobilization of the distal 3/4 of the femur plus knee joint, (c) X-ray 10 months after surgery: solid fusion between femur and tibia, (d) active flexion of "knee joint", (e) active stretching of the special below-knee prosthesis

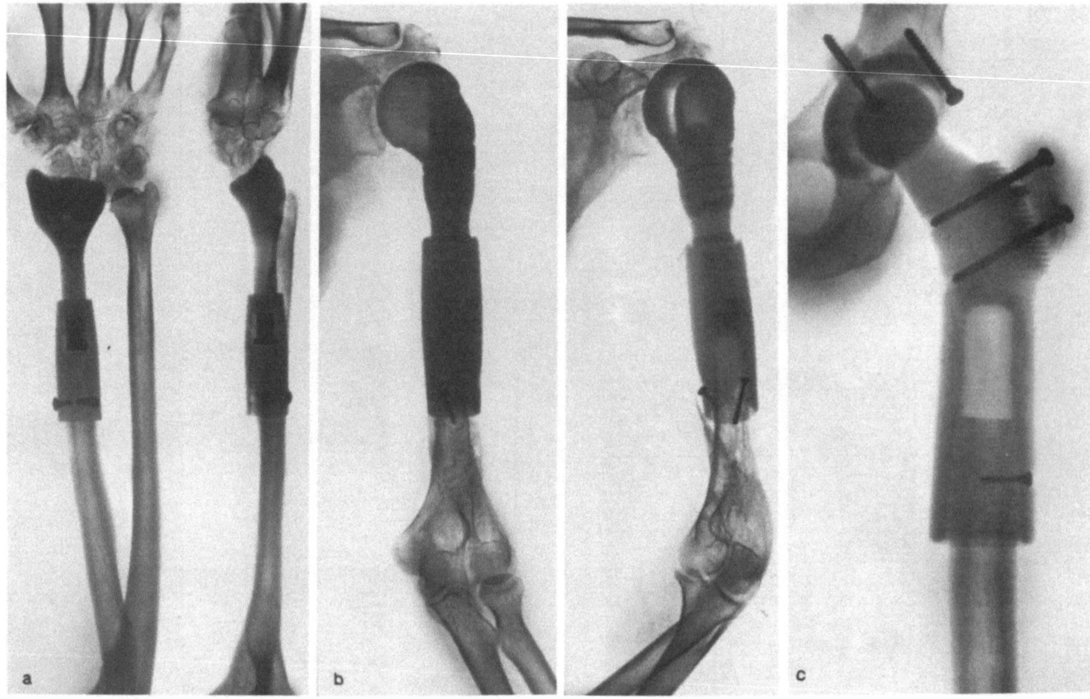

Fig. 11. Endoprosthesis made of "bioceramics", (a) A.V., m., 42 yrs. replacement of distal radius after resection of giant-cell tumor: good function one year after surgery, (b) I.E., f., 16 yrs. replacement of proximal half of the humerus, one year after osteosarcoma resection, (c) Z.R., f., 48 yrs. total hip prothesis 4 months after resection of a hypernephroma metastasis

DISCUSSION

The most serious complication in resection treatment is the possibility of a local recurrence which could have been avoided with an amputation. However, if an operation which is unmistakably radical is performed under the conditions described above, the danger of a recurrence is no greater than after an ablative operation. If, at the time of a meticulous morphologic examination, the tumor is found to extend up to the edge of the resection at any point, the resection no longer qualifies as radical. Appropriate measures such as postoperative irradiation, subsequent operations, or amputation must be performed.

Resection is a more involved and more burdensome operation than amputation. It is nevertheless justifiable with appropriate care of the patients. With respect to this particular topic, it must be stated that there were never any serious postoperative incidents, although some of the patients were quite elderly (as old as 86). Disorders involving wound healing were not infrequent; however, these disorders did not lead to any serious complications such as removal of protheses or secondary amputations in this study.

Use of endoprostheses to make good deficiencies following extensive resections of bone has proved to be propitious. Although experience with aluminium oxide is still limited, numerous advantages have already become apparent: the new style of bindings between prosthesis and tubular bones by means of a conic shield allows cementless, solid fixation of the prosthesis. The compatibility of the material to the body is excellent. Replacement of the proximal humerus, of the distal radius, and of the proximal femur has been greatly standardized. The possibility of adjusting the size of the prothesis according to a building-block principle means that a suitable implant is available at any time for an acute individual case.

Resection treatment should be considered in cases of very large tumors, in which substantially better results can be expected with special reconstruction measures than with amputation. Involvement with radical tumor resections in the extremities presents us with a fascinating task. Successes in the prognostic and functional realms are encouraging with optimal performance of the operation. More tumor clinics should be investigating problems in this area.

SUMMARY

Amputation is an unsatisfactory and depressing measure for the patient as well as for the surgeon. As long as operative removal of tumors in the extremities is indicated, the search for alternative solutions should be the most urgent task for every doctor involved in surgery. Resection would be the most equitable measure as far as demands for radicality and the best possible restoration of function are concerned. In order to warrant the radicality of the operation, meticulous preoperative planning and precise surgical techniques are essential.

Sufficient restoration of function must take into consideration all the factors of the individual case, age and profession of the patient playing a large role. After partial resection of longer tubular bones, fitting of an endo-prosthesis has proved to be advantageous. Implants available at present have various drawbacks; studies directed at the elimination of these drawbacks must be set up.

REFERENCES

1. FUCHS, G.: Resektion des proximalen Oberarmes und Ersatz durch eine Vitallium-Endoprothese. Chir. Prax. 10, 69-75 (1966)
2. GENOVESI, A.: Resezione ed innesto osseo autoplastico per neoplasie primitive dell'estremo prossimale dell'omero. Clin. Orthop. 14, 233-254 (1962)
3. JUVARA, E.: Procédé de Résection de la partie supérieure du tibia. Presse méd. 29, 241 (1921)
4. KNAHR, K., SALZER, M.: Die Endoprothesenversorgung von Metastasen und primär malignen Knochentumoren des proximalen Femurendes. Z. Orthop. 112 (1974) (in press)
5. KOLARZ, G., SALZER, M., SALZER-KUNTSCHIK, M., WILLVONSEDER, R., HÖFER, R.: Die Bedeutung der Knochenszintigraphie für Diagnose und Therapie des Osteosarcoms der langen Röhrenknochen. Arch. Orthop. Unfall-Chir. 76, 333 (1973)
6. LINBERG, B.E.: Interscapulo-thoracic resection for malignant tumors of the shoulder joint region. J. Bone Jt Surg. 26, 344-349 (1928)
7. PACK, G.T., BALDWIN, J.C.: The Tikhor-Linberg resection of the shoulder-girdle: indications for its substitution for interscapulo-thoracic amputation; recent data on endresults of the forequarter amputation. Clin. Orthop. 19, 148 (1961)
8. SALZER, M., ENGELHARDT, A., LOCKE, H., ZWEYMÜLLER, K.: Keramische Endoprothesen der oberen Extremität. Proceedings of the 61st Congress of the DGOT. Z. Orthop. 113, (1975 in press)
9. SALZER, M., ZAUNBAUER, W.: Über Angiographie bei Extremitätentumoren. Wien. klin. Wschr. 77, 930 (1965)
10. SAUERBRUCH, F.: Die Exstirpation des Femur mit Umkipplastik des Unterschenkels. Dtsch. Z. Chir. 169, 1 (1922)
11. ZWEYMÜLLER, K., KRATOCHWIL, A.: Ultraschalldiagnostik bei Knochen- und Weichteiltumoren. Wien. klin. Wschr. (1974, in press)

Giant-Cell Tumor and Chondrosarcomas: Grading, Treatment and Results (Studies of 209 and 131 Cases)

M. CAMPANACCI

We have collected 209 cases of giant-cell tumors. Follow-up ranging from 3 to 42 years is available in 130 cases.

The tumors were graded radiographically as calm (preserved cortex, peritumoral bone sclerosis, slow growth); active (preservation of the periosteum, fuzzy limits, active growth); and aggressive (encroachment on the soft tissues, rapid growth).

Histologically we graded the tumors as typical (which includes Lichtenstein's grades I and II); aggressive (showing some pleomorphic and hypercromatic nuclei and areas of fibrosarcomatous aspect); and sarcomas (generally true fibrosarcomas).

Giant-cell sarcomas are seen occasionally and exceptionally even osteosarcomas. Radiation probably favors transformation to sarcoma.

Radiographically the active form and histologically the typical type are the most frequent. The histologically typical tumors can correspond to a radiographically calm, active or even aggressive variety. Thus radiographically aggressive tumors are by no means consistently malignant (Table 1).

Table 1. Grading of giant-cell tumor according to radiographic and histological aspect. Relationship between radiographic and histological grading

CASES	130	RX PICTURE	HISTOLOGIC PICTURE	CASES	130
"	15%	CALM	TYPICAL	"	86%
"	65%	ACTIVE	AGGRESSIVE	"	6%
"	20%	AGGRESSIVE	SARCOMA	"	8%

Sometimes the tumor, whether histologically typical or aggressive, grows into ligaments, capsula and synovia, thus encroaching on a contiguous bone.

Progression of malignancy was observed radiographically in 40 percent and histologically in 25 percent of 40 recurrent tumors.

All recurrences appeared in less than 3 years, which is why three years was adopted as the minimum follow-up period.

Even the tumors that are seen radiographically and macroscopically to be very aggressive can be cured by conservative treatment, provided that histologic examination shows that they are not sarcomas.

Excision was effective in one quarter of the cases. Mortality was 8 percent.

Results grouped by radiographic grading. Calm type: excision was successful and 58 percent; active type: in 33 percent; aggressive type: amputation was necessary in some cases and metastases were observed in some tumors that were histologically sarcomas, but in about 50 percent cases cure was achieved with resection.

Results grouped by histologic grading. We cannot prove any differences between the typical and the aggressive types. The sample contains very few histologically aggressive tumors, however. Though metastases were not observed in any of these aggressive tumors, we are inclined to consider them as a step toward malignancy and as a dangerous, potentially metastatizing tumor. Sarcoma metastatizes in 82 percent of cases. Various modes of treatment are currently in use.

Radiation is never indicated except in particular sites such as the sacrum.

Curettment is indicated in radiographically calm or moderately active tumors that are histologically typical. It is not indicated for a recurrent tumor, because nine times out of ten it fails. If these conditions are observed curettment can be successful in 40 to 60 percent of cases.

Resection (of the entire or of a large portion of the articular bone) is indicated in the majority of cases: in radiographically active or aggressive tumors, histologically typical or aggressive tumors, in all recurrent tumors, and, rarely in sarcomas. Adequate resection is successful in 90 percent of cases.

Amputation is necessary in two cases: in aggressive, widely expanded tumors where resection is not feasible (in these cases amputation almost always effects a cure), and in most histologically proved sarcomas: success can be predicted in about 20 percent of cases because of the high metastytic rate.

We have also collected 131 chondrosarcomas, 70 of which are central, 50 peripheral, and 11 periosteal. Follow-up ranging from 10 to 32 years is available in 63 cases.

We graded all chondrosarcomas into three radiographic types. Central grade I, in which there is continuity of the cortex; central grade II, with interrupted cortex; central grade III, with wide expansion in the soft tissues. Peripheral grade-I tumors have comparatively well-defined limits and usually heavy radiopacity; in peripheral grade II, the limits are ill-defined, radiopacity is minor and the tumors are larger in volume; peripheral grade-III tumors have no limits and only slight radiopacity; their volume is enormous and there is frequently invasion of the host bone. Histologic grading of the chondrosarcomas into three types is sharper and more meaningful. Grade-I chondrosarcomas have larger nuclei than chondromas of different sizes and frequently double. These aspects do not mean malignancy if the tumor is in the hand. In grade-II tumors the nuclei are larger and hyperchromatic; there is obvious pleomorphism, and double nuclei are very frequent. Grade-III tumors are characterized by extreme cellularitiy and pleomorphism, giant, bizarre, triple or multiple nuclei.

Table 2. Histologic grading, histologic differentiation in cartilage, and progression of malignancy in chondrosarcomas

	Histologic grade I	Histologic grade II	Histologic grade III	Well differentiated	Myxoid	Mesenchymal or fibrosarcoma	Progression of malignancy
	%	%	%	%	%	%	%
central chondrosarcoma	16	60	24	60	30	10	60
peripheral chondrosarcoma	38	56	6	98	2	--	66
periosteal chondrosarcoma	27	63	10	100	--	--	yes

Histologic grade II is the most frequent type of central chondrosarcoma. Grade III is rare amongst peripheral and periosteal tumors. Central chondrosarcomas are frequently myxoid or anaplastic, while peripheral and periosteal chondrosarcomas are almost almays well-differentiated. In all chondrosarcomas progression of malignancy is very frequent (Table 2).

Central chondrosarcomas quite frequently grow in the medullary canal, invading large portions of the bone. Sometimes this invasion is scarcely evident on radiograms. Peripheral chondrosarcomas are always capsulated but, after a previous operation, tumoral nodes may be scattered into the soft tissues.

Recurrences may develop many years after surgery; nineteen years elapsed in one case of central grade-I chondrosarcoma. Both recurrences and progression of malignancy take much longer in the histologic grade-I tumors than in grade-II tumors (Table 3).

Table 3. Time elapsed between surgery and recurrence in chondrosarcomas

	< 1 yr %	1-2 yr %	2-5 yr %	5-10 yr %	10-20 yr %
CENTRAL CHONDROSARCOMA (35 recurrences)	70	15	10	-	5
PERIPHERAL CHONDROSARCOMA (25 recurrences)	52	20	8	20	-

Prognosis in chondrosarcomas depends on the histologic grade and on the possibility or radical removal. Peripheral and periosteal chondrosarcomas have better prognosis than the central ones, because grade III is much rarer and even grade-I and grade-II tumors are less malignant than their central counterparts. Prognosis is favorably influenced by the fact that metastases are often very late.

In central chondrosarcomas, prognosis is very bad if the tumor is located in the trunk. In the limbs, it depends on the histologic grade. The overall survival rate should exceed 20 percent.

In peripheral chondrosarcomas the survival rate is about 25 percent for the tumors in the trunk, 70 percent for those in the limbs. Prognosis seems to be similar in periosteal chondrosarcomas.

In all cases of central chondrosarcoma where the tumor had ruptured the cortex, resection failed. The recurrence quite often showed a progression of malignancy.

Thus treatment of central chondrosarcoma should be radical; resection succeeds almost exclusively when the cortex is not involved by the tumor (Rx grade I); when the cortex is ruptured, amputation is indicated.

The treatment of peripheral chondrosarcoma should be by excision or - more often - resection in radiographically and histologically grade-I and grade-II tumors and even in recurrences. Amputation is necessary in huge tumors (radiographic grade III) and in histologically grade-III tumors.

Periosteal chondrosarcoma can be cured by wide excision or resection; amputation is necessary in histologically grade-III tumors.

As far as surgical techniques are concerned, in total resections of the end of the bone in the knee we prefer arthrodesis by autologous transplant (Putti-Juvara-Merle d'Aubignè). Replacement by homologous articular transplant (of femur or tibia at the knee) almost always fails after varying intervals of time, because of resorption and fracture of the epiphysis. Partial resection of an articular bone (in the knee, the elbow, the ankle), in constrast can be satisfactorily managed by means of an autologous (e.g. iliac bone for an humeral condyle) or homologous transplant. This procedure allows partial preservation of the articular function by a rehabitation of the transplant.

In the resection of proximal humerus an endoprosthesis is indicated, in the resection of proximal femur, an arthroprosthesis. In the resection of the distal radius, we use arthrodesis by means of an autologous transplant. The resected pubis can be substituted by an autologous iliac bridging transplant. In the resection of a metacarpal bone we use an autologous metatarsal bone (the third or fourth).

SUMMARY

The Author reviews 209 cases of giant-cell tumor (follow-up 3-42 years in 130 cases) and 131 chondrosarcomas (70 central, 50 peripheral, 11 periosteal; follow-up 10-32 years in 63 cases). Giant-cell tumors are graded into three radiographic types (calm, active, aggressive) and three histologic types (typical, aggressive, sarcoma). Chondrosarcomas were also graded into three radiographic and three histologic types (grades I, II, III). Incidence and mutual relationships of radiographic and histologic grades are presented. In recurrences it is possible to observe a progression of malignancy in giant-cell tumor and - more often - in chondrosarcomas. Results are related to the radiographic and histologic grading and to the type of treatment. Indications for treatment are given according to the experience gained from this study. The Author enumerates the surgical techniques he has found most suitable for the conservative treatment of these tumors when resection is indicated.

X-Ray Therapy of Primary Bone Tumors

W. HOEFFKEN

GENERAL BASIC DIAGNOSIS PRINCIPLES

Biopsy of bone tumors is essential before tumor therapy can begin. The diagnosis of malignant bone tumors can be established only by accurate histologic examination of the specimen. The risk attendant on biopsy has been widely discussed. MACDONALD and BUDD (4) proved that biopsy does not cause tumor spread or metastasis. As their proof is based on statistical work, prebiopsy irradiation has been recommended as an additional safety measure by v. RONNEN (8), who proposes administration of 400 rads on the day before, and again on the day of biopsy for the devitalization of tumor cells. The effectivity of this method has not yet been demonstrated in a scientific manner. Nevertheless the method has been adopted in many places as a matter of common sense and in parallel to results of experimental tumor research. We have modified this schedule and administer a single dose of 1000 rads (cobalt) immediately before biopsy, thereby avoiding manifestation of cellular changes in the miscroscopic slide and the complication of pathological diagnosis, at least insofar as the morphologic criteria of histopathology are concerned. Histochemical or immunologic patterns may be altered by the procedure.

METHOD OF IRRADIATION

Radiotherapy of bone tumors can now be performed exclusively by megavolt therapy, which means the use of penetrating quants from a cobalt source, a linear accelerator or a betatron. The optimal effective tumor dose depends on the radiosensitivity of the respective type of tumor.

GIANT-CELL TUMOR

The giant-cell tumor is a semimalignant tumor. Opinions on radiotherapy of giant-cell tumors vary considerably. For some decades irradiation of giant-cell tumors has been quite popular and has frequently been used. Every radiotherapist probably knows of cases in which long-term follow-up has revealed regression of the tumor and lasting cure. On the other hand, a fairly large number of cases has been reported in which the tumors showed malignant transformation after irradiation. For this reason, some of the leading clinicians, pathologists and radiologists strictly refuse the irradiation of giant-cell tumors because of the risk of subsequent tumor development (5, 7, 8, 10). We are of the same opinion, but other authors do not accept this view (9, 3, 6, etc.). In spite of many efforts to agree upon a generally acceptable treatment regimen the situation remains embarrassing. The cause of the dissent must be seen not in the inadequate experience of radiotherapists, but in the intricate problems of histologic classification of giant-cell tumors. It is possible that benign tumors always remain so, with or without irradiation, whereas a certain amount of semimalignant tumors become definitely malignant after radiotherapy. Since the optimum degree of certainty in histologic classification and grading is not always possible in every individual case, we propose the following treatment as a compromise for giant-cell tumors of groups I and II:

1. radical surgical resection is indicated for all giant-cell tumors of grades I and II whenever resection implies no functional impairment;

2. if the lesion is not completely resectable, surgery should be followed by cobalt irradiation with a target dose of 3000 rads in 4 - 6 weeks;

3. inoperable giant-cell tumors should be irradiated to a tumor dose of 5000 rads. Patients would have to be followed up closely to ensure the early detection of any recurrence;

4. all giant-cell tumors of group III must be treated like osteosarcomas; in operable cases with no evidence of metastases early amputation or selective later amputation is indicated. The second method comprises primary radiotherapy and - six months later - amputation on condition that operability and absence of metastases have remained unchanged;

5. inoperable giant-cell tumors of grade III should be irradiated with a tumor dose of 8000 rads, like osteosarcomas.

We have to emphasize that important vessels and nerves should be adequately protected to prevent any impairment of function in consequence or irradiation. This is a point of vital importance in every treatment of benign grades in giant-cell tumors.

PRIMARY MALIGNANT BONE TUMORS

Chondrosarcoma and Fibrosarcoma. Tumors of these two types are truly radioresistant. Radical surgery is indicated as a rule, while radiotherapy is reserved to inoperable cases. These would need a very high dosage of at least 8000 rads, a tumor dose that could never be given without subsequent damage to skin, muscle and osseous supporting tissue. Damage to important vessels and nerves can be avoided by technical skill. Subsequent instability caused by osteoradionecrosis should be treated by nailing or other adequate orthopedic procedures.

Ewing's Sarcoma and Reticulum-cell Sarcoma of the Bone. Sarcomas originating from bone marrow are highly radiosensitive. Ewing's sarcoma and reticulum-cell sarcoma can be destroyed totally by a tumor dose of 6000 rads with satisfactory reliability. On the other hand, this dose might occasionally provoke later radionecrosis. Such cases would require stabilizing procedures. Local devitalization and total destruction of a reticulum-cell sarcoma means a good prognosis and often results in survival for years and decades. But in Ewing's sarcoma the chance of cure is next to none, because it is nearly always generalized at the very moment of detection. Amputation would be useless. The only small chance of improvement for patients with Ewing's sarcoma lies in a combination of local irradiation and chemotherapy with multiple drugs (3).

Osteosarcoma. Most osteosarcomas appear in the upper or lower limbs, and they are therefore radically resectable by amputation or exarticulation. But radical surgery comes too late in many cases. In 80 percent of patients their fate has been determined by early distant metastases, e.g. when pulmonary metastases appear within a few months after radical surgery. These patients will die of their primary disease in spite of the mutilating operation they have undergone. They often do not even live to see the projected adaptation of a prothesis (8). We conclude that a mutilating operation may not be totally wrong, but that it appears superflous and useless in the majority of cases, i.e. in 80 percent. Such considerations have led to the proposal of careful selection of cases for amputation (8, 2). It should be performed on condition that no evidence of distant metastases be found after a suitable period of observation. For this type of surgical treatment the primary lesion must be quickly and reliably destroyed. It should at least be sufficiently sterilized to be eliminated as a potential source of danger. Radiologic eradication of the primary tumor is possible with high dosages if we assume sufficient radiosensitivity of osteosarcomas. For a long time osteosarcomas were thought to be radioresistant, but this opinion is wrong, having been conceived in the era of conventional roentgentherapy. Most of the rather soft X-rays then used were absorbed by the calcium in osseous issue, and therefore did not reach the tumor tissue in effective amounts. In supervoltage and in megavoltage therapy, absorption coefficients of osseous tissue and tumor tissue are equivalent. Irradiations of this type allow complete destruction of tumor tissue. Histologic observation of tumor tissue taken after amputation preceded by irradiation with a tumor dose of 8000 - 10.000 rads revealed nothing but necrotic tumor cells (Fig. 1) in numerous cases. Very often no cellular components could be identified in the specimen. Such cases did not allow any conclusions regarding the histologic type of the original tumor. Even if morphologic evaluation of tumor devitalization is still beset with problems, the effectivity of radiation therapy cannot be doubted when histologic patterns before and after radiotherapy are compared (Fig. 2).

Of course, we would not disagree absolutely with amputation in operable cases. Since the possibility of a remainder of tumor cells cannot be excluded (Fig. 3 a, c), this therapeutic method has to be reconsidered. Eradication of the tumor could be obtained by supervoltage therapy, thus replacing amputation by irradiation. But the dosage has to be very high, and resultant damage must be expected. After some 10 to 12 months damaging sequelae in soft tissue and bone will lead to amputation in any case.

Eight years of this treatment policy have enabled us to prove that osteosarcoma can be destroyed totally by a tumor dosage of 8000-10000 rads, adjusted to morphologic criteria. These findings contrast with former opinions. On the other hand, later amputation preceded by irradiation could not be proved to be superior to early amputation without previous irradiation. More investigation is necessary to find out whether a single very-high-dose irradiation for devitalization would be enough to prevent intraoperative mobilization of tumor cells during early amputation. Moreover, a way must be found to prevent further growth of micrometastases that have already disseminated. NEWTON (5) has proposed irradiation of both lungs with a total dosage of 1950 rads given at a rate of 150 rads a day. We shall have to check whether this method is effective, or whether immunosuppressive reactions make it inadvisable.

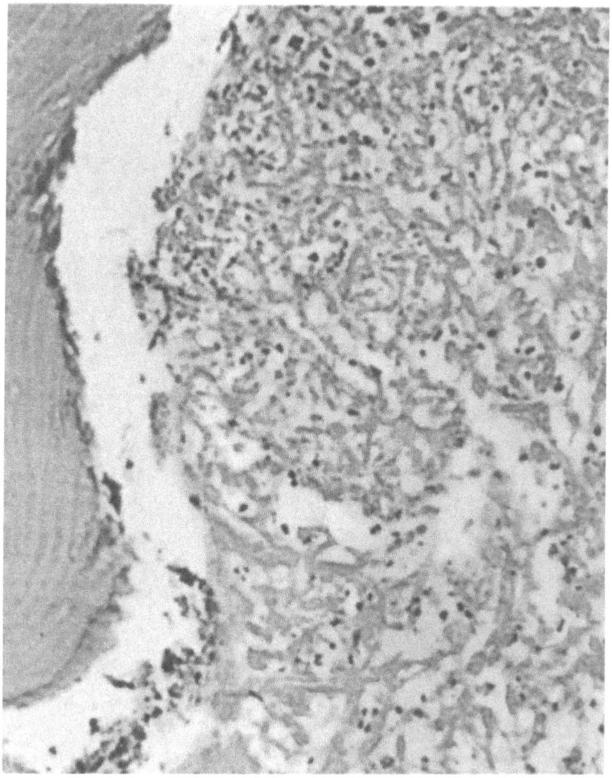

Fig. 1. Osteogenic sarcoma 1 month after irradiation (8000 rads tumor dose applied by cobalt): complete necrosis of tumor tissue, inflammatory reaction. HE, 160 x

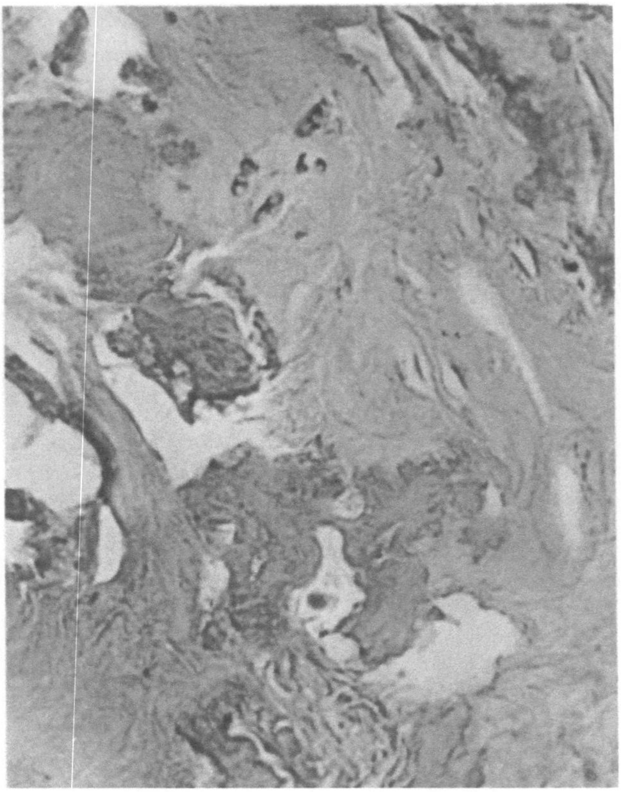

Fig. 2. Osteogenic sarcoma 12 months after irradiation (8500 rads tumor-dose applied by cobalt): strongly marked cell deficiency, development of abundant osteoid substance, no proliferative activity HE, 260 x

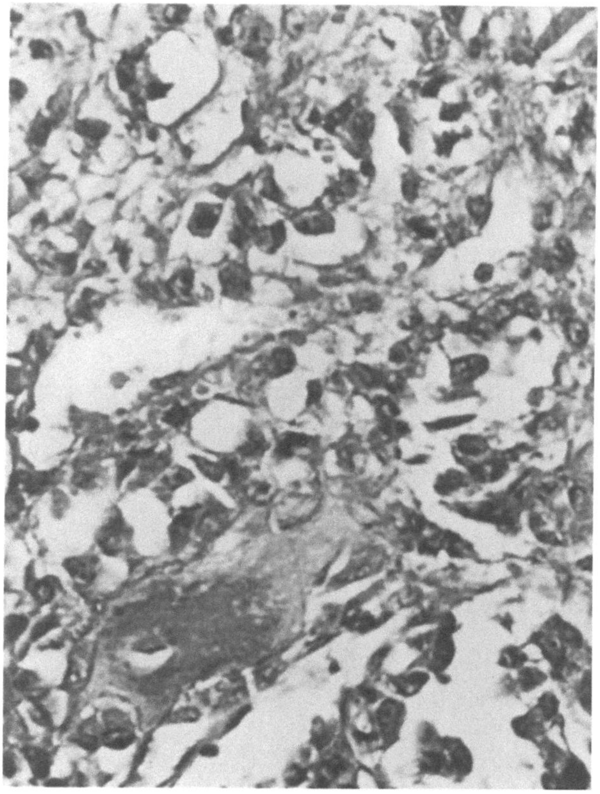

Fig. 3. (a) Before irradiation: moderately differentiated osteogenic sarcoma. HE, 260 x

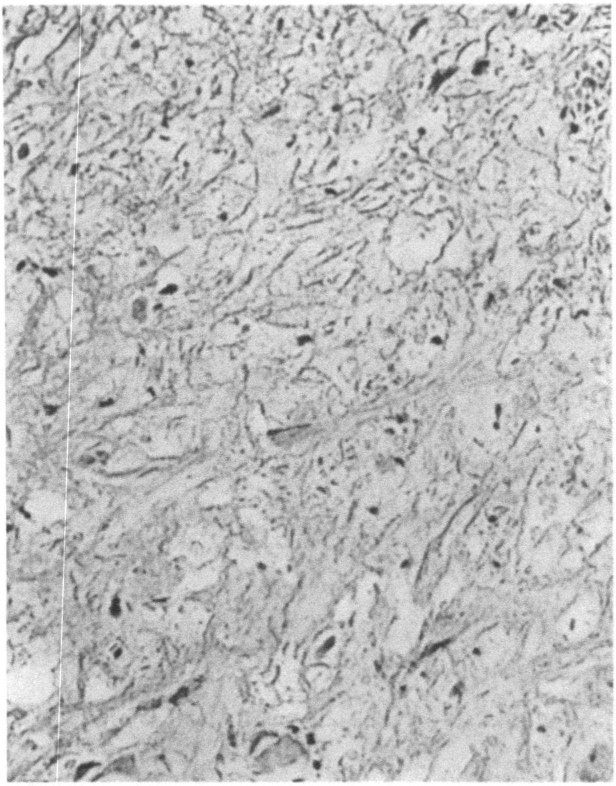

Fig. 3. (b) After irradiation (16,000 rads tumor-dose): vast area of tumor necrosis. HE, 160 x

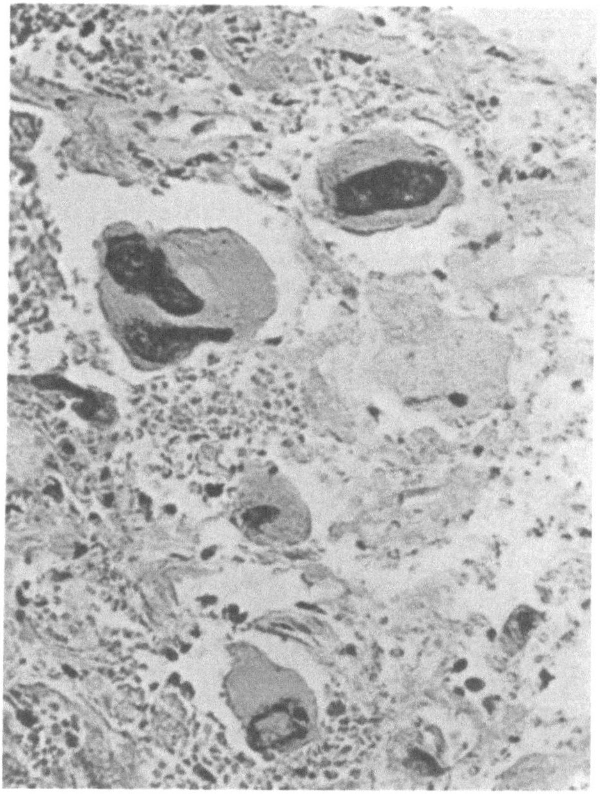

Fig. 3. (c) Detail magnification of 3 b: still sporadic polymorph tumor cells with regressive reaction, lying in the necrotic area. HE, 260 x

For a patient with osteosarcoma, the chances of a cure are still very low. Discussion of various treatment policies must continue.

SUMMARY

Radiotherapy of bone tumors can now be performed exclusively by megavolt therapy. Giant cell tumors should be resected. If the lesion is not completely resectable, surgery should be followed by the administration of a target dose of 3000 rads in 4-6 weeks. Inoperable giant cell tumors are irradiated to a tumor dose of 5000 rads, inoperable giant cell tumors of grade III receive a dose of 8000 rads as do osteosarcomas. Ewing's sarcoma and reticulum cell sarcoma can be totally destroyed by a tumor dose of 6000 rad with sufficient reliability. Combination with chemotherapy may offer a chance of improvement. Osteosarcoma should be resected. If surgery is too late (early distant metastases), a tumor dose of 8000 to 10000 rads would be able to destroy the tumor cells. Histologic control investigations have proved this.

REFERENCES

1. FRIEDMANN, M., PEARLMAN, A.W.: Radiology 91, 1151 (1968)
2. HELLNER, H.: In: Strahlenforschung und Krebsbehandlung Strahlentherapie, Sonderbd. 43, 81 (1953)
3. JAFFE, N.: Treatment of Bone Tumors: Chemotherapy. Proc. XI. Int'. Cancer Congr. Florence 1974 (in press)
4. MACDONALD, I., BUDD, J.W.: Surg. Gynec. Obstet. 82, 81 (1948)
5. NEWTON, K.A.: Prophylactic irradiation of lung in bone sarcoma. In: Bone - Certain Aspects of Neoplasia (Ed. C.H.G. Price, F.G.M. Moss). London: Butterworths 1973
6. PEARLMAM, A.W., FRIEDMANN, M.: Roentgenology 102, 645 (1968)
7. POPPE, H.: 4. Kolloquium über Röntgendiagnostik der Knochentumoren, Rheinisch-Westf. Röntgengesellschaft e.V., Essen, 6.12.1969
8. V.RONNEN, J.R.: Deutscher Röntgenkongreß 1963. Strahlentherapie, Sonderbd. 55, 235 (1964)
9. SCHERER, E.: Strahlentherapie p. 122. Stuttgart: Thieme 1967
10. UEHLINGER, E.: 4. Kolloquium über Röntgendiagnostik der Knochentumoren, Rheinisch-Westf. Röntgengesellschaft e.V., Essen, 6.12.1969

Subject Index

Recent Results in Cancer Research

Sponsored by the Swiss League against Cancer. Editor in Chief: P. Rentchnick, Genève

1 Schindler, R.: Die tierische Zelle in Zellkultur.
2 Neuroblastomas — Biochemical Studies. Edited by C. Bohuon (Symposium).
3 Hueper, W. C.: Occupational and Environmental Cancers of the Respiratory System.
4 Goldman, L.: Laser Cancer Research.
5 Metcalf, D.: The Thymus. Its Role in Immune Responses, Leukaemia Development and Carcinogenesis.
6 Malignant Transformation by Viruses. Edited by W. H. Kirsten (Symposium).
7 Moertel, Ch. G.: Multiple Primary Malignant Neoplasms. Their Incidence and Significance.
8 New Trends in the Treatment of Cancer. Edited by L. Manuila, S. Moles, and P. Rentchnick.
9 Lindenmann, J. and P. A. Klein: Immunological Aspects of Viral Oncolysis.
10 Nelson, R. S.: Radioactive Phosphorus in the Diagnosis of Gastrointestinal Cancer.
11 Freeman, R. G. and J. M. Knox: Treatment of Skin Cancer.
12 Lynch, H. T.: Hereditary Factors in Carcinoma.
13 Tumours in Children. Edited by H. B. Marsden and J. K. Steward.
14 Odartchenko, N.: Production Cellulaire Erythropoïétique.
15 Sokoloff, B.: Carcinoid and Serotonin.
16 Jacobs, M. L.: Malignant Lymphomas and Their Management.
17 Normal and Malignant Cell Growth. Edited by R. J. M. Fry, M. L. Griem, and W. H. Kirsten (Symposium).
18 Anglesio, E.: The Treatment of Hodgkin's Disease.
19 Bannasch, P.: The Cytoplasm of Hepatocytes during Carcinogenesis. Electron- and Lightmicroscopical Investigations of the Nitrosomorpholine-intoxicated Rat Liver.
20 Rubidomycin. A new Agent against Cancer. Edited by J. Bernard, R. Paul, M. Boiron, C. Jacquillat, and R. Maral.
21 Scientific Basis of Cancer Chemotherapy. Edited by G. Mathé (Symposium).
22 Koldovský, P.: Tumor Specific Transplantation Antigen.
23 Fuchs, W. A., J. W. Davidson, and H. W. Fischer: Lymphography in Cancer. With contributions by G. Jantet and H. Rösler.
24 Hayward, J.: Hormones und Human Breast Cancer. An Account of 15 Years Study.
25 Roy-Burman, P.: Analogues of Nucleic Acid Components. Mechanisms of Action.
26 Tumors of the Liver. Edited by G. T. Pack and A. H. Islami.
27 Szymendera, J.: Bone Mineral Metabolism in Cancer.
28 Meek, E. S.: Antitumour and Antiviral Substances of Natural Origin.
29 Aseptic Environments and Cancer Treatment. Edited by G. Mathé (Symposium).
30 Advances in the Treatment of Acute (Blastic) Leukemias. Edited by G. Mathé (Symposium).
31 Denoix, P.: Treatment of Malignant Breast Tumors. Indications and Results.
32 Nelson, R. S.: Endoscopy in Gastric Cancer.
33 Experimental and Clinical Effects of L-Asparaginase. Edited by E. Grundmann and H. F. Oettgen (Symposium).
34 Chemistry and Biological Actions of 4-Nitroquinolin 1-Oxide. Edited by H. Endo, T. Ono, and T. Sugimura.
35 Penn, I.: Malignant Tumors in Organ Transplant Recipients.
36 Current Concepts in the Management of Lymphoma and Leukemia. Edited by J. E. Ultmann, M. L. Griem, W. H. Kirsten, and R. W. Wissler (Symposium).
37 Chiappa, S., R. Musumeci, and C. Uslenghi: Endolymphatic Radiotherapy in Malignant Lymphomas. With contributions by G. Bonadonna, B. Damascelli, G. Fava, F. Pizzetti, U. Veronesi.

38 KOLLER, P. C.: The Role of Chromosomes in Cancer Biology.

39 Current Problems in the Epidemiology of Cancer and Lymphomas. Edited by E. GRUNDMANN and H. TULINIUS (Symposium).

40 LANGLEY, F. A. and A. C. CROMPTON: Epithelial Abnormalities of the Cervix Uteri.

41 Tumours in a Tropical Country. A Survey of Uganda (1964—1968). Edited by A. C. TEMPLETON.

42 Breast Cancer: A Challenging Problem. Edited by M. L. GRIEM, E. V. JENSEN, J. E. ULTMANN, and R. W. WISSLER (Symposium).

43 Nomenclature, Methodology and Results of Clinical Trials in Acute Leukemias. Edited by G. MATHÉ, P. POUILLART, and L. SCHWARZENBERG (Symposium).

44 Special Topics in Carcinogenesis. Edited by E. GRUNDMANN (Symposium).

45 KOLDOVSKÝ, P.: Carcinoembryonic Antigens.

46 Diagnosis and Therapy of Malignant Lymphoma. Edited by K. MUSSHOFF (Symposium).

47 Investigation and Stimulation of Immunity in Cancer Patients. Edited by G. MATHÉ and R. WEINER (Symposium).

48 Platinum Coordination Complexes in Cancer Chemotherapy. Edited by T. A. CONNORS and J. J. ROBERTS (Symposium).

49 Complications of Cancer Chemotherapy. Edited by G. MATHÉ and R. K. OLDHAM (Symposium).

50 Cancer Registry. Edited by E. GRUNDMANN and E. PEDERSEN (Symposium).

51 Gliomas. Current Concepts in Biology, Diagnosis and Therapy. Edited by J. HEKMATPANAH (Symposium).

52 The Ambivalence of Cytostatic Therapy. Edited by E. GRUNDMANN and R. GROSS (Symposium).

54 Malignant Bone Tumors. Edited by E. GRUNDMANN.

Special Supplement: Biology of Amphibian Tumors. Edited by M. MIZELL.

MIX
Papier aus verantwortungsvollen Quellen
Paper from responsible sources
FSC® C105338

If you have any concerns about our products,
you can contact us on
ProductSafety@springernature.com

In case Publisher is established outside the EU,
the EU authorized representative is:
Springer Nature Customer Service Center GmbH
Europaplatz 3, 69115 Heidelberg, Germany

Printed by Libri Plureos GmbH
in Hamburg, Germany